Adult Aphasia Rehabilitation

**Butterworth-Heinemann
Series in Communication Disorders**

Charlena M. Seymour, Ph.D., Series Editor

Battle, D.E. *Communication Disorders in Multicultural Populations* (1993)

Billeaud, F.P. *Communication Disorders in Infants and Toddlers: Assessment and Intervention* (1993)

Huntley, R.A., & Helfer, K.S. *Communication in Later Life* (1995)

Kricos, P.K., & Lesner, S.A. *Hearing Care for the Older Adult: Audiologic Rehabilitation* (1995)

Maxon, A.B., & Brackett, D. *The Hearing Impaired Child: Infancy through High School Years* (1992)

Wall, L.G. *Hearing for the Speech-Language Pathologist and Health Care Professional* (1995)

Wallace, G.L. *Adult Aphasia Rehabilitation* (1996)

Adult Aphasia Rehabilitation

Edited by

Gloriajean L. Wallace, Ph.D., CCC-SLP, BC-NCD

**Professor of Audiology and
Speech Pathology,
University of Tennessee, Knoxville, Tennessee**

Foreword by

Martha Taylor Sarno, M.A., M.D. (honorary), BC-NCD

**Professor of Rehabilitation Medicine,
New York University School of Medicine;
Director, Department of Speech-Language
Pathology, Howard A. Rusk Institute of
Rehabilitation Medicine, New York**

Butterworth-Heinemann
Boston   Oxford   Melbourne   Singapore   Toronto   Munich   New Dehli   Tokyo

Library of Congress Cataloging-in-Publication Data
Adult aphasia rehabilitation / [edited by] Gloriajean L. Wallace ;
    foreword by Martha Taylor Sarno.
        p. cm. -- (Butterworth-Heinemann series in communica-
tions disorders)
    Includes bibliographical references and index.
    ISBN 0-7506-9535-8 (alk. paper)
        1. Aphasia--Patients--Rehabilitation. 2. Aphasia--Patients-
-Rehabilitation.   I. Wallace, Gloriajean L.   II. Series.
        [DNLM: 1. Aphasia--rehabilitation. 2. Aphasia--in adulthood.
    3. Cerebrovascular Disorders--rehabilitation. WL 340.5 A244 1995]
    RC425.A29 1995
    616.8'1--dc20
    DNLM/DLC   95-43137
    for Library of Congress   CIP

British Library Cataloguing-in-Publication Data
A catalogue record for this book is available
from the British Library.

The publisher offers discounts on bulk orders of this book.
For information, please write:

Manager of Special Sales
Butterworth–Heinemann
313 Washington Street
Newton, MA 02158–1626

10 9 8 7 6 5 4 3 2 1

Printed in the United States of America

To the authors' families, extended families, and other significant contacts who in direct and indirect ways influenced and contributed to this consolidated effort

Contents

Contributing Authors

Daniel D. Anderson, Ed.D.
Director, Pacific Basin Rehabilitation Research and Training Center, University of Hawaii at Manoa, Honolulu
18. Planning Rehabilitation Services for Rural and Remote Communities

Rick L. Bollinger, Ph.D., CCC-SLP, BC-NCD
Chief, Audiology and Speech Pathology Service, Miami Department of Veterans Affairs Medical Center, Miami
14. Treatment of Writing Impairment

Mary Boyle, Ph.D., CCC-SLP, BC-NCD
Director, Department of Speech-Language and Audiology, The Winifred Masterson Burke Rehabilitation Hospital, White Plains, New York
20. Resource Guide for Aphasia and Stroke

Martha S. Burns, Ph.D., CCC-SLP
Adjunct Associate Professor of Communication Sciences and Disorders, Northwestern University; Associate Professional Staff, Department of Medicine, Evanston Hospital, Evanston, Illinois
7. Can-Do Therapy: A Positive Approach for Maximizing Recovery During Rehabilitation

Michael P. Cannito, Ph.D., CCC-SLP
Associate Professor, School of Speech-Language Pathology, The University of Memphis, Memphis, Tennessee
12. Treatment of Verbal Apraxia in Broca's Aphasia

Betty Daggett Coleman, M.A., CCC-SLP
Associate Director, Neuropathology Services Program and Clinical Supervisor, Hearing and Speech Center, Department of Audiology and Speech Pathology, University of Tennessee, Knoxville, Tennessee
16. Treatment Efficacy: Reflections and Projections

Maureen H. Fitzgerald, R.N., Ph.D.
Senior Lecturer, School of Occupational Therapy, The University of Sydney, Faculty of Health Sciences, Sydney, New South Wales, Australia
18. Planning Rehabilitation Services for Rural and Remote Communities

Kathryn L. Garrett, Ph.D., CCC-SLP
Clinical Assistant Professor of Communication Disorders, University of

Nebraska-Lincoln, Barkley Memorial Speech-Language and Hearing Clinic, Lincoln, Nebraska
15. Augmentative and Alternative Communication: Applications to Treatment

Lee Ann C. Golper, Ph.D., CCC-SLP, BC-NCD
Director, Department of Speech-Language Pathology, Associate Professor of Audiology and Speech Pathology, and Assistant Professor of Otolaryngology, University of Arkansas for Medical Sciences, Little Rock, Arkansas
4. Language Assessment

Jeffrey S. Hecht, M.D., F.A.A.P.M.R. (Physiatrist)
Medical Director, Patricia Neal Rehabilitation Center at Fort Sanders Regional Medical Center; Associate Professor, Departments of Medicine and Surgery, University of Tennessee Medical Center, Knoxville, Tennessee
1. Medical and Rehabilitation Management; 2. Rehabilitation Funding; Appendix: Commonly Prescribed Drugs and Their Side Effects

Audrey L. Holland, Ph.D., CCC-SLP, BC-NCD
Professor and Department Head of Speech and Hearing Sciences, University of Arizona, Tucson, Arizona
9. Pragmatic Assessment and Treatment for Aphasia

Ronald C. Jones, Ph.D., CCC-A
Audiologist and Chief Associate of RC Jones PHD and Associates, Portsmouth, Virginia
5. Basic Hearing Assessment

Edith Chin Li, Ph.D., CCC-SLP
Professor of Speech Communication, California State University, Fullerton, California
13. Treatment of Naming Impairment

Jon G. Lyon, Ph.D., CCC-SLP
Adjunct Associate Professor of Communication Disorders and Neurology, University of Wisconsin, Madison, Wisconsin; Executive Director, Living with Aphasia, Inc., Mazomanie, Wisconsin
8. Optimizing Communication and Participation in Life for Aphasic Adults and Their Primary Caregivers in Natural Settings: A Use Model for Treatment

Thomas P. Marquardt, Ph.D., CCC-SLP
Professor of Communication Sciences and Disorders, University of Texas, Austin, Texas
12. Treatment of Verbal Apraxia in Broca's Aphasia

Carolyn M. Mayo, Ph.D., CCC-SLP
Director, North Carolina Health Careers Access Program, University of North

Carolina System; Clinical Assistant Professor, Division of Speech and Hearing Sciences, Department of Medical Allied Health Professions, University of North Carolina School of Medicine, Chapel Hill, North Carolina
19. Stroke Prevention: A Health Promotion Approach

Robert Mayo, Ph.D., CCC-SLP
Assistant Professor of Speech-Language Pathology, Division of Speech and Hearing Sciences, Department of Medical Allied Health Professions, University of North Carolina School of Medicine; Director of Speech-Language Services, University of North Carolina Craniofacial Center, School of Dentistry, University of North Carolina, Chapel Hill, North Carolina
19. Stroke Prevention: A Health Promotion Approach

Sharon E. Moss, Ph.D., CCC-SLP, BC-NCD
Clinical Research Speech-Language Pathologist, Department of Rehabilitation Medicine, National Institutes of Health, Bethesda, Maryland; Adjunct Assistant Professor of Communication Sciences and Disorders, Howard University, Washington, D.C.
11. Model-Based Approach to Rehabilitation of Acquired Reading Disorders

Janet P. Patterson, Ph.D., CCC-SLP
Assistant Professor of Audiology and Speech Sciences, Michigan State University, East Lansing, Michigan
10. Treatment of Auditory Comprehension Impairment

William A. Paulsen, M.D., F.A.A.N. (Neurologist)
Associate Professor of Medicine and Chief of Neurology, University of Tennessee Memorial Research Center, Knoxville, Tennessee
1. Medical and Rehabilitation Management

Robert S. Pierce, Ph.D., CCC-SLP
Professor of Speech Pathology and Audiology, Kent State University, Kent, Ohio
10. Treatment of Auditory Comprehension Impairment

John D. Tonkovich, Ph.D., CCC-SLP/A
Speech-Language Pathologist, Shelby Township, Michigan
2. Rehabilitation Funding

Gloriajean L. Wallace, Ph.D., CCC-SLP, BC-NCD
Professor of Audiology and Speech Pathology, University of Tennessee, Knoxville, Tennessee
1. Medical and Rehabilitation Management; 6. Management of Aphasic Individuals from Culturally and Linguistically Diverse Populations; 16. Treatment Efficacy: Reflections and Projections; 18. Planning Rehabilitation Services for Rural and Remote Communities

Robert T. Wertz, Ph.D., CCC-SLP, BC-NCD
VA-Vanderbilt Professor of Hearing and Speech Sciences, Vanderbilt

University School of Medicine; Research Speech Pathologist, Audiology and Speech Pathology Service, Veterans Administration Medical Center, Nashville, Tennessee
3. Clinical Descriptions

Sarah E. Williams, Ph.D., J.D., CCC-SLP
Former Research Speech Pathologist, VA Medical Center, Bay Pines, Florida; Attorney at Law, Carter, Stein, Ford, Schaaf, and Towzey, St. Petersburg, Florida
17. Psychological Adjustment Following Stroke

Herbert K. M. Yee, M.S., P.T.
Director, Department of Physical Therapy, Waianae Coast Comprehensive Health Center, Waianae, Hawaii
18. Planning Rehabilitation Services for Rural and Remote Communities

Foreword

The broad spectrum of timely topics contained in this volume acknowledges both the multifaceted nature of aphasia and the dramatic increase in clinical and research activity in aphasiology in the past three decades. This period has seen a move away from the perception of aphasia as a purely neurologic, linguistic, or neuropsychologic disorder to a multidimensional pathologic state. The problems posed by aphasia are now viewed as a challenge by many disciplines since the disorder has an impact on so many aspects of the human condition.

This book also addresses important areas that are often neglected. Such issues as the management of individuals with aphasia in culturally diverse populations or rural, remote communities are relevant, for they call attention to the cultural and living antecedents and environments of the person as variables warranting consideration in the rehabilitation management scheme. Accounting for an individual's community, cultural history, and values gives both meaning and context to recovery and community reintegration.

The shift in the delivery of health services to more cost-effective policies and practices has posed inevitable limits on the availability and accessibility of services for the majority of those with acquired aphasia. This change, coupled with a rapidly growing aging community, makes it more compelling than ever that creative approaches be developed. Health professionals must weigh what kind of research is needed to counteract the trend toward early, short-term language treatment based on cost rather than long-term need or benefits and quality of care. The inclusion of chapters on rehabilitation funding, treatment efficacy, and medication acknowledge the impact of current health reforms on the more than one million persons who comprise the aphasia community.

Other important and heretofore relatively neglected topics included are stroke prevention and the promotion of wellness. These topics highlight the increasing sophistication that health professionals and consumers alike need to bring to the search for solutions to living with aphasia. The timeliness, scope, and relevance of this volume should stimulate and inspire work that will help empower and improve the quality of life of individuals with aphasia.

Martha Taylor Sarno

Preface

Stroke (also called brain attack) is the third leading killer in the United States, following heart attack and cancer. According to the National Stroke Association, approximately 550,000 individuals are affected each year by stroke, 150,000 of whom will die. A range of outcomes may result for the remaining 400,000 survivors of stroke. Approximately 10% of stroke survivors will be left with mild impairments and are generally able to return to their former life-style. Ten percent will have severe residual impairments that will necessitate long-term care in a nursing facility. Eighty percent will have mild to moderate disabilities in ambulation, swallowing, and/or communication that will require rehabilitation.

This book focuses on the latter group, the 80% who will require rehabilitation. Of particular interest is the group of stroke survivors who have aphasia, language impairments that impede communication. This book contains 20 chapters written by a diverse spectrum of authors on topics of practical relevance to clinicians and advanced graduate students specializing in the rehabilitation of adults who have acquired aphasia.

In Chapter 1, William A. Paulsen, Jeffrey S. Hecht, and I provide the reader with an overview of the medical and rehabilitation experiences encountered by the stroke patient. The chapter opens with the presentation of an actual case, which is used to springboard a discussion of medical and rehabilitation issues in a practical manner. The authors refer the reader to the appendix (prepared by Dr. Hecht) for a listing of medications frequently prescribed for stroke patients and a discussion of the effects of drugs on behavior.

In Chapter 2, Jeffrey S. Hecht and John D. Tonkovich provide an extensive review of funding issues that affect the accessibility and utilization of rehabilitation. This chapter includes a very well thought out and practical section on managed care. Chapter 3, by Robert T. Wertz, discusses major aphasia classification systems and provides a detailed description of patient characteristics according to each of these systems, including correlations between behavior and brain lesion sites. The chapter ends with a practical discussion of the usefulness of aphasia classification systems.

Chapter 4, by Lee Ann C. Golper, is perhaps the most comprehensive chapter on speech-language assessment of aphasic individuals ever written. This chapter includes a discussion of the purpose of assessment, psychometric principles, description of specific language assessments, test selection,

SOAP format report writing, and use of diagnostic information to guide treatment decisions. An extensive listing of neuropsychological assessments is included at the end of the chapter. In Chapter 5, Ronald C. Jones discusses the importance of hearing assessment for aphasic patients. Included is a discussion of common auditory disorders associated with aphasia, the role of the audiologist and speech-language pathologist in assessment, and specific suggestions for conducting an audiologic assessment with individuals who have incurred stroke.

Chapter 6 (my own) provides an introductory discussion of the management of culturally and linguistically diverse patients with acquired aphasia. Specific content includes the epidemiology of stroke in minority populations, definition and discussion of the role of the bilingual and the monolingual speech-language pathologist, and delineation of pressing clinical research needs. This is the first chapter on multicultural issues to be included in an aphasia book.

Chapter 7, by Martha S. Burns, discusses ways to maximize patient performance by using a "can do" approach, in which positive aspects of a patient's performance are identified and incorporated into therapy rather than the traditional model that emphasizes identification and treatment of deficit areas. Dr. Burns also emphasizes the importance of both the clinician and client maintaining a positive attitude during treatment. In Chapter 8, Jon G. Lyon provides a detailed discussion of a cutting-edge model for promoting participation in life after stroke, called "Communication Partners." This model is based on Dr. Lyon's own research and clinical work with individuals with aphasia. The chapter is augmented by the presentation of a case study example that helps demonstrate the Communication Partners approach in a practical way.

In Chapter 9, Audrey L. Holland, who introduced pragmatics to the area of adult aphasia, discusses pragmatic assessment and treatment of aphasic individuals. This chapter presents information about standardized pragmatic assessments, observational approaches, and a very comprehensive coverage of pragmatic treatment approaches, including several developed by Dr. Holland. Chapter 10, by Robert S. Pierce and Janet P. Patterson, discusses treatment of auditory comprehension from the single-word level through the sentence level. The effect of length of utterance, amount of information, speaking rate, memory, context, and other extralinguistic variables on performance, as well as specific strategies to aid comprehension, are discussed. Chapter 11, by Sharon E. Moss, reviews neuropsychological models of reading, specific acquired reading disorder syndromes, and specific treatment approaches for each type of reading disorder discussed. In Chapter 12, Thomas P. Marquardt and Michael P. Cannito discuss the characteristics and assessment of verbal apraxia in preparation for their up-to-date and exhaustive discussion of available treatment approaches.

Chapter 13, by Edith Chin Li, presents models for naming, a description of oral and written naming deficits in aphasia, and specific suggestions for treatment of naming disorders. Much of the treatment information is based on Dr. Li's own work in this area. In Chapter 14, Rick L. Bollinger describes writing errors characteristic of aphasic individuals as well as assessment and intervention approaches. The chapter includes a discussion of a pragmatically based approach to rehabilitation of writing disorders using the media of television, which was developed by Dr. Bollinger. In Chapter 15, Kathryn L. Garrett presents a cutting-edge model for classifying aphasic individuals based on their communication needs and eligibility for augmentative and/or alternative communication systems. Specific information pertaining to the assessment and communication system selection is presented in a very practical manner. Chapter 16, by Betty Daggett Coleman and myself, discusses treatment efficacy from the classical viewpoint, the perspective of the clinician. We then review literature that discusses efficacy from the point of view of aphasic persons and their family members. The ethnographic approach to research is discussed, in terms of its potential to provide greater insight into the issue of efficacy.

In Chapter 17, Sarah E. Williams discusses an important but seldom addressed issue—psychological adjustment after stroke. This very thorough chapter includes a presentation of neuropharmacology, neuroendocrinology, and neuroanatomical models of depression; information pertaining to the diagnosis of depression; and a discussion of current treatment approaches and future directions for the management of depression after stroke. Chapter 18, by Daniel D. Anderson, Maureen H. Fitzgerald, Herbert K. M. Yee. and myself, discusses the "how to" of developing rehabilitation programs for underserved populations who live in rural and remote communities. We walk the reader through the process from the needs assessment stage to program implementation. The chapter closes with two examples, one of which reviews the development of a speech-language program in a rural community. Chapter 19, by Carolyn M. Mayo and Robert Mayo, presents detailed epidemiologic information, followed by an innovative health promotion model that can be implemented by aphasiologists as a part of their routine treatment regimen. This is the first chapter on health promotion pertaining to the aphasia population ever written by speech-language pathologists. Chapter 20, by Mary Boyle, provides resources for information on stroke and aphasia. Addresses and phone numbers are provided for journals, publishers, newsletters and booklets, professional and consumer associations, legislative sources, and sources for grants, assessment and treatment materials.

While this book spans a diverse range of topics, the insightful reader will discover a common tread that unites each chapter. Each emphasizes the importance of individualization and functionality of treatment. Undoubtedly the reader will find these comprehensive, innovative, and very practical chapters a valuable resource.

GLW

Acknowledgments

Special thanks are due to God for giving me strength and discipline; Dr. John Wallace, for his inspiration; Mrs. Gladys Wallace, for her belief in me; and Ms. Christina Joy Hunter, who with great patience and understanding allowed her mom to complete this project in as undisturbed as possible a manner. Christina, as you have watched me work through the process of completing this book, I hope that you have gained the understanding that a seed can become a flower; that there is power in persistence; and that a rainbow still remains the promise for those who are true to themselves.

GLW

Chapter 1

Medical and Rehabilitation Management

Jeffrey S. Hecht, William A. Paulsen, and Gloriajean L. Wallace

Sam Brown (not his real name) was enjoying his retirement. He had always lived hard and played hard, but today he was lying on the couch enjoying the Super Bowl with a six-pack of beer and a carton of cigarettes. Without warning, he saw flashes of light in his left eye. He had noticed the same flashes over the past 2 weeks, but now his vision seemed to come and go in that eye. After 10 minutes his vision returned to normal, but he began to notice it was harder to hold the can of beer in his right hand. When he took a sip, beer dripped from the right side of his mouth. Alarmed, he tried to call out to his wife, but no sound emerged from his mouth. He tried to stand up and fell to the floor. Hearing the crash, his wife ran in, found him on the floor, and called 911. When the paramedics arrived, they found a man with right hemiplegia (paralysis of the right arm and leg) who was unable to talk.

En route to the emergency room, Sam Brown developed sudden movements on the right side of his body associated with loss of consciousness. This was diagnosed as an epileptic seizure. The paramedics quickly started intravenous (IV) lines and gave him a loading dose of phenytoin (Dilantin). Oxygen was given by mask. Fortunately, the patient had a strong heart and cardiopulmonary resuscitation (CPR) was not needed. An indwelling catheter was placed through his penis into his bladder. The physician found Brown unable to move his right arm or leg and unable to speak, though he did understand enough to follow verbal commands. He was diagnosed as having suffered a stroke.

1

MEDICAL MANAGEMENT IN THE ACUTE STAGE
AFTER A STROKE

The acute stroke represents the most common neurologic problem encountered in a general hospital. The resulting neurologic deficit results from occlusion or rupture of cerebral blood vessels. There are three major categories of strokes: cerebral embolus, cerebral thrombosis, and hemorrhage, either subarachnoid (usually due to a ruptured aneurysm or, less frequently, an arteriovenous malformation) or intracerebral. Transient ischemic attacks (TIAs) and reversible ischemic neurological deficits (RINDs) are short-lived cerebral events lasting less than 24 hours and, by definition, are totally reversible. TIAs are significant because 40% of TIA patients go on to develop a functionally significant stroke within 5 years.

Both thrombic and embolic strokes are more likely to be seen in patients with a variety of recognized risk factors (Wolf, D'Agostino, Belanger, & Kannel, 1991): hypertension, heart disease, diabetes mellitus, obesity, inactivity, hyperlipidemia (elevated cholesterol or triglycerides), or cigarette smoking. Additional risk factors may include use of cocaine (Levine et al., 1990), IV drugs, or stimulants such as amphetamines; heavy alcohol consumption (more than three drinks a day); use of birth control pills; or certain systemic diseases, such as systemic lupus erythematosus, that cause vascular abnormalities. Individuals with sickle cell disease are also at risk for stroke (Caplan & Saunders, 1991; Klatsky, Armstrong, & Friedman, 1991). Virtually any disease that leads to the occlusion of cerebral blood vessels can ultimately result in stroke. U.S. populations vary significantly in their incidence of stroke by race, sex, and state (Gasecki & Hachinski, 1993).

Intracerebral hemorrhage is commonly associated with hypertension (Kase, Williams, Wyatt, & Mohr, 1982). Patients develop sudden explosive headache often associated with vomiting. Although mortality is high, some hemorrhages result in a higher degree of functional recovery compared to the initial presentation than is seen in patients with an ischemic stroke. This occurs because with hemorrhage, brain tissue is temporarily damaged by pressure effects rather than being permanently destroyed (Feldmann, 1991, 1990).

Subarachnoid hemorrhages are caused by rupture of an aneurysm (weak place in a blood vessel that causes a ballooning of the vessel). Patients typically experience severe headache, nausea, visual disturbances, fever, or neck or facial pain.

Stroke is a major cause of aphasia—the acquired loss or reduction in language comprehension, production, and related areas due to neurologic impairment (Brust, Shafer, Richter, & Bruun, 1976). (Other neurologically based causes of language impairment include trauma and brain tumor [Recht, McCarthy, O'Donnell, Cohen, & Drachman, 1989].) Strokes affect speech and language if they involve the primary speech and language centers or the descending pathways.

Sam Brown was rushed into radiology for a computed tomography (CT) scan of the head and brain. The results were normal and showed no bleeding within the brain. His physician knew that an ischemic stroke does not show up on CT scan for several hours. However, because there was no bleeding, the patient was started on IV heparin, an anticoagulant.

Faced with an acute stroke patient, one asks the following questions: What is the location of the lesion? Is the stroke ischemic or hemorrhagic? What is the underlying cause? What is the duration of the stroke? Emergency CT scan without contrast will exclude hemorrhage but usually does not show an infarct; however, magnetic resonance imaging (MRI) will usually demonstrate the lesion in the acute phase. MRI allows more exact delineation of brain disease and is rapidly replacing CT in the assessment of patients (Alexander, Naeser, & Palumbo, 1987). Visualization of the infarct can also be enhanced with the use of an agent that concentrates in parts of the brain where there is breakdown of the blood-brain barrier. While MRI has some obvious advantages over CT, such as typically no need for enhancement, avoidance of bony defects, and greater sensitivity, it also has some disadvantages. The test requires a cooperative patient, takes longer to administer, and is inaccessible to many patients on life-support systems. However, new MRI scanners are being developed that are faster and that may overcome some of these problems. Other studies available to further understand the underlying cause of mechanisms of the aphasic condition include electroencephalogram (EEG), lumbar puncture (LP) with studies of the cerebrospinal fluid (CSF), and isotope techniques such as single-photon emission computerized tomography (SPECT) and positron emission tomography (PET) (Grotta, 1993).

Sam Brown was transferred to the neurologic intensive care unit, where he had been admitted by his primary care physician. There the patient was seen by a neurologist (a specialist in brain disorders). Electrocardiogram (ECG) electrodes that had been placed on his chest in the emergency room were now connected to an oscilloscope to monitor his heart rhythms. An oxygen saturation monitor was used to determine the ability of his blood to carry the necessary oxygen. He was continued on nasal oxygen support. His indwelling (Foley) catheter drained into a collection bag, and his urine output was carefully measured. Bags of IV fluids hung at his side. Problems with swallowing required occasional suctioning. An egg-crate mattress was used to help protect his skin. He underwent an EEG to determine the extent of brain injury and the existence of any active seizure foci.

SEIZURES

Patients with brain dysfunction, which also causes aphasia, are at risk for epileptic seizures. Seizures follow thrombolic strokes in 90% of cases

(Black, Hachinsk, & Norris, 1982) and are more common with cortical insults such as subarachnoid hemorrhages, where the risk is 7–14% (Kase et al., 1982). Various types of seizure behavior may occur. Focal motor seizures called *partial seizures* result in jerking movements of the arm, leg, or face; consciousness is not lost. More extensive seizures can originate from an activity near a site of brain damage that spreads across the brain to cause movements in all four extremities. This leads to a complex seizure in which consciousness is lost and frequently results in movements that are tonic (muscle contraction) or clonic (rhythmic contraction and relaxation of muscles leading to jerking movements). In outdated medical terminology, this was called a grand mal seizure. Temporal lobe seizures are somewhat unusual and cause bizarre purposeful activities, behavior changes, and unusual sounds or smells rather than jerking movement. They make up 20% of seizure activity.

Seizures are usually brief. If a brief focal motor seizure occurs, no special measures need to be taken, though the physician should be notified. With generalized seizures, patients should be removed from any danger that might pose a hazard to them. Clothing around the collar must be loosened. Glasses should be removed. Medical personnel should help the patient lie on his or her side or stomach, not on the back (in case of vomiting). The arms and legs should be allowed to move freely. It is no longer judged necessary to put something in the patient's mouth. A physician should be called. If a seizure persists (*status epilepticus*), medical attention should be sought immediately.

During a generalized seizure, the patient may cry out, lose consciousness, and fall. The arms, legs, and face move. Bowel and bladder control is often lost. Breathing may be irregular. Following the seizure, the patient will stop moving and will resume breathing normally. The patient usually awakens in a few minutes to complain about sore muscles or headache. Confusion or fatigue can persist for hours after a seizure.

Whereas medications are used both to prevent and to treat seizures, alcohol and certain medications can cause seizures by irritating the brain tissue. Besides raising the risk of seizures by lowering the seizure threshold, alcohol is a toxin to the recovering brain and should be avoided following a stroke. Antiepileptics may be sedating and may impair performance in therapy. See the Appendix for a full review of medications and their side effects (Wiebe-Velazquez & Blume, 1993).

Mr. Brown suffered transient enlargement of the left pupil. His physician felt it represented increased intracerebral pressure on the brain stem. It quickly responded to treatment with hyperventilation, mannitol, and dexamethasone (Decadron). When he developed a fever, a chest x-ray showed an infiltrate in the right lower lobe of his chest. His physician suspected pneumonia, and Brown was seen by a pulmonary specialist. She started appropriate antibiotics. When stable for 48 hours, Brown began physical therapy to increase range of motion in his extremities. A physiatrist (physician specializing in physical medicine and rehabilitation) was consulted to evaluate bodily functions and nutrition and to initiate appropriate therapies.

ASSOCIATED PROBLEMS

The importance of delineating aphasia and related disorders lies in determining the site of the lesion (Berthier et al., 1991; DeRenzi, Colombo, & Scarpa, 1991; Mori, Yamadori, & Furumoto, 1989). The speed of onset, associated symptoms, and other factors help establish the specific cause (Brust et al., 1976; Recht et al., 1989; Tyrrell, Warrington, Frackowiak, & Rossor, 1990). The patient with aphasia may be referred to as aphasic or may present with symptoms that are interpreted as something else, such as confusion. Likewise, the patient with assumed aphasia may in fact have some additional communication impairments, such as dysarthria. In either case, aphasia can usually be diagnosed by simple bedside tests: spontaneous speech, naming, language comprehension, repetition, reading, and writing. This testing usually excludes disorders such as mutism or dysarthria. Depending on the responses to these bedside tests, the patient's aphasia may be characterized as Broca's, Wernicke's, anomic, conduction, mixed nonfluent, global, one of the transcortical aphasias, or as an unclassifiable aphasic language impairment (see Chapter 3).

It is important to remember that the language centers of the brain lie near areas associated with feeling, sensation, and vision (DeRenzi et al., 1991; Mori et al., 1989). An alert clinician can discern clues to the site of the lesion by noting the presence of any of a variety of types of functional impairment. For example, because areas controlling movement are located in anterior parts of the brain, an insult to the Broca's area, which causes a motor aphasia, is often associated with paralysis of the mouth, tongue, lips, face, thumb, fingers, hand, and arm, and, to a lesser extent, the hip and leg. Limb apraxia, or the inability to volitionally control movement of the limb, may also result from a lesion to this area. Wernicke's type, sometimes called receptive aphasia, involves sensory pathways located in the posterior brain.

Stroke involving the superior division of the middle cerebral artery or prerolandic and rolandic arteries causes expressive problems associated with motor dysfunction, while insults involving the inferior division of the middle cerebral artery and anterior and posterior parietal arteries cause receptive language deficits and sensory loss. Insults involving the posterior temporal branches or the middle cerebral stem may cause visual loss. Involvement of branches of the anterior cerebral artery is more likely to cause expressive language deficits and problems with motor dysfunction or sensory loss to the foot, leg, and sometimes bladder. Posterior cerebral artery involvement is associated with contralateral blindness (hemianopsia) and receptive language problems. Involvement of the superior division of the middle cerebral artery causes a dense sensory motor deficit in the contralateral face, arm, and leg, with less involvement of the leg. As recovery occurs, the patient can often walk with a hemiplegia but little recovery occurs in the arm. There is global aphasia with subsequent improvement in verbal and written comprehension, but motor aphasia is likely to persist. Small focal infarcts involving branches of this division may produce motor deficit in the right arm called ideomotor apraxia, while sparing language. Ideomotor limb apraxia is often bilateral.

The small branches from the middle cerebral artery penetrate to the internal capsule and corona radiata (lenticulostriate arteries), and occlusion causes a lacunar infarct. These lacunes, which are typically seen in patients with long-standing diabetes or hypertension, may be multiple and deeply scattered in the hemispheres, and are often about the size of a BB or match head. The clinical deficit tends to recover well with fairly minimal sequelae. However, lacunes may accumulate to cause pseudobulbar palsy (a spastic paralysis of cranial nerve–innervated junctions, that imitates a brain stem stroke), dysphagia, and dementia. Occlusion of the dominant anterior cerebral artery may produce a transcortical motor aphasia characterized by inability to repeat words and sentences and much-reduced spontaneous speech. There may be involvement of the frontal cortex with change in personality—decreased spontaneity, flatness of affect, distractibility, perseveration, and decreased reasoning skills. There may be loss of strength and sensation in the right leg and foot with relatively minor involvement of the face and hand. It is not uncommon to see problems with bladder control.

Vertebrobasilar syndromes are strokes involving the posterior circulation to the brain via the vertebral and basilar arteries that supply the brain stem, cerebellum, and deep brain structures. Common symptoms relevant to the speech-language pathologist (SLP) include dysarthria, perioral numbness, ataxia of speech, ataxic swallowing, or more severe dysphagia. In fact, the most severe dysphagia is often seen with brain stem strokes, which may cause lower motor neuron flaccid paralysis. Unilateral cortical strokes cause less impairment than strokes affecting the lower motor neurons that provide bilateral innervation. However, bilateral cortical strokes may cause severe dysphagia as part of the pseudobulbar palsy profile.

Bulbar palsy refers to brain stem involvement. Nausea is an associated symptom (the prepared clinician will always have an emesis basin in the room); the nature of bulbar palsy is to emulate gastrointestinal dysfunction. In fact, the patient with a posterior fossa brain tumor may present with this and an episodic vertigo primarily, even before an ataxia is noted. Other associated symptoms may include diplopia, bilateral limb or arm weakness or numbness, and gait ataxia. There may be a decrease in arousal due to ischemia of the reticular activating system in the midbrain and pons. Bulbar palsy may be associated with "drop attacks" in which ischemia to this area leads to loss of leg strength and falls without associated loss of consciousness. Occlusion of the basilar artery causes quadriparesis, ataxia, sensory loss, and depression of arousal. A brain stem infarct confined to the basal pons, leaving tegmental structures intact, causes a "locked-in" syndrome in which consciousness is preserved but no voluntary movement or speech is possible. Eye movements may be the only means by which patients can communicate. Stroke involving the lateral medulla caused by involvement of the posterior inferior cerebellar artery causes dysarthria and dysphagia with loss of pain sensation in the face on the side of the lesion and on the opposite half of the body. There is also incoordination or ataxia on the opposite side.

Patients with posterior cerebral involvement may have deficits in visual field on the opposite side; they may complain of blurred vision rather than recognizing loss of an entire half of their visual field. Patients may show confusion. In a TIA, this confusion may represent a *transient global amnesia* that may cause the patient to be transiently uncertain of their relationship to other persons or to their environment unassociated with other visual, motor or sensory deficits. This may be related to disturbed function of hippocampal and medial temporal structures and in posterior circulation stroke patients may be associated with a receptive aphasia. This carries a relatively poor prognosis for new learning and rehabilitation, but patients are able to carry out well-learned automatic activities. Receptive aphasia may be associated with a loss of feeling on the opposite side of the body, or pain as the sense of feeling returns. Patients with posterior cerebral occlusion may have difficulty in naming objects or colors or in reading.

MEDICAL MANAGEMENT IN THE SUBACUTE TO CHRONIC STAGE

Because of swallowing difficulties, Sam Brown began feeding through a nasogastric tube. Occupational therapy was consulted for splinting the paralyzed extremity and beginning upper-extremity activities. A speech-language pathologist was consulted to assess communication and swallowing. After the initial assessment, a modified barium swallow was recommended by the speech-language pathologist. The study showed slowness of the oral phase, delay in initiating the swallow reflex, and some collection of contrast material in the valleculae space. No aspiration was noted. Tube feedings were continued due to concerns about the inadequacy of nutritional intake (attributed to his very slow rate of eating).

The physical problems and deficits associated with the aphasia play a significant role in a patient's adaptation and coping with the language disturbance. For example, patients may be less concerned about their language impairment than they are about swallowing problems; loss of feeling, pain, or strength; inability to use an arm or to walk; facial weakness; loss of vision; or inability to perform prestroke activities such as walking, driving, working, or enjoying hobbies. It is critical to rehabilitation that the SLP help the patient realize how treating aphasia will help the patient achieve his or her personal goals (Hecht, 1991).

Now stable, Sam Brown was transferred from the intensive care unit to an acute neurology floor. Heparin was stopped, and he was started on ticlopidine on the third day. On the fifth day, his right leg showed swelling. A Doppler study of the venous circulation revealed phlebitis (blood clot) in the leg. Ticlopidine was stopped, and he was begun again on IV heparin and later switched to warfarin (Coumadin). After 5 days of bed rest, he appeared once again to be stable. He progressed rapidly in sitting and developed endurance. He was discharged from the acute hospital and transferred to a rehabilitation center, where he began a program of comprehensive rehabilitation.

Brown was admitted by the physiatrist, who requested consultations with physical therapy, occupational therapy, speech pathology, recreational therapy, psychology, social services, and rehabilitational nursing. The patient's wife was involved in family stroke education programs. The speech-language pathologist felt that the patient's communication was sufficient to understand visual and most verbal information, so Brown was also involved in patient stroke education groups.

Brown's caregivers identified numerous risk factors for vascular disease: he was obese, he was a three-pack-a-day smoker, and he drank a six-pack of beer daily. In addition, he had elevated cholesterol and triglyceride levels, and had a low high-density lipoprotein (HDL) cholesterol. His blood pressure was elevated at 160/95. He started a low-cholesterol, low-fat, weight-reduction diet and alcohol was prohibited. He was started on an antihyperlipidemic, and his antihypertensives were increased. Within 3 weeks, his cholesterol, triglycerides, and blood pressure were all within the normal range, and he had lost 5 lb. A withdrawal reaction from cigarettes prompted a nicotine patch to reduce his craving, after which he tolerated the withdrawal adequately.

Initially the patient resisted rehabilitation. He later became a willing participant and made substantial progress in mobility, self-care, and communication skills. At 3 weeks, his progress appeared to slow, his appetite decreased, and he began to have trouble waking early in the morning. He was diagnosed as having depression, started on an antidepressant, and his progress again improved within a week. He was discharged from the rehabilitation center at 5 weeks, with communication skills adequate to support his interactions with family members and friends. Mr. Brown no longer experienced difficulty with eating. He was independent in wheelchair transfers and mobility, upper-body dressing, and hygiene. He required standby assistance for walking with a brace and cane and required minimal assistance to don his shoe and sock on the right side. He required moderate assistance for advanced transfers such as to a bathtub and required mini-

mal assistance for climbing the three steps into his home. He started out-patient therapy, continued to make progress after discharge, and found a new hobby—painting—that added zest to his life.

A physician's training emphasizes two stages of care. The first, prevention (Asymptomatic Carotid Atherosclerosis Study Group, 1989; North American Symptomatic Carotid Endarterectomy Study Group, 1987), may involve risk factor reduction by, for example, lowering blood pressure through smoking cessation and a low-sodium diet. The second stage, diagnosis and curative treatment, might entail radiologic imaging and the removal of a blood clot responsible for ischemia (Canadian Cooperative Study Group, 1978; Fields, Lemak, Frankowski, & Hardy, 1977; Fisher, 1958; Gent, Blakely, Easton, et al., 1989; Hass et al., 1989; Keith, Phillips, Whisnant, Nishimaru, & O'Fallon, 1987; Putman & Adams, 1985; Steering Committee of the Physicians' Health Study Research Group, 1989; Sze, Reitman, Pincus, Sacks, & Chalmers, 1988).

But there is a third phase of medical care: rehabilitation. For a stroke patient with aphasia, rehabilitation can involve language therapy, management of eating difficulties, and a host of other tasks. These activities take time, and SLPs can find their roles misunderstood by physicians, who do not receive training in rehabilitation, and by others, including family members. The case study of Sam Brown shows that, when pursued with alertness and patience, the rehabilitation process can make a significant difference in the patient's quality of life.

THE REHABILITATION TEAM

Many patients with stroke have such mild or transient deficits that they can be managed in the acute-care setting and discharged directly to home with home health, outpatient, or no services. Other patients may have such severe neurologic problems, perhaps superimposed on other medical conditions, that they participate in an intensive stroke rehabilitation program. (Nearly half of the patients who leave a rehabilitation unit of a hospital do so with an additional medical diagnosis.) These patients require a maintenance-level program or lower-intensity program that can be provided in a skilled nursing facility. However, about 50% of patients fit into an intermediate category and will benefit from intensive stroke rehabilitation.

Once the stroke has stabilized without further neurologic progression and superimposed medical conditions are controlled, the need for comprehensive inpatient rehabilitation can be considered. A decision is made about whether to transfer the patient to a rehabilitation hospital or stroke rehabilitation unit of an acute-care hospital. Although these facilities may resemble other hospitals, they embody a different philosophy. Instead of supportive "convalescent" care, rehabilitation implies an active and interactive program with patients, who are out of bed most of the day and participate in therapy at least 3 hours per day, according to Medicare criteria. The Commission on Accreditation of Rehabilitation Facilities (CARF) (1993), established by rehabilitation professionals to certify rehabilitation facilities according to commonly accepted and uniform standards, defines rehabilitation as follows: the process of providing coordinated, comprehensive, appropriate services to a person with a disability, to achieve improved health, welfare, and the person's maximum physical, social, psychological, and vocational potential for useful and productive activity.

Therapists' Roles

Physicians

CARF defines two roles for physicians in the rehabilitation setting. They can be addressed by the same or by different physicians. The first role is to scrutinize medical needs, prevent complications, and address problems as they arise. Medical status must be optimized for patients to fully participate in therapy. Problems may be addressed using medications for pain or phenol blocks to relieve spasticity. Nutrition must be optimized. The second role is to act as medical team leader, balancing various medical nursing, therapy, and psychosocial issues, particularly when there is a conflict between rehabilitative and medical needs.

According to CARF standards for "physician rehabilitation services," the physician responsible for the patient's program should be a physiatrist or a comparably qualified physician by virtue of training and experience; this should be reflected in the privileges granted by the institution. CARF goes on to say that this physician "should provide active management, direction and supervision of the person's rehabilitation program so that it is consistent with the diagnoses, functional limitations and prognosis of the person. . . There should be regular, direct individual contact with the person served by the rehabilitation physician (no less than once per day on any day that the person being served is receiving full interdisciplinary therapy services)." Interdisciplinary team conferences are required no less than every other week (CARF, 1992, pp. 44–45; Ferguson, 1990).

Nurses

Nursing plays a major role in rehabilitation. CARF sets specific standards for nursing services and identifies the best organizations as those that incorporate rehabilitative nursing into the entire rehabilitative program, including attendance and active participation in team conferences. Nurses spend many hours with patients when not involved in other structured therapy programs. Because many family members visit in the evenings, the primary nurse may be the main source of information for family members regarding the sharing of team goals and development of discharge plans. Registered nurses (RNs) may acquire special certification in rehabilitation providing a certified rehabilitation registered nurse (CRRN). Some units may be staffed with RNs, licensed practical nurses (LPNs), or nurses' aides, depending on the levels of care needed. The focus of nursing in rehabilitation certainly differs from that in the acute care setting. In rehabilitation, the focus is not what the nurse should do for the patient but, rather, how the nurse can help the patient learn and do things independently. Nursing therefore provides continuity and carryover of information learned in rehabilitation programs to practical applications on the unit—i.e., the nurse ensures that progress made is incorporated into daily care in the unit. It is important that the SLP share relevant information with nurses regarding such issues as a means to facilitate communication, the use of adaptive communication devices, how best to use hearing aids, and suggestions for swallowing programs. Nurses can share this information with family members. Because of their close personal role and 24-hour availability, nurses are the team members best able to share educational materials with families (Josephs, 1992; Prazich, 1985).

Physical Therapists

Physical therapists (PTs) teach mobility skills. This involves expanding the range of motion of extremities; developing positioning, strengthening, balance, endurance, and coordination training; and helping to teach techniques to overcome pathologic reflexes (Taub, Miller, Novack, & Cook, 1993). Also, the therapist should optimize positioning to reduce pain in the neck, back, bottom, and shoulder so that patients can concentrate during speech and language treatment sessions. One important PT role is to determine, along with the physician, the patient's highest level of potential motor function. Together, the two define whether the patient may need a wheelchair, walk with assistance, or walk alone.

The PT is responsible for making suggestions about or arranging for appropriate mobility equipment at the patient's discharge. This includes wheelchairs, assistive devices such as canes or walkers, braces or orthotics (in conjunction with the physician), elevated commode seats, shower chairs, hand-held showers, wheelchair-lift devices for cars, and so forth. The PT, in conjunction with the occupational therapist, may suggest how to modify homes that have stairs, narrow doorways, and inaccessible bathrooms. PTs play a key role in training the family to assist with mobility skills.

Of course, patients' communication skills play an important role in their ability to participate in therapy. Patients with severe aphasia may have difficulty comprehending the necessary tasks and therapy. Newly trained PTs may not understand how to work with aphasic patients by using gestures and pantomime. Many of the techniques developed for PTs focus on motor skills but may not prepare them to deal with the cognitively impaired patient. SLPs can help PTs communicate with their patients and therefore make the most progress in the briefest amount of time. For example, at the Patricia Neal Rehabilitation Center, our Cognitively Directed Imitation (CDI) draws on intact right-brain strengths (sparing of perceptual and visual learning functions) to overcome cognitive deficits from left-brain insults that stand in the way of learning motor skills. PTs have 2 years of undergraduate training. There are bachelor of arts degree programs and even master's degree programs in physical therapy.

Occupational Therapists

Traditionally, occupational therapists (OTs) provide strengthening and coordination to the upper extremities (arms and upper body). OTs are also involved with assessing perceptual and visual functions in right-brain skills. The extent to which these functions are spared affects a patient's ability to learn new skills following a stroke (Chensea, Henderson, & Cermak, 1993).

OTs also address activities of daily living (ADL) such as feeding, grooming, personal hygiene, dressing, and toileting. OTs help patients who have lost the use of a dominant extremity transfer the skills to the other limb. This is relevant to the SLP's work on expressive language functions. OTs help design and obtain special adaptive equipment, including specially designed forks and spoons for eating, long-handled aids for dressing, and special cushions and supports to maintain good posture and position a paralyzed limb. Splints to support paralyzed upper extremities may be provided or fabricated by an OT. OTs often work with PTs to teach transfer skills (moving a patient from one place to another). Where there are severe problems with spasticity, the two therapists may work together on casting a spastic limb, sometimes using a new cast every week to improve range of motion.

Many patients have suffered more than one stroke. Multiple cortical strokes commonly lead to a *multi-infarct dementia* (MID). Where patients have cognitive deficits in addition to aphasia, the OT works with a SLP to address compensatory techniques for deficits in memory, attention, and functional living skills such as managing money, completing household tasks, and working with tools. OTs can help identify relevant pictures to place on a communication board. Good positioning developed by PTs and OTs facilitates swallowing, good breathing, and communication. The OT is an excellent resource person to answer questions about what the patient will be able to do at home. Occupational therapist training is comparable in length to that of PTs.

Speech-Language Pathologists

The entire rehabilitation team looks to the SLP to enhance its effectiveness in working with aphasic patients and their families. A prompt screening assessment by the SLP can identify problems with swallowing and lead to interventions that will prevent pneumonia, maximize nutrition, and prevent unneeded interruptions of the rehabilitative stay (Sliwa & Liss, 1993). Additionally, the well-functioning team looks to the initial SLP screening assessment for information on hearing deficits that can interfere with rehabilitation and simulate dementia or depression. The team needs the SLP to be sure the patient has his or her prostheses for hearing (aid) or communicating. If the patient has none but needs a temporary assistive listening device to succeed in rehabilitation, it should be provided. The screening evaluation can determine the best approach for the team to communicate with the aphasic patient, whether through gestures, single words, or sentences. If sentences, the team needs to know the optimal rate and intensity of speech and the optimal sentence length. The team needs to know how much is aphasia and how much is apraxia. The team needs to know if nodding and smiling by the patient represents true comprehension of language, or good social skills and understanding of pragmatic body language in the absence of comprehension. Important information from the screening cannot wait several days for the initial team conference but must be communicated promptly.

After screening and communicating initial impressions with the team, the SLP should complete detailed evaluations of the areas of identified deficit and strength. Information on swallowing is also important to the nurse and physician. A modified barium swallowing study may be needed to help with the prognosis and treatment (Johnson, McKenzie, & Sievers, 1993). Information on the best means of communicating so the patient can express basic needs (like toileting, thirst, hunger, and pain) is vital to nursing and therapy. How best to help the patient learn is often the key to success in OT and PT. The physician needs information on the type and extent of deficits, whether there is a pattern, and the prognosis (Nicholas, Helm-Estabrooks, Ward-Lonergan, & Morgan, 1993). The social worker and psychologist need to know the severity of the aphasia to assist with family counseling (Williams, 1993). The psychologist also needs this information to decide whether detailed psychological testing is possible or likely to not be reliable.

The family needs the help of the SLP but may be resistant to accepting suggestions and to hearing prognostic information if negative. Family members may need reminders that aphasia is not the same as hearing loss and that they need not yell. Others may think aphasia equals dementia and that their loved one is now retarded. On the other hand, families may think the smiles and head nods of their aphasic loved one means that he or she understands everything. They must be cautioned, as some have taken meaningless social head nods as permission to proceed with business deals and personal decisions. Educational materials on aphasia or other deficits should be shared with the family.

For patients who have had more than one stroke, the SLP needs to ascertain whether there are superimposed problems of nondominant parietal lobe syndrome with poor pragmatic communication skills, impaired judgment, problems in time awareness, and a loss of sensitivity to body language. Some left-handed patients who suffer a left-brain stroke may have shared brain dominance, and have some of these features with aphasia in a single unilateral stroke. It is also helpful for the SLP to assess whether there is a general decline in cognitive functions superimposed on the major event. A careful history focused on SLP problems from a knowledgeable family member may supplement information obtained by the physician and nurse. This may be extremely helpful for determining prognosis and setting rehabilitation goals. The SLP can provide such helpful tools as passey-muir valves for communication through a tracheostomy, assistive listening devices, and nonverbal communication devices.

Treatment of the aphasia, apraxia, dementia, dysphagias, and other problems make the SLP a key part of the team. It is helpful to let families and the team know whether your treatments will be one-on-one or group, employ written materials or the computer, and what "homework" is required. Creativity is a helpful asset for the SLP, as is tenacity, since treatment of aphasia can be a long-term and therefore challenging process. It is certainly important to take some time at first to develop a good therapeutic relationship with the patient.

SLPs should not be shy about letting family members know they have 2 years of master's level specialty training and a year-long clinical fellowship experience that have provided them with special expertise in dealing with communication and swallowing problems. Families should also be assured that a solid knowledge base in these areas has been confirmed by the SLP's successful performance on the National Examination of Speech Pathology and Audiology and by certification through the American Speech-Language-Hearing Association, and perhaps by status as being state-licensed to practice. In addition, board certification for adult and/or pediatric neurologic communication disorders is offered through the Academy of Neurologic Communication Disorders and Sciences (ANCDS). Finally, one should remember that the family will be more sensitive to body language and innuendos from their loved one than the SLP will, and that they are more likely to elicit the emotions that will lead to the first communication efforts by the patient. It should be remembered that even if family members do not accept all suggestions at first, sharing ideas without making family members "lose face" will make it easier for them to accept helpful suggestions later. It should also be remembered that prognosis in an individual cannot be certain within the first few weeks (Pashek & Holland, 1988).

Psychologists

Not all rehabilitation centers have their own licensed psychologist, neuropsychologist, and counselors. However, CARF requires that all such centers at least be affiliated with these professionals.

Psychologists help patients and family members adjust to the disability. Depression is commonly seen following dominant hemisphere stroke and is best approached using behavioral techniques as well as medications. Psychologists can help other therapists deal with a patient's behavioral problems. It is important to realize that many patients (as many as 15% or more) have underlying psychological problems that existed before the stroke. These range from such disabling conditions as schizophrenia or bipolar depressive disorder (manic depression) to depression, anxiety disorders, agoraphobia (fear of strange places or open places), claustrophobia (fear of enclosed spaces, such as a SLP's office), compulsive disorders (tendency to wash hands, chew fingernails, or perform other tasks repeatedly and frequently), and personality disorders ranging from hysteria to sociopathy. Additionally, patients may have addictions that in some cases are risk factors for stroke. For example, cocaine is a cause of stroke in young people; alcohol and cigarette smoking are other risk factors. The psychologist can help with these disorders or help with appropriate referrals. Additionally, psychologists can assist in providing additional testing to determine the extent of cognitive, intellectual, or behavioral impairment from stroke or underlying conditions.

For example, for a patient who appears depressed and demented, one condition can imitate the other. Distinguishing between them can be helpful therapeutically and a psychologist can play a role in this regard. On the other hand, severe aphasia can make neuropsychological testing very difficult, particularly when combined with motor dyspraxia. A SLP's input can help a psychologist or neuropsychologist avoid wasting time and dollars by attempting neuropsychological testing that will be of little value. In conjunction with other team members, psychologists often address sexuality issues as well (DeBoskey, et al., 1987).

A psychology department may employ psychology examiners, master's degree psychologists, and/or Ph.D.'s (Finlayson & Upton, 1987).

Recreational Therapists

Recreational therapists evaluate the patient's prestroke leisure interests, life pattern, and coping styles in an attempt to involve patients in structured activities during free time. This may vary from arts and crafts to individual activities to planned meals, group outings, and sports. The goals of recreational therapy dovetail with those of other therapies—encouraging arm functions, building endurance, developing socialization skills, reducing depression and developing coping skills, and helping integrate patients with the community. Recreational therapists can be an important resource to the SLP in developing communication books and in keeping therapy meaningful to the patient. A SLP's insight into communication and swallowing disorders can help recreational therapists in program planning. Recreational therapists study for 4 years to obtain the therapeutic recreation specialist (TRS) degree.

Social Workers and Rehabilitation Counselors

Social workers and rehabilitation counselors are an important communication link between patients, family, and the rehabilitation team. Their mandate is to obtain a detailed personal history, family history, work history, and social history, as well as to determine past psychological or social problems such as legal confrontations or abuse of alcohol or drugs. This information is extremely important in determining proper rehabilitative goals. Early discharge planning should begin before admission to the rehabilitation center. Social workers play a key role in coordinating the program and helping to prepare family members for discharge. It is important that all team members involve family in educational programs, and that whatever their financial status, a family member or significant other (in addition to the patient himself or herself, as feasible) be trained to be a "case manager." While some would argue that a third party can play this role, we feel that the family can best be its own watchdog for resources over the long term. Social workers can help family members learn this role, and during the acute rehabilitative stay, can actually take over much of the communication between patient, family, rehabilitation team, and insurance carrier. Nevertheless, it is important to develop the ability of the family to deal with these and other demands. Social workers may be trained as licensed clinical social workers (a 4-year degree) or may be graduates of an additional 2 years of training, earning a master of social work (MSW) degree. Rehabilitation counselors go through a 4-year graduate training program in that field.

Chaplains

Spiritual issues are often of great concern to patients following stroke. In fact, the concept of stroke as a "stroke of God" dates to Roman times. The Roman physician Galen described the futility of expecting a physician to effect recovery in someone who has suffered apoplexy (stroke) "from the gods." Patients bring individual, and sometimes unconventional, spiritual beliefs into the rehabilitation center. Some may relate a stroke to having engaged in an activity that, from a health professional's point of view, is medically unrelated. Some patients may consider a stroke as punishment that they deserved or as a cause for feeling guilt or blame. The hospital chaplain or patients' own personal spiritual leaders can help them maintain their "spiritual integrity." Patients and family members often feel great comfort in being able to discuss their spiritual needs.

Other Services

One out of three stroke patients is under the age of 65. Many were working before the stroke and are interested in the potential for ultimately returning to gainful employment. As a consultant to the rehabilitation team, certified vocational evaluators (CVEs) may assess interests and capabilities and may perform a job site analysis. This specialist can help the rehabilitation team determine if it is feasible for the stroke patient to return to work and, if so, when. Factors other than severity of stroke that are associated with a greater rate of return to work include age less than 65, professional or managerial occupation (as opposed to blue-collar or farm), higher education, and extent of language deficit. Twelve percent of those with initial aphonia returned to work—half the rate of nonaphasics (Howard, Till, Toole, Matthews, & Truscott, 1985).

Stroke patients may or may not be able to return to driving. Factors important in this determination include the percentage of paralysis and the presence of balance, cognitive skills, visual field loss, and language functions. Various driver's assessment tools have been developed; some programs even have simulators like those of driver's training schools. The Cognitive Behavioral Driver's Inventory (CBDI) was developed by Dr. Eric Engum and others at the Patricia Neal Rehabilitation Center to specifically examine the cognitive skills that may play a role in the successful return to the road. The CBDI uses certain standardized psychological tests performed by a neuropsychologist (to assess perception and attention) and other specific motor skills (such as visual skills and reaction time) assessed by an occupational therapist. Following a successful or borderline score on the CBDI, a road test is offered to the patient. CBDI has proven extremely useful in predicting patients' success in returning to driving and has excellent correlation with driving records (Engum et al., 1988a, 1988b).

Roles of all Treating Professions

As noted above, many professionals besides the SLP become involved in caring for patients with aphasia. There may be a need for frequent informal contacts between professionals, sometimes as often as daily, in addition to the requirement to assemble formally on a weekly basis to share opinions and expertise. These formal and informal team conferences help develop common goals in conjunction with patient and family input. Whatever the leadership and whatever the team members, the most important rule is that they work together to allow all to participate and thus obtain maximum benefits for the patient. It is important that all treating therapists obtain patient and family goals and adjust their goals in conjunction with patient and family input as treatment proceeds. Never should there be unilateral development of goals and plans by a treatment team without involvement of patient and family.

REFERENCES

Alexander, M.P., Naeser, M.A., & Palumbo, C.L. (1987). Correlations of subcortical CT lesion sites and aphasia profiles. *Brain, 110*, 961–991.

Asymptomatic Carotid Atherosclerosis Study Group. (1989). Study design for randomized prospective trial of carotid endarterectomy for asymptomatic atherosclerosis. *Stroke, 20*, 844–849.

Berthier, M.L., Strakstein, S.E., Leiguarda, R., Ruiz, A., Mayberg, H.S., Wagner, H., Price, T.R., & Robinson, R.G. (1991). Transcortical aphasia. *Brain, 114*, 1409–1427.

Black, S.E., Hachinsk, V.C., & Norris, J.W. (1982). Seizures after stroke. *Canadian Journal of Neurological Science, 9*, 291.

Brust, J.C.M., Shafer, S.Q., Richter, R.W., & Bruun, B. (1976). Aphasia in acute stroke. *Stroke, 7*, 167–173.

Canadian Cooperative Study Group. (1978). A randomized trial of aspirin and sulfinpyrazone in threatened stroke. *New England Journal of Medicine, 299*, 53–59.

Caplan, L.R., & Saunders, E. (1991). Strokes in African-Americans, hypertension in African-Americans, from cardiovascular diseases and stroke in African-Americans and other racial minorities in the United States. *AHA Medical Scientific Statement, 83*, 1462–1480.

Chensea, M.J., Henderson, A., & Cermak, S.A. (1993). Patterns of visual spatial inattention and their functional significance in stroke patients. *Archives Physical and Medical Rehabilitation, 74*, 355–360.

Commission on Accreditation of Rehabilitation Facilities [CARF]. (1992).

Commission on Accreditation of Rehabilitation Facilities [CARF]. (1993).

DeBoskey, D.S., et al., (1987). *Actions and reactions: A stroke manual for families.* Tampa, FL: Hillsborough Co. Hosp. Authority.

DeRenzi, E., Colombo, A., & Scarpa, M. (1991). The aphasic isolate. *Brain, 114*, 1719–1730.

Engum, E.S., Cron, L., Hulse, C.K., Pendergrass T.M., et al. (1988a). Cognitive behavioral driver's inventory. *Cognitive Rehabilitation, 6*, 34–50.

Engum, E.S., Lambert, E.W., Womac, J. & Pendergrass, T.M. (1988b). Norms and decision making rules for the cognitive behavioral driver's inventory. *Cognitive Rehabilitation, 6*, 12–18.

Feldmann, E. (1990, 1991). Intracerebral hemorrhage. *Current Concepts in Cerebrovascular Disease and Stroke, 25*, 31–35; *26*, 1–6.

Ferguson, S.G. (1990). After stroke—Rediscovering yourself. *The Neal Report, 2*, 4–8.

Fields, W.S., Lemak, N.A., Frankowski, R.F., & Hardy, R.J. (1977). Controlled trial of aspirin in cerebral ischemia. *Stroke, 8*, 301–135.

Finlayson, M.A., & Upton, A.R. (1987). Neuropsychological assessment and treatment of stroke patients. In M.E. Brandstate & J.V. Basmajian (Eds.), *Stroke Rehabilitation.* Baltimore: Williams & Wilkins.

Fisher, C. (1958). The use of anticoagulants in cerebral thombosis. *Neurology, 8*, 311–332.

Gasecki, A.P., & Hachinski, V.C. (1993). Risk factors and atherothrombotic stroke. In R.W. Teasell (Ed.), Long-term consequences of stroke, *PMR:STARS, 7*, 43–46.

Gent, M., Blakely, J.A., Easton, J.D., et al. (1989). The Canadian American Ticlopidine Study (CATS) in thromboembolic stroke. *Lancet, 1*, 1215–1220.

Grotta, J.C. (1993). Acute stroke management. *Stroke Clinical Updates, 3*, 1–24.

Hass, W.K., Easton, J.D., Adams, H.P., Jr., Pryse-Phillips, W., Molony, B.A., Anderson, S., & Kamm, B. (1989). A randomized trial comparing ticlopidine hydrochloride with aspirin for the prevention of stroke in high risk patients. *New England Journal of Medicine, 321,* 501–507.

Hecht, J.S. (1991). Inpatient rehabilitation. In D.S. DeBoskey, J.S. Hecht, & C.J. Calub (Eds.), *Educating families of the head injured.* (pp. 45–64). Gaithersburg, MD: Aspen.

Howard, G., Till, J.S., Toole, J.F., Matthews, C., & Truscott, B.L. (1985). Factors influencing return and work following cerebral infarction. *Journal of American Medical Association, 253,* 226–232.

Johnson, E.R., McKenzie, S.W., & Sievers, A. (1993). Aspiration pneumonia in stroke. *Archives Physical and Medical Rehabilitation, 74,* 973–976.

Josephs, A. (1992). *Stroke: An owner's manual.* Long Beach, CA: Amadeus Press.

Kase, C.S., Williams, J.P., Wyatt, D.A., & Mohr, J.P. (1982). Lobar intracerebral hematomas: Clinical and CT analysis of 22 cases. *Neurology, 32,* 1146.

Keith, D.S., Phillips, S.J., Whisnant, J.P., Nishimaru, K., & O'Fallon, W.M. (1987). Heparin therapy for recent transient focal cerebral ischemia. *Mayo Clinic Proceedings, 62,* 1101–1106.

Klatsky, A.L., Armstrong, M.A., & Friedman, G.D. (1991). Racial differences in cerebrovascular disease hospitalizations. *Stroke, 22,* 299–304.

Levine, S.R., Brust, J.C., Futrell, N., Brass, L.M., Blake, D., Fayad, P., Schultz, L.R., Millikan, C.H., & Welch, K.M. (1990). Cerebrovascular complications of the use of the "crack" form of alkaloidal cocaine. *New England Journal of Medicine, 2,* 699–703.

Mori, E., Yamadori, A., & Furumoto, M. (1989). Left precentral gyrus and Broca's aphasia: A clinicopathologic study. *Neurology, 39,* 51–54.

Nicholas, M.L., Helm-Estabrooks, N., Ward-Lonergan, J., & Morgan, A.R. (1993). Evolution of severe aphasia in the first two years post onset. *Archives Physical and Medical Rehabilitation, 74*(8), 830–836.

North American Symptomatic Carotid Endarterectomy Study Group. (1987). Carotid endarterectomy: Three critical evaluations. *Stroke, 18,* 987–989.

Pashek, G.V., & Holland, A.L. (1988). Evolution of aphasia in the first year post onset. *Cortex, 24,* 411–423.

Prazich, M. (1985). *A stroke patient's own story.* Danville, IL: Interstate Printers and Publishers.

Putman, S.F., & Adams, H.P., Jr. (1985). Usefulness of heparin in the initial management of patients with recent transient ischemia attacks. *Archives of Neurology, 42,* 960–962.

Recht, L.D., McCarthy, K., O'Donnell, B.F., Cohen, R., & Drachman, D.A. (1989). Tumor-associated aphasia in left hemisphere primary brain tumors: The importance of age and tumor grade. *Neurology, 38,* 48–50.

Sliwa, J.A., & Liss, S. (1993). Drug-induced dysphagia. *Archives Physical and Medical Rehabilitation, 74,* 445–447.

Steering Committee of the Physicians' Health Study Research Group. (1989). Final report on the aspirin component of the ongoing Physicians' Health Study. *New England Journal of Medicine, 321,* 129–135.

Sze, P.C., Reitman, D., Pincus, M.M., Sacks, H.S., & Chalmers, T.C. (1988). Antiplatelet agents in the secondary prevention of stroke: Meta-analysis of the randomized control trials. *Stroke, 19,* 436–442.

Taub, E., Miller, N.E., Novack, T.A., & Cook, E.W. (1993). Technique to improve chronic motor deficit after stroke. *Archives Physical and Medical Rehabilitation, 74*, 347–354.

Tyrrell, P.J., Warrington, E.K., Frackowiak, R.S.J., & Rossor, M.N. (1990). Heterogeneity in progressive aphasia due to focal cortical atrophy. *Brain, 113*, 1321–1336.

Wiebe-Velazquez, S., & Blume, W.T. (1993). Seizures. *Physical Medicine and Rehabilitation: State of the Art Reviews*, Vol. 7, Number 1, February.

Williams, S.E. (1993). The impact of aphasia on marital satisfaction. *Archives Physical and Medical Rehabilitation, 74*, 361–367.

Wolf, P.A., D'Agostino, R.B., Belanger, A.J., & Kannel, W.B. (1991). Probability of stroke: A risk profile from the Framingham Study. *Stroke, 22*, 312–318.

Chapter 2

Rehabilitation Funding

Jeffrey S. Hecht and John D. Tonkovich

While more dollars ($666 million—12.2% of our gross national product—in 1990 alone) are reportedly spent on health care in the United States than in any other country, 15% of Americans—more than 30 million—do not have sufficient health insurance. Many of those lack coverage for rehabilitation in the event of catastrophic events such as head injury or stroke. Marcia Angel, M.D. (1992), Executive Editor of the *New England Journal of Medicine*, has written that six criteria must be satisfied to create a workable and reformed health care system. These criteria are elaborated where relevant.

1. A health care system should be coherent. Our present system is hopelessly complex, chaotic, and often contradictory. We have multiple payers and forms of delivery, each with different rules and incentives, and we have a burgeoning administrative bureaucracy devoted in large part to shifting costs.
2. It should be universal. Health care should be regarded as a benefit of citizenship, like education, not as a commodity. Every American should therefore be covered according to medical need, not ability to pay. Just as an educated citizenry benefits us all, so does a healthy citizenry.
3. It should be comprehensive. All medically indicated health care should be provided, including long-term care and preventive services. At present, even those of us with "good" private medical insurance are, in fact, underinsured.
4. It should be *structured* to contain costs. Our present system is wildly inflationary. We have no cap on overall spending for health care, and we reward providers and health care facilities, mostly on a piecework basis, for expanding their volume—that is, for providing more services to more patients more often. We have reacted to these inflationary features by overlaying burdensome, often misguided, cost-containment measures.
5. It should be paid for fairly.
6. It should foster the morale of doctors and patients. A health care system cannot work well if doctors and patients are dissatisfied. Today, doctors

and other health care professionals are subjected to frustrating regulations that occupy a growing fraction of their time and interfere with their ability to provide optimal care for each patient. Patients, in turn, feel vulnerable to what at best might seem like capricious limitations in their care. Both groups are drowned in paperwork. The doctor-patient relationship needs to be free from micromanagement and red tape.

FUNDING SOURCES

Traditional Private Insurance Plans

Private insurance can be confusing. There are over 1,200 private health insurers in America, each with its own rules and plans and most with many types of policies. Traditional medical insurance plans often include a certain deductible, after which the patient is expected to pay a certain percentage (say, 10–30%) of "coinsurance," while the insurance company pays the remaining larger percentage up to a certain limit. Beyond the limit, insurance pays 100% in most cases up to a certain cap. The cap can be surprisingly low, so many consumers purchase "major medical policies" to provide a larger cap, such as $1 million or more. Some people purchase "umbrella" policies that will cover them if they incur bills beyond the coverage limit of their major medical insurance. Some states allow insurers to sell policies that cover only specific conditions, such as cancer or heart disease. Some insurers sell policies with ridiculously low caps, such as $59 or $100 a day for inpatient hospitalization—well below market costs.

Rehabilitation coverage is likewise variable, from nonexistent to comprehensive. While insurers compete to offer low deductibles and fringe benefits such as dental care or eye care at a low cost to the public, the fine print often excludes rehabilitative services such as speech pathology in the event of a catastrophic illness or accident. Many policies offered by Blue Cross, for example, exclude rehabilitation or cover only physical therapy. Insurers also review patients' hospital stays, and not uncommonly dictate to hospitals and physicians that payment will no longer be provided after a certain date. At times, this leads to frightening circumstances.

Consider the case of a 38-year-old widow and mother of two teenage daughters who was the solo driver in a motor vehicle crash. She suffered brain trauma and multiple fractures, including a pelvic fracture that made her unable to bear weight. After the initial medical condition was stabilized, her orthopedic and trauma surgeons referred her for comprehensive rehabilitation to address mobility and cognitive deficits relating to her orthopedic injuries and brain injury. Unfortunately, the insurer claimed that her policy covered neither rehabilitation nor skilled nursing care. Further, the company insisted that since she was "stable," it would no longer pay for inpatient acute hospitalization and suggested that she be immediately discharged.

Chaos ensued. Her 16-year-old daughter dropped out of high school to care for her mother, who was then discharged to home with the only covered services being home health physical therapy and home health nursing.

Another case demonstrating the same point is that of a 32-year-old woman who suffered a left-brain infarct. This individual, who was in her eighth month of pregnancy, acquired right hemiplegia and aphasia. She was stabilized and the child was delivered by cesarean section—a healthy boy. Unfortunately, her husband was "between jobs" and her state Medicaid system did not cover rehabilitation. As the husband could not care for his severely disabled wife and new baby, the state's funding system was essentially pushing this woman into a long-term nursing home situation, where continued care was covered. Instead, her physicians and therapists felt that she was such a good rehabilitation candidate that it would have been tragic to miss the critical opportunity for successful rehabilitation. The Stroke Rehabilitation Center and its physicians accepted her with no funding whatsoever. She made excellent progress, and was discharged home in 6 weeks, independent in mobility and most self-care skills. After 12 weeks of outpatient therapy, she was able to care for herself, her baby, and her home. Her outpatient speech-language pathology services were provided for free as the state does not cover this service. Her language likewise improved to a functional level. This rehabilitation allowed her husband to look for a job. Today, he has a well-paying job with the city with full medical benefits for his family. If not for rehabilitation, she would continue to depend on taxpayer funds for the rest of her life while her husband could not become a taxpayer for several years. With rehabilitation, she has achieved the outcome noted.

Coverage for speech-language pathology services can be specifically limited by maximal reimbursement of some policies (such as a specific cap on speech-language pathology or other therapy services). Coverage can also be limited by a percentage cap on charges (for example, a 50% cap is frequently established for psychology services). It can also be limited by specific exclusions, such as in the example above. Policies may also provide for only a limited number of visits by speech-language pathologists individually, or can lump their visits with physical therapy and occupational therapy, allowing only a certain number of total therapy visits per year.

Managed Care Organizations

As health care costs continue to rise, and as spending per capita for health care services increases, many Americans now participate in managed care organizations for their health care needs. This type of insurance coverage differs from traditional private insurance plans. The features of managed care plans include the following:

- Linkage of specific providers and service delivery based on a contractual agreement

- Providers who are paid by the managed care plan
- Continuum of services including primary care, prevention, wellness, and health education
- Systematic assessment of quality of care through resources management
- Information systems to monitor costs, processes and outcomes (Cornett, Klontz, & White, 1994). The underlying assumptions of managed care organizations are that resources can be used in a cost-effective manner and that these resources can be used to produce better patient outcomes.

There are four basic types of managed care plans: health maintenance organizations (HMOs), preferred provider organizations (PPOs), exclusive provider organizations (EPOs), and point-of-service (POS) plans (Cornett, Klontz, & White, 1994). Patients enrolled in PPOs and HMOs may face limitations on rehabilitation services. PPOs provide medical services through a group of affiliated physicians and other health care providers. Patients who use this network of providers receive a certain rate, such as 90% insurance coverage, while the patient is asked to pay 10% coinsurance. An EPO is a type of PPO that requires patients to receive all services from affiliated providers. Patients who choose to use a provider outside of the group must pay the entire cost of the services.

HMOs also operate with a group of designated "preferred" physicians and providers but in a different manner. In an HMO, the group is paid a fixed amount whether or not the patient comes for any services. Thus, it is in the interest of the HMO to limit services. Open-ended HMOs (or POS plans) enable patients to select providers outside the network, although there are strong financial disincentives for using providers outside the network of affiliated providers. These disincentives may include higher copayments or increased use of coinsurance to receive services from out of network providers.

HMOs may restrict the setting in which rehabilitation is provided. Some HMOs, for instance, do not cover rehabilitation in an acute rehabilitation hospital but insist that such services be dispensed in nursing facilities, home health care, or outpatient settings. In these instances, providers may negotiate for out-of-contract benefits so that services may be provided in other settings. HMOs may also limit services by placing caps on the allowable days or by reviewing the need for ongoing care every 3–7 days, and/or by having an implicit rather than an explicit cap. Often, an advisor or case manager is called into the case as an employee of the insurance company to monitor outcomes. Occasionally, there is disagreement between case managers and rehabilitation teams about the adequacy of outcomes, and reimbursement might be denied. When this has occurred, the courts have been reluctant to reprimand HMOs for their role in restricting access to care (American Medical Association, 1993).

Sometimes, legal assistance may be needed to determine coverage levels. It is not uncommon for an insurance company to misrepresent its policies. Brabham (1992) writes, "At one time or another each of us has helped persons with disabilities with a question: Does my health insurance policy cover medical rehabilitation services? In the end, services may be covered, but this is often dependent upon how the insurance company interprets their own vague policy language rather than by any clear coverage statements in the policy." An organization called the Medical Rehabilitation Education Foundation (MREF), a branch of the National Association of Rehabilitation Facilities (NARF), is helping to make consumers, employers, legislators, and physicians aware of the value of medical rehabilitation and the need for more specific language in policies. Brabham notes that "the lack of clearly stated coverage of medical rehabilitation services in insurance policies is a genuine roadblock to increasing utilization of medical rehabilitation among insured patients." One helpful route for the uncovered patient and family is to contact the state insurance commissioner or member of the state legislature. Sometimes this helps insurance companies recognize that they made "a simple mistake."

Unfortunately, legal decisions encourage such unscrupulous behavior among insurance companies. When patients and families sue insurance companies that have withheld medically necessary benefits, courts have merely forced the company to pay the amount due without allowing meaningful punitive awards. In addition, from a business standpoint, it behooves insurers to withhold payments as long as possible so that interest can be collected on the large sums of money that are held in investment accounts. These are among the many ways some insurers place their customers—customers without whom insurers could not exist—at a distinct financial and emotional disadvantage.

On the other hand, many insurance companies are cognizant of the important role of rehabilitation in reducing the overall cost of health care by returning a patient to a maximum level of function and independence in as short a time as possible. In fact, intensive rehabilitation has been shown to pay a handsome return on the investment. When contacted by rehabilitation providers, some insurance companies will make "out-of-contract" arrangements for medically necessary rehabilitation services. A case manager working with a rehabilitation facility or with the insurance company can help with these arrangements.

In the event of trauma occurring in a motor vehicle accident, coverage may be available through automobile insurance. Policy limits vary greatly from state to state. In some states, they are as low as $10,000, a sum that does not go far in a catastrophic event. Other states have innovative systems to fund catastrophic care. Michigan, New Jersey, and Pennsylvania set aside general catastrophic funds to be used for rehabilitation for those injured in automobile accidents. Florida has a particularly creative system whereby those most involved with causing trauma—drunk and drugged drivers and speeders—contribute to the rehabilitation of patients with brain injuries through a set-aside portion of state funds collected from tickets issued for driving under the influence and speeding.

Private Payment

Surprisingly, some individuals pay, either in part or in total, for the rehabilitation services they receive, without additional funds being provided by insurance companies or governmental funds. There are several different sets of circumstances in which this occurs.

Some individuals either have no health insurance or have policies that exclude coverage for rehabilitation services. These individuals must pay out-of-pocket for the services they receive. In some cases, fees for services may be adjusted according to the family income of individual patients. This type of financial arrangement is more commonly available in settings where services are provided through community agencies, or in university clinics where students provide services under supervision.

Some individuals, once they have achieved maximum therapeutic benefit from restorative rehabilitation services, want to continue treatment to maintain a particular level of performance. Since maintenance therapy is not covered by the vast majority of insurance policies, these individuals must pay for maintenance therapy out-of-pocket.

Some individuals want to have their services provided in settings other than those covered by their insurance policies. For example, someone may want to receive speech-language pathology services in the home, when the individual's health insurance policy provides for such services on an outpatient basis only. These persons would be required to pay privately for such services, unless they were able to negotiate with the insurance company for out of contract benefits.

Medicare

Medicare is a federally funded and administered program. It is complicated but does not represent the quagmire associated with private insurance. Medicare, the federal government's health insurance program for the elderly, covers persons over age 65. For those who have worked for 8 quarters and have a disability, coverage is available before age 65 after they have received 2 years of disability checks. A special program also provides Medicare services at the time of diagnosis to patients with chronic renal disease, such as those who need hemodialysis.

There are two basic parts to Medicare: Part A and Part B (Phillippi, 1991). Part A services cover inpatient hospitalization. Part B services cover health care in the nursing home; home health physician fees and therapy services; equipment such as wheelchairs, hospital beds, and bedside commodes; maintenance of this equipment; and outpatient therapy services.

TABLE 2.1 Medicare Underlying Policy Coverage: Superimposed on This Is the Diagnostic Related Group (DRG) System in Acute Hospitals (1995 figures)

Hospitalization coverage

$696 deductible, then 100% coverage	Patient or co-insurance pays $169/day	Patient or co-insurance pays $338/day	Medicare coverage ends
0–60 days	61–90 days	91–150 days	Beyond 150 days
Renewable 90 days if out of hospital or SNF for 60 days in a row	Renewable 90 days if out of hospital or SNF for 60 days in a row	These 60 lifetime reserve days are forever lost once used	—

Speech-language pathologist coverage

80% of "approved amount" covered after $100 deductible; patient responsible for 20%

Skilled-nursing facility (SNF or SNU)

100% coverage	80% coverage
20 days	21–100 days

Immediate-care facility (ICF)

no coverage by Medicare

80% coverage: No limit on days; limit on number of treatments per fiscal year can be imposed by fiscal intermediary. Appeals for more coverage can be filed based on medical necessity.

Medicare recipients pay nothing for Part A coverage. Part B coverage is optional, and costs $41.10 per month (1993 figures). These payments can be deducted from a person's Social Security check. The recipient must have Medicare before the onset of the disability to qualify for services; coverage cannot be retroactive. Hospitalization coverage includes a deductible that in 1993 was $696 for the first 60 hospital days. After the deductible, the patient's share increases to $169 a day for the next 30 days, and $338 a day for the ninety-first to one-hundred-fiftieth hospital day (Table 2.1). Physician and therapy services are covered by Medicare at 80% after a $100 deductible. Patients often purchase coinsurance to cover the 20% not covered by Medicare. These policies vary greatly and are called Medicare supplemental policies or Medigap insurance (Health Care Financing Administration, 1993). There have been discussions of standardizing these policies so that patients will have a better understanding of what they are buying and what their coverage represents. Medicare covers care in a skilled-nursing facility (SNF or SNU), but not in an intermediate-care facility (ICF). The significance of this is discussed below.

For inpatient hospitalization, Medicare has two policies that take effect simultaneously. Under an underlying policy, a patient has 100% coverage under Medicare for the first 2 months after meeting the deductible, then has a 20% coinsurance requirement from the sixty-first through ninetieth day, and a 40% coinsurance requirement from the ninety-first through one-hundred-fiftieth day. The first 90 days are "renewable" if a person is out of the hospital (and not in a skilled nursing facility) for 60 uninterrupted days. At the end of the 90 days are 60 nonrenewable "lifetime reserve" days that the person has only once in a lifetime. For those who are severely ill, secondary policies often provide coverage after the one-hundred-fiftieth day.

The above discussion has been made less relevant for acute hospitalization in the last few years because of a superimposed system called diagnostic-related groups (DRGs). Under this system, a hospital is paid a lump sum for a patient's primary and associated diagnoses no matter what the length of the hospital stay. This system is somewhat confusing. For example, a hospital is paid the same amount for a patient with an intracranial hemorrhage who dies after 2 days as for one who lives, has intensive interventional therapies, and who makes substantial progress after a 2-week hospitalization. The hospital has financial incentives in the first case and disincentives in the second. However, the system does make some allowances for unusual situations, such as particularly long hospital stays, and for medical complications.

Rehabilitation centers (whether free-standing or units of hospitals) are exempt from the DRGs and therefore are reimbursed based on their costs. Additionally, they are subject to the time and coverage limitation of the "underlying" Medicare policy described above. In recent years, rehabilitation hospitals have been under a "TEFRA cap" (Tax Equity and Financial Reform Act). This law affects how rehabilitation centers are funded by defining an optimal charge per day for the diagnosis. If a hospital's average charges to Medicare for the year per case is higher than the capitated rate, it must refund some of the money to Medicare; if its average charges are lower than the TEFRA cap (i.e., shorter lengths of stay), the hospital receives incentive payments from Medicare.

Part B services are covered throughout the inpatient hospital stay at an 80% Medicare pay and 20% coinsurance payment once the patient's annual deductible is met. There is no cap. The need for a coinsurance payment continues indefinitely. Inpatient speech-language pathology services and other therapies are provided under Part A, whereas outpatient and home health services are provided under Part B. Medicare covers outpatient speech pathology services but operates with a review organization (Medical Fiscal Intermediary) that screens the need for such services. Unfortunately, clinicians often do not discover until several months after treatment that their bills for services have been denied as not medically necessary. The screens often impose service limits that are reported to be remarkably short. While it is essential that the speech-language pathologist abide by ethical proscriptions and treat patients who are showing objective responses to treatment and improvement, the speech pathologist is challenged to document such improvement on a month-to-month basis in language that the reviewing organization can understand. Details of such documentation lie beyond the scope of this discussion. Home health services have similar reviews and caps but are less stringently reviewed.

Nursing facility care is covered under Medicare Part B. Medicare covers 20 days in a skilled nursing facility at 100% for those who need intensive rehabilitation and for those with feeding tubes and severe decubitus ulcers (bed sores). After 20 days, the patient is then covered for 80 days, with Medicare paying 80% and the patient (or his or her coinsurance) being responsible for the remaining 20%. The skilled nursing facility must show regular progress in physical therapy to continue in the rehabilitation phase. Medicare requires the skilled nursing facility patient to have once daily physical therapy but does not define the length of that contact. Occupational therapy and speech pathology services are also reimbursed beyond the fixed room rate.

Other Public Insurance Systems

Medicaid is a federally funded program administered by the states. States provide some funds and receive matching federal funds that are often greater than the state's contribution. Medicaid varies from state to state, with different rules regarding care in the hospital, rehabilitation center, nursing facility, outpatient, and home health settings. Programs vary depending on the state's financial stability and its awareness of the facts regarding the favorable cost-benefit ratio of rehabilitation. Most state Medicaid systems cover inpatient rehabilitation. The few states that do not cover inpatient rehabilitation through their Medicaid systems do provide rehabilitation coverage through their vocational rehabilitation programs (DVR). DVR has a federal-to-state dollar match even more favorable than the amount contributed by the state. In 1991, Tennessee became the first and only state to systematically exclude the newly disabled from inpatient rehabilitation services. Coverage of young disabled individuals under Medicaid in Tennessee is effectively allowed only in nursing homes. Some states limit Medicaid reimbursement for speech-language pathology outpatient services.

Medicaid covers SNF care in many settings and also covers intermediate care. In fact, care in nursing facilities is the greatest share of Medicaid cost in every state. ICFs allow physical therapy services as frequently as three times weekly, usually to provide services geared towards maintenance rather than the intensive programs that lead to progress. Speech-language pathology and occupational therapy are usually not covered in the ICF setting.

Worker's compensation, an insurance plan with mandated federal requirements, is administered on a state-by-state basis. It is provided through employers and protects those who are injured on the job. There are various types of worker's compensation, with different systems covering injuries on land, injuries on water, and injuries that occur in federal jobs. Worker's compensation pays for intensive hospital services and later ongoing rehabilitation and provides reimbursement for a percentage of lost wages, which is determined on a state-by-state basis. In some states, a case manager is provided to help the patient and family members with worker's compensation. This insurance can provide for such reimbursements as medication, mileage for family members driving to and from a facility, and housing during therapy programs that are far from where the family members reside. It may also cover items that are not in traditional policies.

State vocational rehabilitation is established through a federal mandate and administered on a state-by-state basis. Again, state dollars are set aside and are "matched" by federal dollars. The match is often an even greater federal percentage than it is under Medicaid. The goal of vocational rehabilitation in most cases is to return people to the workforce. There may be other mandates, such as allowing people to live more independently or allowing a homemaker to return home so a spouse can work. This can be problematic in severely aphasic patients, who often continue to have severe and persisting vocational disabilities. If patients are accepted, vocational rehabilitation will pay for any needed service, including speech-language pathology, audiology, cognitive rehabilitation, psychology, occupational and physical therapies, vocational evaluations, occupational medicine programs (specific efforts to get people ready to re-enter the workplace), job placement, driver's evaluation, medications, and equipment.

States often are more generous in coverage of special programs for children with disabilities. These programs apply to people under age 21. Parents must meet financial guidelines, which are usually similar to Medicaid guidelines, to receive coverage under these programs. Coverage varies from state to state, with differences in the lengths of stays allowed for inpatients. Services are covered for both inpatients and outpatients.

Public assistance, another source of funding, varies among cities, counties, and states. A governing board usually administers funds. These may be set aside for certain diagnoses or disabilities, and patients must meet strict standards regarding need. Many communities have volunteer organizations, such as Sertoma, Easter Seals, and Goodwill Industries, with funds to help with needed care. Other service organizations may provide help or equipment for different disabilities (for example, Sertoma for hearing aids and communication devices, Lions for the visually impaired, Elks for cerebral palsy, Scottish Rite for equipment loans, and Shriners for burns and orthopedic injuries). Communities, churches, or newspapers may have special funds for those in poverty who need services. Charities are rarely adequate sources of sufficient coverage for comprehensive rehabilitative services. In cases that involve litigation, an attorney may be able to provide a guarantee of payment to a facility that provides treatment to an individual who does not have other funds. This is called a "letter of protection" and guarantees that rehabilitation costs will be paid once a court reaches a final settlement. However, the rehabilitation provider runs the risk of not being paid for services if the case is not settled in favor of the patient. Increasingly, courts are establishing structured settlements to provide ongoing needs for injured patients rather than giving a lump sum. These funds can be designated for speech-language pathology or other necessary rehabilitation services.

MAXIMIZING THE LIKELIHOOD OF REIMBURSEMENT FOR SPEECH-LANGUAGE PATHOLOGY SERVICES

Documentation

In both the public and private sectors, payment for rehabilitation services is typically contingent on the receipt of timely, concise, and accurate documentation of treatments provided and patient outcomes. Therefore, speech-language pathologists should pay careful attention to the manner in which diagnostic reports, treatment plans, progress summaries, and discharge reports are written. Documentation sometimes does not accurately reflect what has occurred in treatment sessions, and payment for the treatments subsequently may be denied. Speech-language pathologists may find the following guidelines regarding documentation useful.

1. *Avoid using professional jargon.* Many speech-language pathologists are accustomed to writing reports that are filled with terminology that is only intelligible to other speech-language pathologists! Consider the following excerpt from a diagnostic report by a speech-language pathologist, who wrote, "Mr. Kelly has both phonemic and verbal paraphasias in the context of fluent verbal output. His attempts at word retrieval often result in circumlocutions, and he is prone to perseveration." Most reviewers from insurance companies or federal agencies are not speech-language pathologists, and entries such as this one are baffling and confusing to reviewers. Simple language should be used in reporting. For instance, "Sometimes sounds and syllables slip out of sequence in Mr. Kelly's speech, and he sometimes substitutes words. While he is able to speak in complete sentences, he often gets stuck on a word and perseverates on that word, even though he attempts to say something else." When it is important to use professional jargon in a report, it may be useful to define the term or provide parenthetical examples.

2. *Attempt to describe how the patient's communication disorder affects daily living communication.* While it may be worthwhile to note that a patient scored at the forty-first percentile overall on the PICA (*Porch Index of Communicative Ability*, 1981), claims reviewers are apt not to care. They may be interested in knowing whether or not this patient possesses sufficient communication skills to be able to live independently and safely, or that while she understands about 80–90% of what is said to her, she is able to communicate successfully by talking about 10–25% of the time. That is not to say that test scores are unimportant or should be excluded from speech-language pathology reports. Claims reviewers often look for objective measures of progress, but they also need to gain insight into the functional abilities of aphasic individuals.

3. *Avoid using terminology that can be interpreted to suggest that speech-language pathology services are making the patient stay the same or get worse.* Certainly not deliberately, but sometimes speech-language pathologists write things in reports that send up "red flags" to claims reviewers. Some terms and phrases to avoid in reports include "regressing," "no change," "verbal expression is deteriorating," "no progress," "patient not motivated," "patient uncooperative," "patient has plateaued," and "maintenance therapy." Many providers will not reimburse services geared toward rehabilitating cognitive aspects of communication, so the speech-language pathologist may want to avoid using the word *cognitive*, particularly in goals outlined in treatment plans. Use of a single word may mean the difference between reimbursement and denial. Consider the case of a 48-year-old man who became aphasic subsequent to herpes encephalitis. CT scannning revealed a large area of infarction in the left temporal-parietal area and a small infarction in the right temporal area. When the man was seen for a speech-language evaluation, he was found to have severe word-finding difficulties in the context of fluent output and good auditory comprehension, and he had some minor difficulties with abstract language (e.g., interpretations of proverbs and idioms). In her evaluation report, the speech-language pathologist wrote that the man had anomic aphasia and a cognitive-communication disorder. Despite the fact that the aphasia was the man's predominant communication problem, the claims reviewer initially denied payment for services because it was the insurance company's policy not to reimburse for cognitive retraining.

4. *Documentation should be timely and should accurately reflect patient outcomes.* Speech-language pathologists should complete documentation of services provided as the services are provided or shortly thereafter. For example, it is much easier to remember what a patient did in a treatment session 5 minutes ago than what he may have done in a treatment session 5 weeks ago! Documentation should reflect, as closely as possible, what the patient has become able to do as a result of treatment. Consider the following case example. A speech-language pathologist

had been working with a woman with conduction aphasia on role playing telephone conversations. The clinician provided extensive verbal and nonverbal cueing during the role playing exercises, and the aphasic woman performed adequately. In a treatment progress note, the clinician documented that the patient was successful in 100% of her attempts to engage in telephone conversations. Reimbursement for speech-language pathology services beyond that session were denied initially by a claims reviewer, who asked "if she can talk on the telephone successfully 100% of the time, why does she need more therapy?" When appropriate, clarify reports by providing examples, especially in instances when an aphasic patient's performance is related to extensive external cueing provided by the clinician.

5. *Reports should be neat, well-organized, succinct, and easy to read.* When reports are handwritten, the handwriting should be legible. Reports should be well-organized and have some logical order. They need not be long. In fact, claims reviewers often prefer shorter reports, as long as pertinent information has been included.

Working with Case Managers

As health care reform progresses, speech-language pathologists will see rapid growth in managed care programs, not only in the private sector, but in the public sector as well. In advocating for services for aphasic adult clients, speech-language pathologists will need to develop proactive strategies for working with case managers. Case managers are the link between the health care provider and the insurance carrier, so it is essential that speech-language pathologists foster positive relationships with them.

Many case managers have backgrounds in nursing or social work, and although they may have general knowledge about aphasia and the work that speech-language pathologists do, they may require additional information and education about specific aphasia management strategies and procedures. The following guidelines may be useful for speech-language pathologists in providing this information to case managers.

1. *Develop goals that are reasonable and that are based on the patient's medical diagnosis and likely recovery.* Ischemic and hemorrhagic strokes have different courses of recovery (Brookshire, 1992), and speech-language pathologists should take this into account when developing treatment plans for their aphasic clients. Those who have suffered ischemic strokes will likely show greatest recovery during the first few weeks post-onset, while those who have suffered hemorrhagic strokes often show little improvement until 8 or more weeks post-onset. By working with the case manager, the speech-language pathologist might use knowledge of the recovery from stroke to shape the treatment plan. For instance, the intensity of intervention for aphasias resulting from

ischemic strokes might be greater immediately post-onset, while more intensive intervention efforts for aphasias resulting from hemorrhagic strokes might be delayed until at least 2 months post-onset. Speech and language rehabilitation efforts should capitalize on the patient's recovery from stroke. During the so-called "spontaneous recovery period," a period typically 3–6 months post-onset of stroke, the speech-language pathologist should attempt to provide patients and their families with education about aphasia and temporary communication strategies, while monitoring and documenting recovery. Strategies that facilitate communication successes and those that compensate for communication deficits should most likely be included during intervention efforts that lie beyond what is considered the spontaneous recovery period.

2. *Develop goals that are realistic and that are based on the patient's aphasia severity.* Those aphasic individuals with profound aphasic deficits immediately following a stroke will likely have persisting aphasic deficits, even after spontaneous recovery and speech-language intervention. For these individuals, intervention efforts should be directed toward helping them cope with aphasia and communicate by whatever means possible. Novice clinicians are often far too eager to attempt to restore the communication behaviors of such individuals to premorbid levels. Case managers, on the other hand, are likely to accept less, as long as the intervention efforts attempt to restore the individual to his or her maximum level of communicative functioning, whatever that might be. Those aphasic individuals with mild aphasic deficits immediately post-onset are likely to show almost complete recovery and may not need much speech-language intervention.

3. *State goals in terms of functional outcomes.* Case managers need to know the effects of speech-language interventions on aphasic patients' functional abilities. Many speech-language pathologists have little if any training in determining the functional implications of the services they provide. Clinicians may find the American Speech-Language-Hearing Association's (1995) *Functional Assessment of Communication Skills (ASHA FACS)* a useful tool for evaluating functional communication abilities and for planning interventions for aphasic clients. The *ASHA FACS* consists of behavioral descriptors in four communication domains: social communication, communication of basic needs, reading/writing/number concepts, and daily planning. By observation, caregiver report, and/or direct testing, speech-language pathologists rate patient performance for each of the instrument's items on a 7-point scale, which is provided in Table 2.2. Some of the items that are rated are the patient's ability to understand what's heard on television and radio, request help when necessary, write messages, and dial telephone numbers. The items on the *ASHA FACS* are exactly the kinds of functional outcomes case managers look for in prospective treatment plans, and speech-language pathologists may find these items a useful springboard for aphasia treatment planning and goal setting.

TABLE 2.2 Scale Used to Rate Communication Behavior on the ASHA FACS (American Speech-Language-Hearing Association, 1995).

Rating	Descriptor	Definition
7	Can do	Client performs behavior; needs no assistance and/or prompting
6	Can do with minimal assistance	Client performs behavior, rarely needing assistance and/or prompting
5	Can do with minimal to moderate assistance	Client performs behavior, occasionally needing assistance and/or prompting
4	Can do with moderate assistance	Client performs behavior, often needing assistance and/or prompting
3	Can do with moderate to maximal assistance	Client performs behavior, very frequently needing assistance and/or prompting
2	Can do with maximal assistance	Client performs behavior only with constant assistance and/or prompting
1	Cannot do	Client cannot perform behavior, even with maximal assistance and/or prompting
0	No basis for rating	Circumstances in which a behavior cannot be observed, directly tested, or available from other sources

Assistance/prompting includes but is not limited to repeating, rephrasing, simplifying language, slowing rate of speech, providing help in using assistive/alternative devices, using gestures, writing/drawing pictures, giving additional time for response, asking yes/no questions, and giving a limited choice.

4. *Negotiate with case managers for patient-specific needs.* Speech-language pathologists have become accustomed to providing services without interruption from the time shortly after the onset of aphasia until a time when the patient achieves treatment goals. In managed care organizations, it may not be necessary to provide services continuously and without interruption. For instance, highly motivated patients may benefit from several sessions of treatment to learn a new strategy, followed by a break from treatment so that they can practice using the strategy, followed by several more sessions to learn more advanced strategies, and so forth.

Sometimes, particularly after the onset of aphasia, patients become depressed and are unable and/or unwilling to participate in speech-language pathology services. Namnum (1995), in a personal account of his recovery from aphasia, stated that while he received 9 weeks of therapy immediately post-onset from obviously trained and dedicated therapists, nothing happened in the therapy because he could not relate to it. It was not until he became emotionally ready to recognize the implications of his aphasia that he felt he could benefit from speech-language intervention. Case managers often have some flexibility regarding authorization for the rate and frequency of delivery of speech-language pathology services, and in situations such as Namnum's, it is not unusual for managed care organizations to delay the onset of treatment.

5. *Invite case managers and other insurance company representatives to interdisciplinary team conferences.* Case managers often welcome the opportunity to participate in interdisciplinary team conferences to ensure that the most appropriate care is being provided to their insured patient, to contain costs, and to plan long-term costs. In team conferences, participants should provide functional patient information, particularly as it relates to the attainment of goals set for the patient. Participants should avoid saying things such as "This isn't my patient" or "I really don't know too much about this patient," as these kinds of remarks do little to instill confidence about the quality of the services provided. The case manager and/or insurance representatives should be provided with opportunities to ask questions and to obtain clarification. Payment and duration of treatment are often tied to what occurs in interdisciplinary team conferences, so when patients continue to show potential for improvement, this should be stated directly, even in instances where patient progress is at a temporary plateau.

Case managers are often willing to accommodate patient needs, and it is essential to establish positive working relationships with these individuals. Many of them do not know a lot about specific aphasia types and interventions and often appreciate information speech-language pathologists can provide them for sound decision-making.

THE FUTURE OF REIMBURSEMENT FOR SPEECH-LANGUAGE PATHOLOGY SERVICES

It is clear that in the years ahead, the health care industry must dramatically overhaul the health care delivery system to make it more efficient and to reduce costs. Certain changes in the ways that speech-language pathology services are delivered to aphasic patients are likely.

One aspect of delivery that is likely to change is that payers are likely to begin looking for lower cost alternatives for the delivery of services to aphasic patients. It is likely that a new level of speech-language pathology provider will emerge—paraprofessionals who will serve as speech-language pathology assistants. These individuals will likely provide much of the speech and language rehabilitation to aphasic individuals, and in turn, will reduce costs to payers.

It is also likely that family members and other caregivers will play an increasingly important role in delivering speech-language pathology services. Speech-language pathologists, with a minimal number of visits, may choose to use them by training family members and other caregivers to provide the training and instruction in communication strategies to their aphasic person. This will also reduce costs associated with service delivery.

Because there will undoubtedly be persons other than speech-language pathologists delivering speech and language services to aphasic patients, there will be increased competition among speech-language pathologists for clients. This may also drive down costs, as speech-language pathologists adjust their fees downward to stay competitive.

Because so many individuals will be uninsured or underinsured, it is likely that not all consumers will be eligible for the same level of intervention efforts. For instance, aphasic individuals who have afforded lofty premiums and out-of-pocket expenses may be eligible to receive a full array of speech-language pathology services, while those with federally funded insurance may be eligible for an evaluation and a minimal number of sessions. Because of literature that suggests poor prognoses for recovery for some types of aphasia (e.g., global aphasia), individuals with these diagnoses may be excluded from receiving speech-language pathology services at all.

Payers may begin reimbursing for specific outcomes and may deny reimbursement for services that did not result in desired outcomes. This will enable them to reduce costs and to ensure a quality standard simultaneously.

How health care reimbursement will change is uncertain, but there is little dispute that the entire health care industry will see many major changes as we move into the twenty-first century.

Rehabilitation funding can be an extremely challenging undertaking. It is helpful to have allies in social service and hospital financial departments to help. Speech-language pathologists must keep abreast of the continual changes in health care funding and financing and should continually develop strategies that provide for the most efficacious rehabilitation at the lowest cost. Speech-language pathologists should be proactive in this area and should advocate for their patients' needs.

REFERENCES

American Speech-Language-Hearing Association. (1995). *Functional assessment of communication skills for adults* (ASHA FACS). Rockville, MD: American Speech-Language-Hearing Association.

American Medical Association. (1993). Gatekeeper is agent of IPA-model HMO. *AMA News, 36,* 9.

Angell, M. (1992). The presidential candidates and health care reform. *New England Journal of Medicine, 327,* 800–801.

Brabham, R.E. (1992). Needed: Model insurance language for rehabilitation services. NARF Rehabilitation Report, 1, 7. In *Caring for a person with dysphasia.* Dallas: American Heart Association, 1990.

Brookshire, R.H. (1992). *An introduction to neurogenic communication disorders.* St. Louis: Mosby-Year Book.

Cornett, B.S., Klontz, H., & White, S.C. (1994). Managed care: An overview. In American Speech-Language-Hearing Association. *Managing managed care: A practical guide for audiologists and speech-language pathologists.* Rockville, MD: American Speech-Language-Hearing Association.

Health Care Financing Administration. (1993). *Medicare Q & A.* Baltimore: Health Care Financing Administration.

Namnum, A. (1995). Readiness for therapy: Aphasia patient offers insights into rehab process. *ADVANCE for Speech-Language Pathologists and Audiologists, 5,* (26), 11, 38.

Phillippi, L. (1991). *The ABC's of Medicare Part A and Part B for clinicians.* Racine, WI: M.J. Therapy and Association, Inc.

Porch, B.E. (1981). *Porch index of communicative ability.* Palo Alto, CA: Consulting Psychologists Press.

Chapter 3

Clinical Descriptions

Robert T. Wertz

B. Ganglia, M.D., of the Neurology Service, wrote the following consultation request: "W.B., a 72-year-old white male, suffered a left hemisphere infarct in the middle cerebral artery with extension into the angular gyrus. There is no indication of hemiplegia. He is 2 weeks postonset. Please evaluate and consider treatment." Dr. Ganglia received the following response.

W.B. displays severe aphasia crossing all communicative modalities, including auditory comprehension, reading, oral-expressive language, and writing. There is no indication of coexisting apraxia of speech or dysarthria. His auditory comprehension is limited to 40% correct understanding of single words and short sentences. His reading ability is reduced to 30% correct for single words and short phrases. Oral-expressive language indicates normal prosody, six- to seven-word phrase length, no impairment of articulation, and a variety of grammatical constructions. W.B. produces numerous phonological errors (e.g., "mather" for "mother") and frequent semantic errors (e.g., "chairs" for "table"). His connected speech is inaccurate and inappropriate— for example, when asked to describe the use of a toothbrush, he replied, "I use it to scratch my sand." Repetition is impaired for both single words (e.g., "hippo face" for "caterpillar") and short phrases. W.B.'s writing resembles his oral-expressive language. It is intelligible but abounds with misspellings and incorrect words. Writing to dictation is impossible for W.B. He is 70% accurate in copying words and geometric shapes. Evoking accurate responses in any modality requires a repetition of instructions and auditory and visual cues.

W.B.'s aphasia could be described as receptive aphasia, fluent aphasia, or Wernicke's aphasia. Obviously, there is more than one way to describe aphasia. Some are more informative than others.

Some believe aphasia is a general language disorder that crosses all communicative modalities, and they eschew the use of adjectives to modify or describe it (Darley, 1982). Others (Goodglass & Kaplan, 1983; Helm-Estabrooks & Albert, 1991; Kertesz, 1979) believe there are sufficient differences among aphasic patients to permit the use of a taxonomy for classifying the "aphasias."

How one describes aphasia or the aphasias depends on the purpose. For example, one can describe to facilitate patient management, communicate among medical and allied health professionals, group patients for research, or counsel the patient and his or her family and friends. This chapter discusses different descriptive systems for aphasia and how one's definition of aphasia influences the description.

THE DILEMMA OF DEFINITIONS

There are several systems for describing aphasia, and each is influenced by the way aphasia is defined.

Aphasia is One

Marie (1906) postulated "aphasia is one." Even though he went on to list several types—"anarthria . . . anarthria with aphasia . . . temporal aphasia . . . angular gyrus aphasia . . . global aphasia"—his position was a reaction to the localizationists of his day who classified aphasia into different types. Marie believed that people with aphasia differed primarily in severity and in the presence of a coexisting disorder—for example, anarthria with aphasia.

Darley (1982) and Schuell and her colleagues (Schuell, Jenkins & Jimenez-Pabon, 1964) represent Marie's position today. Schuell (1965) used adjectives—simple aphasia, aphasia with visual involvement, aphasia with sensorimotor involvement, etc.—to classify aphasic patients into prognostic groups. However, she, like Darley, suggested that aphasia is "a reduction of available language that crosses all language modalities and may or may not be complicated by perceptual or sensorimotor involvement, by various forms of dysarthria, or by other sequela of brain damage" (Schuell, 1965, p. 4).

Similarly, Darley's (1982) definition makes it clear why he would never use an adjective to modify aphasia. For him, aphasia is:

> impairment as a result of brain damage, of the capacity for interpretation and formulation of language symbols; multimodality loss or reduction in efficiency of the ability to decode and encode conventional meaningful linguistic elements (morphemes and larger syntactic units) disproportionate to impairment of other intellective functions; not attributable to dementia, confusion, sensory loss, or motor dysfunction; and manifested in reduced availability of vocabulary, reduced efficiency in application of syntactic rules, reduced auditory retention span, and impaired efficiency in input and output channel selection (Darley, 1982, p. 42).

Rosenbek, LaPointe, & Wertz (1989) suggest that Darley and Schuell represent the "ands" approach to aphasia—deficits in auditory comprehension, reading, oral-expressive language, *and* writing. Neither require equal impairment in all modalities, but each modality must be impaired for the patient to be considered aphasic. The patient who could do everything but write would not be considered aphasic by Darley or Schuell. This contrasts with an "any or all" position by those who classify aphasia into types.

Aphasia is All or Part

Those (Albert, Goodglass, Helm, Rubens, & Alexander, 1981; Benson, 1979; Damasio, 1981; Goodglass & Kaplan, 1983; Helm-Estabrooks & Albert, 1991; Kertesz, 1979) who classify aphasia into types have formulated definitions consistent with this practice. Goodglass and Kaplan's (1983) definition is representative:

> Aphasia refers to the disturbance of any or all of the skills, associations and habits of spoken or written language, produced by injury to certain brain areas that are specialized for these functions (Goodglass & Kaplan, 1983, p. 5).

Albert and his colleagues (1981) elaborate by specifying that:

> The assessment of language function must deal with this aspect of dysphasia—its possible selectivity for particular modalities of input or output and—in some instances—for specific input-output combinations (Albert et al., 1981, p. 12).

Thus, people with aphasia need not show deficits in all modalities. Disproportionate involvement among modalities, the "all or part" advocates suggest, permits classification.

Aphasia as Impaired Access

Kreindler and Fradis (1968) and McNeil (1982) provide definitions of aphasia that emphasize *why* language deficits exist more than the *kind* of language deficits that exist. For example, McNeil's definition indicates:

> Aphasia is a multimodality physiological inefficiency with greater than loss of verbal symbolic manipulations (e.g., association, storage, retrieval, and rule implementation). In isolated form it is caused by focal damage to cortical and/or subcortical structures of the hemisphere(s) dominant for such symbolic manipulations. It is affected by and affects other physiological information processing and cognitive processes to the degree that they support, interact with, or are supported by the symbolic deficits (McNeil, 1982, p. 693).

One might infer that this position—aphasia as impaired access—permits description of language deficits in some or all communicative modalities.

However, any description based on this definition would speculate why the language deficits exist (for example, physiological inefficiency, increased fatiguability, increased sensory thresholds, decreased speed of reaction, fluctuation of attention and effort allocation, or inertia of neurophysiological excitation and inhibition).

Aphasia as a Cognitive Deficit

Others (Brown, 1977; Chapey, 1981; Martin, 1981) define aphasia as a disruption of cognitive processes or language and cognitive processes. For example, Martin (1981) uses Neisser's (1966) definition of cognition to refer "to all processes by which sensory information is transformed, reduced, elaborated, stored, recovered, and used." Thus, for Martin, aphasia is "the reduction, because of brain damage, of the efficiency of the action or interaction of the cognitive processes that support language" (Martin, 1981, p. 65).

Similarly, Chapey (1981) defines aphasia as

> an acquired impairment in language and the cognitive processes which underlie language caused by organic damage to the brain. It is characterized by a reduction in and dysfunction of language content or meaning, language form or structure and language use or function and the cognitive processes which underlie language, such as memory and thinking (Chapey, 1981, p. 31).

This position is similar to those who espouse that aphasia results from impaired access. However, the primary deficit in aphasia is believed to result from impaired cognitive processing. Thus, description of aphasia may be general—aphasia is a general language deficit—or specific—aphasia may be all or part. But the description must include some reference to the cognitive processes assumed to "underlie" or support language.

A Clinical Definition

As indicated earlier, there are a variety of purposes for describing aphasia—clinical management, interdisciplinary communication, research, and communication with patient and family. Since one's definition of aphasia directs one's description of aphasia, a definition that meets all of the purposes seems preferable. The definition provided by Rosenbek et al. (1989) may do that:

> Aphasia is an impairment, due to acquired and recent damage of the central nervous system, of the ability to comprehend and formulate language. It is a multimodality disorder represented by a variety of impairments in auditory comprehension, reading, oral-expressive language, and writing. The disrupted language may be influenced by physiological inefficiency or impaired cognition, but it cannot be explained by dementia, sensory loss, or motor dysfunction (Rosenbek et al., 1989, p. 53).

This definition appears to encompass a variety of viewpoints. Aphasia does affect all communicative modalities, especially if one probes each with sufficiently difficult tasks to determine where performance begins to break down. However, the variety of impairments in different modalities permits some patients to be classified into aphasic syndromes. Why language is disrupted in aphasia is ascribed to central nervous system damage, but this damage may reduce physiologic efficiency and normal cognition.

Even this general, all-purpose definition can be challenged. For example, "recent damage" does not account for slowly or primary progressive aphasia (Duffy & Peterson, 1992) or for the position held by some (Au, Albert, & Obler, 1988) that language deficits in dementia are best described as aphasia. Perhaps no single definition will ever satisfy everyone. But Rosenbek et al.'s (1989) appears to satisfy most of the purposes for describing aphasia.

CLASSIFICATION SYSTEMS

Again, one's definition of aphasia influences one's description of aphasia. If one believes "aphasia is one," there is no need for classification. Conversely, if one believes aphasia may disrupt communication in different modalities differently, one formulates a taxonomy to differentiate among different type of aphasia. The labels applied to the different types provide the description.

Over the years, classifications have come and gone. Many have been modified by time. Recently, a few new types have emerged. The following represent classifications that continue to be popular.

Aphasia Without Adjectives

"Aphasia without adjectives" represents a refusal to classify. Marie's (1906) position has been perpetuated by Darley (1982), who makes that position very clear:

> Little clinical purpose is served by proliferating adjectives, which are presumed to designate different "types" of aphasia. These adjectives emerge because they are based on different, at times incomplete or biased, observations; they reflect what people look for and believe in (Darley, 1982, p. 42).

Thus, an aphasia-without-adjectives description elaborates an aphasic patient's language impairment in each communicative modality—auditory comprehension, reading, oral-expressive language, and writing. Differences in severity within each modality are noted, as is the presence of any coexisting disorders—apraxia of speech, dysarthria, and so forth.

For the patient who has prosodic problems, short phrase length, articulatory difficulty, disruption of grammatical form, some literal or phonemic paraphasias in running speech, difficulty repeating words and phrases, difficulty in word finding, and relatively good auditory comprehension, advocates of aphasia without adjectives would list symptoms and assign a severity rating. For example, this patient's grammatical form deficits might be called "telegraphic" and described as consisting primarily of content words. The relatively intact auditory comprehension might be noted as 80% intact for understanding conversation but dropping to 60% correct when the auditory message increases in length and complexity. The patient's abnormal prosody, articulatory difficulty, and repetition problems probably would be identified as a coexisting disorder, apraxia of speech.

The aphasia-without-adjectives approach works well for clinical management and patient and family communication. It is appropriate for research, if the research questions are limited to overall severity of aphasia or severity within specific communicative modalities. It is adequate and, perhaps, preferable for interdisciplinary communication among disciplines charged with rehabilitation (physiatry, physical therapy, occupational therapy, etc.). It may be shunned by disciplines (neurology, neurosurgery, neuropsychology) whose focus is on diagnosis, lesion localization, and brain and behavior relationships. Describing aphasia without adjectives is less cumbersome in explaining changes in aphasia, because improvement or the lack of it is described as a change in severity or the waxing or waning of a coexisting disorder.

Expressive-Receptive Dichotomy

Another general system for classifying aphasia is the expressive-receptive dichotomy popularized by Weisenberg and McBride (1935). It is a step away from the motor-sensory division that has dominated since the work of Broca (1861) and Wernicke (1908). The expressive-receptive division was influenced by Head's (1926) classification into verbal aphasia (Weisenberg and McBride's predominately expressive aphasia) and syntactic aphasia (Weisenberg and McBride's predominately receptive aphasia).

Actually, Weisenberg and McBride's classification was fourfold:

1. *Predominately expressive*, where the most severe deficits are in writing and speech.
2. *Predominately receptive*, where the most severe deficits are in understanding spoken and printed language.
3. *Expressive-receptive*, where there are severe deficits in all modalities—auditory comprehension, reading, oral-expressive language, and writing.
4. *Amnestic*, where the primary deficit is in word-finding.

Weisenberg and McBride observed that aphasia is first and foremost a language disorder. Moreover, they criticized the practice of classifying aphasia into types as arbitrary and unsatisfactory, because their patients did not show that one form of language—understanding, reading, speaking, writing—was affected to the exclusion of the others. For example, patients with predominately expressive aphasia were not free of receptive deficits.

Weisenberg and McBride's expressive-receptive dichotomy persists. It is not uncommon to receive a consultation request that states, "Please evaluate this 67-year-old patient with expressive aphasia." One must remember that the adjective "predominately" is important. It signifies the most obvious deficit but does not exclude others.

Fluent Versus Nonfluent

The concept of fluency is included in several examinations for aphasia: the Boston Diagnostic Aphasia Examination (BDAE) (Goodglass & Kaplan, 1983), the Aachen Aphasia Test (Huber, Poeck, & Wilmes, 1984), the Western Aphasia Battery (WAB) (Kertesz, 1982), and the Shewan Spontaneous Language Analysis System (SSLA) (Shewan, 1988). Initially, it was suggested by Howes' (1964) psycholinguistic research on word frequency distributions and emission rate. He suggested two types of aphasia, a fluent type A and a nonfluent type B. Goodglass, Quadfasel, and Timberlake (1964), however, developed a system for rating fluency based on the "longest occasional uninterrupted strings of words that are produced" (Goodglass & Kaplan, 1983, p. 6). Fluency is typically rated today by phrase length.

The relationship between fluency and articulation is debatable and confusing. In nonaphasic disorders—stuttering and apraxia of speech—fluency signifies hesitations, repetitions, and prolongations. In aphasia, fluency is concerned with phrase length and grammatical complexity. However, in aphasia, articulatory ability is frequently, but not always, associated with phrase length and grammatical complexity (Goodglass & Kaplan, 1983).

Typically, fluency is appraised during conversation and picture description. The BDAE (Goodglass & Kaplan, 1983) uses a 7-point scale to rate fluency in several areas—articulatory agility, phrase length, and melodic line. However, in the BDAE's Subtest Summary Profile, verbal agility (0–14) is included in the appraisal of fluency. Patients who score 1 through 4 on the 7-point rating scale in melodic line ("absent" through "limited to short phrases and stereotypes"), phrase length ("one word" to "four words"), and articulatory agility ("always impaired or impossible" through "normal only in familiar words and phrases") are considered nonfluent. Typically, verbal agility performance would be scored from 0 to 6 out of the possible 14 points. Conversely, patients who rate 5–7 in articulatory agility, phrase length, and melodic line would be considered fluent. Verbal agility scores would measure 8 and above out of the possible 14 points, but they may drop below 8 for fluent patients with severe auditory comprehension deficits, probably because they fail to understand the instructions.

Other areas of the BDAE's Rating Scale Profile of Speech Characteristics must be examined, however, to solidify the fluent-nonfluent label. For example, nonfluent patients would need to score in the 1 ("none available") through 4 ("limited to simple declaratives and stereotypes") range in grammatical form. Fluent patients would score 5 and above. Further, nonfluent patients would be rated 5 through 7 ("speech exclusively content words") on word finding ("informational content in relation to fluency").

The WAB (Kertesz, 1982) uses a 0- to 10-point rating scale to separate aphasic people into fluent and nonfluent groups. It incorporates phrase length, a variety of grammatical constructions, the presence of jargon, word-finding difficulty, and circumlocution. As with the BDAE, fluency is rated on the basis of performance in conversation (answering questions) and picture description.

Nonfluent patients are rated from 0 ("no response or short meaningless utterances") through 4 ("predominately single words, often appropriate, with occasional verbs or prepositional phrases. Automatic sentences only: 'Oh, I don't know.' "). Fluent patients are rated 5 ("predominately telegraphic, halting speech, but some grammatical organization. Paraphasias may be prominent; few propositional sentences") to 10 ("sentences of normal length and complexity, without perceptible word-finding difficulty").

Feyereisen, Pillon, and DePartz (1991) observe that fluency is used in two ways—to refer to an aphasic syndrome and to describe a speech symptom. Fluency is the interaction between phrase length and grammatical form (the syndrome) and articulatory agility (the symptoms).

The fluency-nonfluency classification is also confounded by severity. Nonfluent patients range from the most severe, globally aphasic patients, to patients with mild Broca's or transcortical motor aphasia who are classified as nonfluent because of impaired articulatory agility and melodic line, short phrase length, and restricted grammatical form. Fluent patients may range from severe Wernicke's patients to very mild anomic patients.

Wertz, Kitselman, and Deal (1981) report that clinicians are reliable—95% agreement—in classifying aphasic people into fluent and nonfluent groups. At 1 month postonset, nonfluent patients are more severely aphasic than fluent patients, and this difference persists at 1 year postonset. Both groups make essentially the same amount of improvement during the first year postonset. However, approximately half of the nonfluent patients at 1 month postonset were fluent at 1 year postonset. None of the fluent patients, as one might expect, became nonfluent.

How well does the fluent-nonfluent dichotomy meet the purposes of description? It is not very useful for patient management, because the classification provides little information on anything other than oral-expressive language and articulation. Thus, it does not assist in focusing treatment. The classification has meaning for interdisciplinary communication, but it is not as informative as a more elaborate taxonomy. As indicated above, grouping patients into fluent and nonfluent groups is problematic for research purposes, because the nonfluent group will typically be more severe than the fluent group. Finally, the fluent and nonfluent labels carry little information for the patient and his or her family and friends.

Brain-Behavior Taxonomies

Kertesz (1979) observed that clinical experience with patients who are apha-sic dictates the following:

1. Indeed there is a need for classification.
2. Patients and their symptomatology are complex yet similar enough to the experiences of others.
3. Many classifiers describe the same phenomena from a different angle and in fact complement rather than contradict each other (Kertesz, 1979, p. 1).

Goodglass and Kaplan (1983), Damasio (1992), and others (Albert et al., 1981; Benson, 1979; Helm-Estabrooks, 1992) agree.

Historically, classification of aphasia into the aphasias has been based on assumed brain-behavior relationships—that a lesion in one part of the brain results in a complex of symptoms that differ from those that result from a lesion in another part of the brain. Contemporary taxonomies for classifying the aphasias are consistent, with a few exceptions, and are repre-sented by the types of aphasia shown in Table 3.1.

Notice that symptoms used to classify are confined to oral-expressive language, auditory comprehension, and repetition. These taxonomies do not ignore reading and writing, but they do not use these modalities to classify people who are aphasic.

Typically, classification results from performance on a battery of tasks contained in an aphasia test such as the BDAE (Goodglass & Kaplan, 1983) or the WAB (Kertesz, 1982). The former uses a rating scale of speech charac-teristics to evaluate patient performance in conversation and picture description, repetition, and auditory comprehension. The resulting profile is used to classify. The latter uses the aphasia quotient sections—fluency, auditory comprehension, repetition, and naming. Performance in each area is compared with discrete cutoff scores to identify a specific type of aphasia. Helm-Estabrooks (1992) has developed a system that uses cutoff scores for use with the BDAE. The following is a brief listing of the salient symptoms for the classical, contemporary types of aphasia listed in Table 3.1.

Global Aphasia

Global aphasia is the most severe type of aphasia and is characterized by impairment in all modalities. Oral-expressive language is nonfluent and reduced to a few words; recurring utterances, often verbal stereotypes; emotional exclamations; and, sometimes, a few serial utterances. Repetition, naming, and auditory comprehension are also severely impaired. Global aphasia is believed to result from large lesions in the left perisylvian region.

TABLE 3.1   Types of Aphasia

Type	Speech	Comprehension	Repetition	Localization
Global	Nonfluent	Impaired	Impaired	Massive left perisylvian region
Broca's	Nonfluent	Generally preserved	Impaired	Left lower, posterior frontal
Transcortical motor	Nonfluent	Generally preserved	Generally preserved	Anterior or superior to Broca's area
Wernicke's	Fluent	Impaired	Impaired	Left posterior, superior temporal
Transcortical sensory	Fluent	Impaired	Generally preserved	Posterior or inferior to Wernicke's area
Conduction	Fluent	Generally preserved	Impaired	Left supramarginal gyrus
Anomic	Fluent	Generally preserved	Generally preserved	No localizing significance

Source: Modified from A. Damasio. (1992). Aphasia. *New England Journal of Medicine 326*, 531–539.

Broca's Aphasia

Broca's aphasia is characterized by the difference between relatively better auditory comprehension than the restricted, nonfluent, oral-expressive language. Deficits in auditory comprehension may be noted when the auditory stimulus is longer or more complex. Expressive language is characterized by prosodic deficits, articulatory agility problems, short phrase length, and restricted or absent grammatical form. Repetition is typically impaired, as is naming. Broca's aphasia is believed to result from a lesion in the left-posterior frontal area.

Transcortical Motor Aphasia

Transcortical motor aphasia resembles Broca's aphasia, but it is differentiated by the relatively spared performance in repetition. Transcortical motor patients repeat better than one would expect based on the impairment in other aspects of their nonfluent, oral-expressive language. Transcortical motor aphasia is believed to result from a lesion that is anterior or superior to the Broca's area.

Wernicke's Aphasia

Patients with Wernicke's aphasia display fluent, "empty" oral-expressive language and marked deficits in auditory comprehension. While there is relatively good prosody, good articulation, longer phrase length, and evidence of grammatical form, Wernicke's patients produce literal and semantic paraphasias, sometimes jargon and neologisms, and paragrammatic syntax. Repetition and naming are impaired. Wernicke's aphasia is believed to result from a lesion in the left-posterior, superior temporal area.

Transcortical Sensory Aphasia

Patients with transcortical sensory aphasia resemble Wernicke's aphasic patients. However, they differ in their relatively intact ability to repeat. Performance on repetition tasks is essentially better than one would expect based on their deficits in auditory comprehension. Transcortical sensory aphasia is believed to result from a lesion that is posterior or inferior to the Wernicke's area.

Conduction Aphasia

Patients with conduction aphasia are typified by inordinate difficulty in repetition compared with their relatively intact auditory comprehension and fairly good oral-expressive language. Naming is impaired, and articulatory errors—substitutions, additions, and omissions—are present. Conduction aphasia is believed to result from a lesion in the left supramarginal gyrus.

Anomic Aphasia

Some (Damasio, 1981) suggest that pure anomic aphasia is rare. It is the least frequently observed aphasia on the BDAE, but it is fairly common on the WAB. These patients are fluent with relatively good auditory comprehension and repetition. Their primary problem is in naming. Anomic aphasia has no localizing significance.

Conflicts in Classification

Differences between the BDAE and WAB classifications are the BDAE's use of a "mixed nonfluent" type of aphasia and an "unclassifiable" category. The former lies somewhere between global and Broca's aphasia. Oral-expressive language is sparse, as in the Broca's aphasic patient, but impairment of auditory comprehension is too severe to be classified as Broca's aphasia. The latter type of aphasia, unclassifiable, is reserved for those patients whose performance does not fit the profiles for the other types.

Kertesz (1982) includes "isolation" aphasia in his taxonomy. It is rare and characterized by severe nonfluency and auditory comprehension and naming deficits, but only mild to moderate disruption of repetition. Except for better performance in repetition, these patients would be classified as globally aphasic. The lesion is reported (Geschwind, Quadfasel, & Segarra, 1968) to surround, but spare, the perisylvian speech area.

How useful are these taxonomies? Clinicians show significant agreement in classifying patients using both the BDAE and the WAB criteria (Wertz et al., 1981). However, agreement for the BDAE was 63%, and agreement for the WAB was 90%. Moreover, while correlations for auditory comprehension, fluency, repetition, and naming performance between the BDAE and the WAB are significant, +.90, agreement in classification between the two measures is 27% (Wertz, Deal, & Robinson, 1984). This results from the BDAE classifying approximately 60% of the sample as unclassifiable, while the WAB classified essentially every patient into an aphasia type.

The labels—global, Broca's, transcortical motor, and so forth—are useful for patient management if everyone knows what the labels imply. However, the implications of these labels are general. For example, Broca's aphasia signifies nonfluent, oral-expressive language; relatively intact auditory comprehension; impaired repetition; and impaired naming. The labels only suggest direction for treatment, and a clinician needs a more elaborate description that specifies specific symptoms and the severity of involvement on specific tasks within each language modality.

Taxonomies facilitate interdisciplinary communication because, as Kertesz (1979) suggests, most disciplines are familiar with the current classification systems. Similarly, for purposes of research, patients can be grouped according to type. However, there will be considerable heterogeneity within each group, because there is considerable heterogeneity within each type. Some (Caramazza & Badecker, 1989) suggest that research, especially treatment research, be confined to single-subject designs, because heterogeneity within types of aphasia makes group results misleading.

Finally, classifying patients according to aphasia type is not very useful for describing a patient's condition to him or her or family members and friends. For them, the labels are meaningless. Saying "You have Broca's aphasia" is no more useful than telling the patient he or she has aphasia. Both require elaboration.

Recent Classifications

Time renders nothing static. Modern technology—advances in neuroradiology—and refined behavioral methods have added to the ways aphasia may be described and classified. Recent classifications include the subcortical aphasias and primary progressive aphasia. Both challenge traditional beliefs.

Subcortical Aphasias

For years, aphasia was believed to result from damaged cortex. More recently, Alexander and LoVerme (1980) and Naeser, Alexander, Helm-Estabrooks, Levin, Laughlin, and Geschwind (1982) have identified subcortical aphasias resulting from damage in the internal capsule, putamen, or thalamus. The lesions vary in size and location, and both influence the types and severity of the speech and language deficits observed.

Goodglass and Kaplan (1983) describe three subcortical aphasias. One results from anterior damage in the internal capsule and the putamen and is characterized by severely impaired dysarthric articulation, adequate phrase length (four to six words), mild repetition problems, moderate difficulty in naming, mild auditory comprehension deficits, moderate reading problems, and severe writing deficits. The second subcortical aphasia results from posterior capsular-putamenal lesions. These patients display fluent speech, severe auditory comprehension and naming problems, mild repetition errors, and moderate reading and writing problems. The third results from anterior and posterior damage that involves the internal capsule and putamen and extends into the thalamus. These patients are globally aphasic. Spontaneous speech is nonfluent and limited to stereotyped monosyllables, one-word phrase length, and severely impaired articulation. Auditory comprehension, reading, naming, repetition, and writing are severely impaired.

While subcortical damage can result in aphasia (Alexander & LoVerme, 1980; Goodglass & Kaplan, 1983; Naeser et al., 1982), many aphasic patients suffer cortical lesions that extend into subcortical areas. This complicates classification and description, as does the presence of dysarthria, a non-aphasic disorder. Taxonomies for classifying aphasia are designed to demonstrate brain-behavior relationships—where the lesion is should result in a specific set of symptoms that can be grouped under a specific label (type of aphasia). However, classification is perceptual, based on observation of a patient's auditory comprehension, reading, oral-expressive language, and writing. If the perceived symptoms do not relate to the specific location of the assumed lesion, clinicians must accept that fact or be prepared to say that they really did not see and hear what they actually saw and heard.

Primary Progressive Aphasia

Traditionally, aphasia has been believed to erupt—to have a specific onset. Except for aphasia resulting from neoplasms, this has been one means for differentiating aphasia from the communicative deficits seen in dementia—a disorder that creeps. However, in recent years, a number of patients have been reported to display gradual deterioration of language skills without generalized cognitive impairment or a readily identifiable cause—vascular, neoplastic, metabolic, infectious, or traumatic. Because language disturbance is the primary complaint in these patients, it has been labeled slowly progressive aphasia or, more commonly, primary progressive aphasia.

Duffy and Peterson (1992) provide an extremely thorough review of 54 cases reported in 24 papers. They also provide a tentative definition, adopted from Duffy (1987), of primary progressive aphasia as a language deficit:

> of insidious onset, gradual progression, and prolonged course, in the absence of generalized cognitive impairments (at least for a substantial period of time), due to a degenerative condition, predominantly and presumably involving the left perisylvian region of the brain (Duffy, 1987, p. 349; Duffy & Peterson, 1992, p. 2).

Localization of brain damage in these patients from neuroimaging ranges from normal—no evidence of brain damage—to diffuse and bilateral. Similarly, symptoms range from Broca-like, nonfluent language disturbance to Wernicke-like, fluent language disturbance. Weintraub, Rubin, and Mesulam (1990) conclude that primary progressive aphasia can result in any of the traditional types of aphasia.

The course of the disease is mixed. For example, the duration of isolated (language) symptoms ranges from 1 to 15 years in some patients. About half of the reported cases eventually show nonaphasic cognitive deficits (dementia) (Duffy & Peterson, 1992).

Certainly, primary progressive aphasia differs from the typical aphasias. Because it does, the way we describe it requires additional rigor. And, because the deficits are progressive, management—prognosis and treatment—is likely to differ from that used with the typical aphasias.

CLINICAL DESCRIPTION

How one describes aphasia depends on one's purpose. For clinical management, the aphasia-without-adjectives approach is preferable. This does not preclude use of a classification system—expressive-receptive, fluent-nonfluent, or a taxonomy. However, Goodglass and Kaplan's (1983) caution that 40–60% of people with aphasia cannot be classified validly and reliably is wise. Labels should inform, not misinform.

For interdisciplinary communication, classifying aphasia into the aphasias is useful. It provides a shorthand that saves time and, usually, meets the purposes of interdisciplinary communication. Typically, practitioners in neurology, neurosurgery, and neuropsychology will not take time to peruse an elaborate description. A label—Broca's, Wernicke's, and so forth—will suffice. However, it may be necessary to check assumptions: "Are we really talking about the same thing?" Moreover, it is essential to revise a label when change in patient performance dictates it. Approximately 50% of aphasic patients change from one type of aphasia to another during the first year after onset (Kertesz & McCabe, 1977; Wertz et al., 1981).

The descriptive system used for research depends on the research question. Some questions require selecting patients based on overall severity of aphasia. Others may dictate selecting patients based on severity within a specific language modality. One must ensure that the selection criteria do not confound the results. For example, classifying patients into fluent and nonfluent groups will create overall differences in severity between groups if patients with global aphasia (most severe) are included in the nonfluent group and patients with anomic aphasia (least severe) are included in the fluent group.

Patients, families, and friends require a brief, useful description of the aphasia. A label or labels—aphasia or even Broca's aphasia—may be used, but no one should be expected to remember them or know what they mean. What follows the label provides the meaning. Most important, we soothe concern: "You have a language problem. You have not lost your mind." Then, we tell the patient much of what he or she already knows: "When what you hear gets long and complicated, you are going to miss some of it." And, "Knowing what you want to say and not being able to say it is part of this thing we call aphasia." But, we avoid telling aphasic persons and their families more than they want to know.

Technical jargon can be a tool for precise communication. However, it may be a barrier for outsiders. Feeling good about being "in the know" does not justify creating confusion. Using a classification system is one thing. Making it all add up is another. Clinical description of the aphasias must contain appropriate proportions of the parts and the overall appearance, depending on the purpose description is attempting to achieve.

REFERENCES

Albert, M.L., Goodglass, H., Helm, N.A., Rubens, A.B., & Alexander, M.P. (1981). *Clinical aspects of dysphasia.* New York: Springer-Verlag.

Alexander, M.P., & LoVerme, S.R. (1980). Aphasia following left hemisphere intracerebral hemorrhage. *Neurology, 30,* 1193–1202.

Au, R., Albert, M.L., & Obler, L.K. (1988). The relation of aphasia to dementia. *Aphasiology, 2,* 161–174.

Benson, D.F. (1979). *Aphasia, alexia, and agraphia.* New York: Churchill Livingstone.

Broca, P. (1861). Remarques sur le siège de la faculté du langage articulé, suives d'une observation d'aphemie. [Comments on the disruption of the faculty of articulated language, continued observation of aphemia.] *Bulletin de la Société d'Anthropologie* (2nd series), 330–357.

Brown, J.W. (1977). *Mind, brain, and consciousness: The neuropsychology of cognition.* New York: Academic Press.

Caramazza, A., & Badecker, K.W. (1989). Patient classification in neuropsychological research. *Brain and Language, 10,* 256–295.

Chapey, R. (1981). The assessment of language disorders in adults. In R. Chapey (Ed.), *Language intervention strategies in adult aphasia* (pp. 31–84). Baltimore: Williams & Wilkins.

Damasio A. (1981). The nature of aphasia: Signs and syndromes. In M.T. Sarno (Ed.), *Acquired aphasia* (pp. 51–65). New York: Academic Press.

Damasio, A.R. (1992). Aphasia. *New England Journal of Medicine, 326,* 531–539.

Darley, F.L. (1982). *Aphasia.* Philadelphia: W.B. Saunders.

Duffy, J.R. (1987). Slowly progressive aphasia. In R.H. Brookshire (Ed.), *Clinical aphasiology* (pp. 349–356). Minneapolis: BRK Publishers.

Duffy, J.R., & Peterson, R.C. (1992). Primary progressive aphasia. *Aphasiology, 6,* 1–16.

Feyereisen, P., Pillon, A., & DePartz, M.P. (1991). On the measures of fluency in the assessment of spontaneous speech production by aphasic subjects. *Aphasiology, 5,* 1–21.

Geschwind, N., Quadfasel, F., & Segarra, J. (1968). Isolation of the speech area. *Neuropsychologia, 6,* 327–340.

Goodglass, H., & Kaplan, E. (1983). *The assessment of aphasia and related disorders* (2nd ed.). Philadelphia: Lea & Febiger.

Goodglass, H., Quadfasel, F.A., & Timberlake, W.H. (1964). Phrase length and the type and severity of aphasia. *Cortex, 1,* 133–153.

Head, H. (1926). *Aphasia and kindred disorders of speech.* New York: Macmillan.

Helm-Estabrooks, N. (1992). *Aphasia diagnostic profiles (ADP).* Chicago: Riverside Publishing Co.

Helm-Estabrooks, N., & Albert, M.L. (1991). *Manual of aphasia therapy.* Austin, TX: PRO-ED.

Howes, D. (1964). Application of the word frequency concept to aphasia. In A.V.S. De Reuck & M. O'Connor (Eds.), *Disorders of language* (pp. 47–75). London: Churchill.

Huber, W., Poeck, K., & Wilmes, K. (1984). The Aachen aphasia test. In F.C. Rose (Ed.), *Progress in aphasiology* (pp. 291–303). New York: Raven Press.

Kertesz, A. (1979). *Aphasia and associated disorders: Taxonomy, localization, and recovery.* New York: Grune & Stratton.

Kertesz, A. (1982). *The Western Aphasia Battery.* New York: Grune & Stratton.

Kertesz, A., & McCabe, P. (1977). Recovery patterns and prognosis in aphasia. *Brain, 100,* 1–18.

Kreindler, A., & Fradis, A. (1968). *Performances in aphasia: A neurodynamical, diagnostic and psychological study.* Paris: Gauthier-Villars.

Marie, P. (1906). Révision de la question de l'aphasie: La troisième circonvolution frontale gauche ne joue aucun rôle spécial dans la fonction du langage. [Revisiting the question of aphasia: The third frontal convolution plays no special role in language function.] *Semaine Médicale, 21,* 241–247.

Martin, A.D. (1981). The role of theory in therapy: A rationale. *Topics in Language Disorders, 1,* 63–72.

McNeil, M.R. (1982). The nature of aphasia in adults. In N.J. Lass, L.V. McReynolds, J.L. Northern, & D.E. Yoder (Eds.), *Speech, language, and hearing: Volume III. Pathologies of speech and language* (pp. 692–740). Philadelphia: W.B. Saunders.

Naeser, M.A., Alexander, M.P., Helm-Estabrooks, N., Levin, H.L., Laughlin, S.A., & Geschwind, N. (1982). Aphasia with predominantly subcortical lesion sites: Description of three capsular/putamenal syndromes. *Archives of Neurology, 39,* 1–14.

Neisser, U. (1966). *Cognitive psychology.* New York: Appleton-Century-Crofts.

Rosenbek, J.C., LaPointe, L.L., & Wertz, R.T. (1989). *Aphasia: A clinical approach.* Austin, TX: PRO-ED.

Schuell, H. (1965). *Differential diagnosis of aphasia with the Minnesota test.* Minneapolis: University of Minnesota Press.

Schuell, H., Jenkins, J.J., & Jimenez-Pabon, E. (1964). *Aphasia in adults: Diagnosis, prognosis, and treatment.* New York: Hoeber Medical Division, Harper & Row Publishers.

Shewan, C.M. (1988). The Shewan spontaneous language analysis (SSLA) system for aphasic adults: Description, reliability, and validity. *Journal of Communication Disorders, 21,* 155–169.

Weintraub, S., Rubin, N.P., & Mesulam, M. (1990). Primary progressive aphasia: Longitudinal course, neuropsychological profile, and language features. *Archives of Neurology, 47,* 1329–1335.

Weisenberg, T.H., & McBride, K.E. (1935). *Aphasia.* New York: Commonwealth Fund.

Wernicke, C. (1908). The symptom complex of aphasia (1874). In A. Church (Ed.), *Diseases of the nervous system* (pp. 265–324). New York: Appleton.

Wertz, R.T., Deal, J.L., & Robinson, A.J. (1984). Classifying the aphasias: A comparison of the Boston diagnostic aphasia examination and the Western aphasia battery. In R.H. Brookshire (Ed.), *Clinical Aphasiology Conference Proceedings* (pp. 40–47). Minneapolis: BRK Publishers.

Wertz, R.T., Kitselman, K.P., & Deal, L.A. (1981). *Classifying the aphasias: Contributions to patient management.* Paper presented to the Academy of Aphasia. London, Ontario.

Chapter 4

Language Assessment

Lee Ann C. Golper

She tries to find the word for glasses. She shines the light of her mind into the store of words and looks in the place where she sees the image of her glasses. There is no word there to go with the picture. Darkness. What was the storehouse of her words, stocked, overflowing, is a dusty emptiness. There are no words that name the things she sees. She shines the light of her mind backwards and forwards on the shelves of objects she means to name. The light searches. Backwards and forwards. There is nothing.

Mary Gordon, *The Other Side*, 1990

Language assessments quantify and delineate aphasic behavior. Darley (1982) reminded us that what we find in testing will come logically from what we expect to find, or "how we ask the questions" (p. 55). We ask questions to suit our purposes. Speech-language pathologists generally use assessments to measure and characterize a communication deficit (including its motor and linguistic characteristics and other cognitive processes affecting communication), to assess the suitability of language therapy, and to find avenues for treatment. Neurologists and neuropsychologists test to determine a disorder "type." Researchers in aphasiology and cognitive-linguistic psychology assess aphasia to find clues to the structure of mental processes underlying normal and deficient communicative behavior. Aphasic patients and their families measure aphasia in terms of its impact on the everyday use of language: "I can't write and I don't get anything out of television any more."

This chapter focuses on the practical side of assessment. It emphasizes evaluation of patients in an acute care and subacute settings where assessment guides treatment decisions. Assessment is discussed as a part of the differential diagnosis of communication deficits, which includes determining primary features and severity. This chapter is not a test-by-test review of the psychometric features of test and measurement instruments and methods available for aphasia evaluation. Rather, it examines the relationship between clinical problems and aphasia assessment. The assessments and tests mentioned in this review are mainly those published or commonly used in North America. The discussion covers how assessment in the early stages of recovery from aphasia should be approached and ways to expand on standardized testing when evaluating input and output processes.

In speech-language pathology, clinical assessment of aphasia is directed toward six purposes:

1. *Making a differential diagnosis,* to determine if aphasia is indeed present or the extent to which language deficits contribute to reduced communicative capacity.
2. *Determining syndrome or "type,"* to determine if the major features represent a distinctive form of aphasia.
3. *Establishing level of severity,* to measure the relative severity of the input and output deficits and the severity of the overall impairment.
4. *Determining suitability for treatment,* to look for indicators of a prognosis for effective response to language treatment.
5. *Identifying appropriate avenues for treatment,* to analyze the aphasic behavior across input and output domains and establish the focus of the therapy.
6. *Measuring changes in communicative status,* to analyze the effects of any spontaneous improvement, and of medical, surgical, pharmacologic, or behavioral therapies.

PSYCHOMETRIC CONSIDERATIONS IN TESTING

Before applying published test procedures to clinical practice or devising an eclectic battery to evaluate aphasia, it is important to understand how tests are constructed and what one needs to consider when using assessment methods (Skenes & McCauley, 1985). To this end, some basic psychometric principles—validity, reliability, normative samples, and standardization—are reviewed below.

Validity

The single most important consideration in assessment tasks is *validity.* One needs to consider: *Does this test or task measure what it purports to measure?* Authors of published tests often compare the performance of "normal" on their tests to performance on similar tests. This comparison is one way to establish a *validity coefficient.* When reporting validity coefficients, the authors are claiming that their tasks appear to measure the same constructs as an established test.

Validation is an important aspect of test construction. But even when a test is considered valid, it behooves the user to ask: *What are we asking this patient to do?* or *What does this test, or task, measure?* For example, we may think we are testing auditory comprehension when asking a patient, "Point to the ceiling and then the floor," but we are also testing attention, initiation, limb praxis, short-term memory, spatial orientation, and audition. Linguistic-cognitive abilities are highly associated, integrated processes. One cannot test auditory comprehension, reading, naming, oral expression, and so forth, without directly or indirectly tapping associated processes. Consider the example of tests or subtests routinely used to assess naming ability in aphasia. Most published naming tasks involve presenting line drawings of objects to the patient and asking him or her to name the object. Errors in naming line drawings can be due to visuoperceptual deficits, hemispatial inattention, cultural differences, and verbal motor deficits, as well as lexico-semantic processing deficits. Consider what is required when naming a picture from the *Boston Naming Test* (BNT) (Kaplan, Goodglass, & Weintraub, 1983):

1. The ability to see all of the drawing.
2. The ability to perceive, recognize, and integrate pertinent details.
3. The ability to interpret what the line drawing represents (picture semantics).
4. The ability to relate the picture to stored associations (verbal semantics).
5. The ability to target and retrieve the correct label for the picture from the mental lexicon.
6. The ability to organize mentally a correct phonologic sequence and to articulate the motoric expression of the name.

Errors can be elicited from "glitches" within and between any of the processes involved. Thus, in this example, the BNT can be viewed as a test *of* naming line drawings as a general process but not a test *for* aphasic anomia.

In general, any given assessment is valid only for the population it was designed to test. Clinicians who use a test for any reason other than its intended purpose must qualify their findings and be cautious in interpretation. For example, tests of mental status are designed to be bedside screenings to examine for dementia or confusion. They generally employ tasks that require verbal processing, such as orientation questions, memory questions, calculations, naming, and following directions. Thus, given the demand on verbal processing, aphasic patients are likely to appear "demented" on such tests. Similarly, patients with Alzheimer's-type dementia may make errors on the *Western Aphasia Battery* (WAB) (Kertesz, 1982) and could presumably be given an "aphasia quotient" score, when the score of the verbal processing errors reflected a pervasive cognitive deficit rather than a nested deficiency in language. In this same light, we should remember that tests designed to be administered to neurologically stable aphasic persons might not be valid instruments to use at bedside with poorly responsive, acutely ill patients.

Reliability

Reliability of test findings refers to the repeatability, or consistency, of the results. During early post-acute recovery from aphasia, reliability of test findings is predictably poor. Depending on the cause and extent of the brain lesion, there may be dramatic physiologic changes in the central nervous system during the first few days after the event.

Reliability between observers is another crucial factor. Tests have little use if findings are not consistent across examiners. In published tests, one looks for reports of *reliability coefficients* that indicate the test delivers the same results when administered by different examiners or when repeatedly administered to the same person or population. Widely used tests have reliability coefficients of around .80 (Carmines & Zeller, 1981). Some authors will provide reliability coefficients for individual subtests. One may find that there tends to be more subjectivity and, thus, less reliability, within specific subtests.

Normative Samples and Standardization

When interpreting findings from tests or assessment tasks, it is usually helpful to know if the results indicate deficiencies compared to a "normal" standard. The normal sample may come from performances of healthy subjects, perhaps selected by some factor (such as age, sex, or education) that the developers felt should be "controlled." Controlling for a particular variable ensures that the results are not influenced by that variable. Occasionally, the normative sample comes from populations of subjects that possess a particular characteristic. The *Porch Index of Communicative Ability* (PICA) (Porch, 1981), for example, is referenced against normative findings from left-hemisphere and bilaterally damaged aphasic persons. Tasks such as those found on the PICA, and in many aphasia tests, ought to be easily performed by literate, non-neurologically impaired persons. One might expect, for example, that most healthy adults can name the 20 objects used in the WAB naming subtest. However, when assessment tasks measure efficiency, normative data are needed for the interpretation of findings. Picture description, word-retrieval, and timed word fluency measures are examples of assessment tasks for which performance norms are especially helpful.

Normative data are usually presented with some sort of "derived table" whereby the raw data are examined against a normal performance curve. The scores can therefore be compared by using derived scoring methods, such as those illustrated in Figure 4.1.

Standardization of assessment procedures refers to the administration methods used when developing the test and gathering the normative statis-

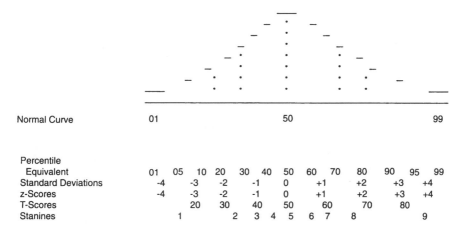

FIGURE 4.1 *Normative scores and scaling referents. (Adapted from L.E. Tyler. (1971). Tests and measurements (2nd ed) Englewood Cliffs, NJ: Prentice-Hall.)*

tics. Some tests have rather rigid administration procedures while others offer more latitude. For example, the PICA has very specific administration guidelines and only certain statements and cues are permissible. You need to be familiar with and to carefully follow the directions in the test manual to apply the norms that were derived from those procedures. When using what are sometimes called "supplemental tests" (assessments of a particular ability, such as the *Token Test* [DeRenzi & Vignolo, 1962] for auditory comprehension) that come from published research studies, it is helpful if the authors have provided descriptions of how they administered these assessments and the subject characteristics (age, gender, severity of aphasia, lesion location, handedness, and so forth).

Test Bias

Any test that presumes to assess a human trait is subject to cultural bias. In the United Kingdom, if one is shown a picture of a hardware store and asked to name it, the correct response could be "ironmonger." A highway rest stop is a "layby." A bus is a "coach"; soccer is "football"; and a posted sign saying, "No football coaches allowed" means a bus full of soccer fans would not be welcome.

Vocabulary, gestures, facial expressions, and body proxemics are part of a cultural vernacular. Some test forms in countries outside of the United States contain blanks for a patient's surname and "Christian name." Asking the patient for a "Christian name" might be acceptable in one culture and offensive in another. Tests can therefore be biased by the cultural orientation of their authors. This bias can affect how they design the methods of testing, what they ask the patients to do, and how they devise the structure of the content of the test questions. *Criterion-referenced testing* may be useful in instances when culture or language differ from that of the standardization population. (Assessment in multicultural communities is discussed in Chapter 6.)

Test bias is present whenever aphasic patients are tested in their second, or non-native, language. One standardized aphasia test battery explicitly designed with versions in multiple languages is the *Multilingual Aphasia Examination* (MAE) (Benton & Hamsher, 1978), which has comparable forms in English, French, German, Italian, and Spanish. If the patient was notably less than fluent in English (for reading and writing as well as speaking), then tests using English to test for aphasic reading deficits, for example, would not be valid.

ASSESSMENT DURING EARLY RECOVERY

Shorter hospital stays for treatment following neurologic injuries, and earlier consultation by rehabilitation, neuropsychology, and speech-language personnel, are increasingly common in the United States. The speech-language pathologist's first contact with an aphasic patient may come within days, and sometimes hours, after the admission. Today, many aphasic patients may undergo their initial speech-language pathology evaluation during the early post-acute stage (from 1 to 14 days). While it is difficult and usually inappropriate to make a differential diagnosis with a poorly responsive, sick patient, the speech-language pathologist's assessments during the early recovery course can serve several useful purposes.

Language Assessments and Functional Outcomes

When assessing recovery or treatment outcomes, standardized functional assessment scales and inventories are often used. These scales are more appropriately applied in subacute and rehabilitation settings than acute care settings. There usually is included some measurement of *language*, or cognitive-communicative abilities, as part of these inventories. Thus, the speech-language pathologist is often the professional best able to characterize communication status. Probably the most widely applied outcome index among the dozens of functional scales available is the *Functional Index Measure* (FIM) (Granger & Hamilton, 1987). Data from this index are increasingly included in "uniform data sets" to establish benchmarks for functional outcomes comparisons. The FIM includes an examination of "expression" and "comprehension" as well as social interaction, memory, and problem-solving. Typically, assessments are made at intake and at discharge from a program or facility. A subsequent adaptation to the FIM, termed the *Functional Assessment Measure* (FAM) (Hall, Hamilton, Gordon, Zasler, & Johnston, 1988), expands the FIM's cognitive areas with 12 additional items related to thinking processes, behavior, communication, and community functioning.

Instruments like the FIM, or FIM+FAM, are not thought to be sensitive to changes in language behavior; consequently, data from other functional language inventories or scales can provide a better sense of the functional effects of treatment. Clinicians can test for functional communicative abilities using a formal assessment, like the *Communicative Abilities of Daily Living* (CADL) (Holland, 1980), or examine across the functional domains and behaviors suggested by Frattali et al. (1995) in the American Speech-Language-Hearing Association's *Functional Assessment of Communication Skills* (FACS) (Frattali, Thompson, Holland, Wohl, & Ferketic, 1995).

Initial Examinations

Assessment in the early post-acute stage of recovery is obviously predicated on the physical and mental status of the patient. In some cases, patients are alert and anxiously await the arrival of the visitors the day after their admission to the hospital. Other patients may be too weak and unresponsive to allow even a gross differential diagnosis for several days. When patients are acutely ill, they lack the attention and mental vigilance to participate in much more than a few minutes of cursory examination. Generally, clinicians can make only a screening assessment of the patient's expressive and receptive abilities during the initial visit and will state their observations with qualifiers, acknowledging the limited sample and the fluctuations expected when patients are neither medically nor neurologically stable. Experienced clinicians understand that they can make only a cursory assessment of patients in the early post-acute stage of recovery, and that it may be wise neither to commit to a diagnosis nor to predict the potential for a response to language rehabilitation.

With these cautions, bedside assessments can be valuable indicators of the aphasic patient's cognitive status, including responsiveness, communicative ability, and ability to be stimulated. Bedside assessments in the early post-acute stage of recovery from aphasia address different problems from those in assessments of neurologically stable patients with chronic aphasia. During the first week or so after neurologic damage, the prominent issues are the medical status of the patient and response to any medical therapies. Consequently, the fact that a patient displays impaired syntax mapping, for example, is not likely to be terribly interesting to the other hospital ward staff members or the family. However, it is important for all concerned to look for indicators that the patient's condition is improving, worsening, or stabilizing. Assessments of responsiveness and verbal output can be part of this database.

Contributing to the Differential Diagnosis

In most cases, no other staff member can differentially assess communicative status as well as a speech-language pathologist. Thus, speech-language pathologists may be able to establish or correct the admitting diagnosis of the communication deficit. If a patient comes to an emergency room apparently having suffered a stroke and is not speaking, he or she is likely to be described as "aphasic." But the speech-language pathologist should know what to expect from patients who are aphasic, and the bedside assessment may find evidence to challenge the admitting diagnosis. If the patient produces linguistically well-formed verbal expression, demonstrates generally intact auditory or reading comprehension, and can write grammatical sentences, or can demonstrate intact spelling with an alphabet communication board, then the admitting diagnosis of "aphasic" becomes suspect and deserving of further analysis.

Consider the example of patient J.H., a 72-year-old right-handed man with a history of parkinsonism, admitted with upper-extremity right hemiparesis, right-side facial weakness, and aphasia. In the admission notes, J.H. was described to demonstrate no evidence of comprehension of simple directions, and he was said to be unable to name or repeat; thus, according to the admitting notes, he was "aphasic." On the morning after admission, when asked by the speech-language pathologist how he was feeling, J.H. whispered, after a delay of several seconds, "I don't know, I'm waiting for the doctors to tell me."

Subsequent questioning indicated that he required several seconds to elicit a motoric response of any sort, but the latencies of hand movements were not as long as those for speech. He was asked to use a "thumbs up/down" sign to indicate yes and no. Assessment of his comprehension in a manner that required only "thumbs up/down" responses proceeded relatively quickly and indicated good auditory comprehension. Similarly, he was able to identify his name from three choices and could indicate yes and no in response to written questions entirely accurately. He accurately indicated yes and no to auditory comprehension questions that were both long and linguistically complex, such as: "Would you normally have dinner before you brush your teeth in the morning?" Verbal responses, including those that followed after long delays (5 or more seconds), were accurate but questioning was tediously slow. He correctly answered questions from the *Mini-Mental State* (MMS) (Folstein, Folstein, & McHugh, 1975), but his responses were slow and one had to listen carefully to understand his barely audible and minimally intelligible speech. Follow-up bedside assessment visits included providing a voice amplifier to make his speech more audible. Over the course of three evaluation days, the clinician had gathered sufficient data to feel confident diagnosing a mixed (hypokinetic/spastic) dysarthria, with no grossly notable problem understanding or formulating language. Although cerebral computed tomography (CT) scans at admission revealed only an old right basal ganglia calcification, follow-up studies were interpreted to demonstrate a left subcortical (internal capsule) infarct. His more recent subcortical lesion had produced additional motor deficits overlaid upon pre-existing parkinsonism.

Speech-language pathologists are expected to contribute to the differential diagnosis of neurologically impaired patients. Even the most experienced clinicians, however, may find it difficult to determine with certainty if communication deficits after acute infarction reflect frank aphasia, motor speech impairments, generalized cognitive disturbances, or (and more likely) some combination of language, motor, and mental status deficits. Patients sometimes present with a history of previous strokes, dementia, or other neurologic diseases. Some patients are reported to have fallen after their stroke, with risk of head injuries. Some patients have an aspiration pneumonia resulting from their stroke and are both sick and aphasic. Some patients arrive at the hospital without their glasses, hearing aids, or dentures, making a valid assessment of communication more difficult.

Standardized Tests

Most standardized test batteries and published supplemental tests for aphasia are *not* intended for use at bedside. Individuals too ill to leave the ward are not likely to have been subjects in normative samples. Some standardized tests have subtests that are adaptable to bedside assessments, but only a couple of published tests are specifically intended for use in bedside screening and assessment. One such test that has been in use for a number of years and continues to enjoy some popularity with clinicians is the *Aphasia Language Performance Scales* (ALPS) (Keenan & Brassel, 1975). This test assesses severity of impaired language performance across modalities (reading, writing, listening, and talking) with 10 items for each subtest progressing from simple to more complex tasks. Very little paraphernalia aside from a packet of reading cards and typical pocket items (key, coins, etc.) is required to administer this test, and the patient is required to sit up for only one subtest (writing tasks). Another more recent test designed for administration at the bedside is the *Bedside Evaluation and Screening Test* (BEST) (West & Sands, 1987). This test comes in a self-contained kit with items easily transported to the bedside. The BEST was field-tested with patients who were seen on their wards. Thus, items (such as writing tasks) impractical for bedside administration were eliminated.

The WAB (Kertesz, 1982) and the *Boston Assessment of Severe Aphasia* (BASA) (Helm-Estabrooks, Ramsberger, Morgan, & Nicholas, 1989) are two of the more comprehensive tests for aphasia that, with some patients, may be used at bedside. The BASA is designed especially for severely aphasic persons. Along with verbal responses, the examiner notes gestural and affective communicative attempts. The tasks are best suited for the patient who has a severe verbal output impairment and moderately severe language comprehension deficit. Patients who are severely, globally aphasic can respond to very few items from the BASA or any other standardized test. The WAB is relatively easy to administer in the early post-acute stage of recovery. It requires real objects for part of the naming subtest that need to be brought to the patient. This test is reasonably short and could be used with patients who might not be able to tolerate more extensive testing. The WAB is used to determine the type of aphasia syndrome and the severity of aphasia. Clinicians sometimes use the 20 yes or no questions from the WAB in a nonstandard manner (that is, they deviate from standard procedures by administering only a part of a test) to assess comprehension. Experienced clinicians routinely tend to use an amalgam of test protocols, subtests, and parastandardized or nonstandardized probe assessments when conducting bedside screenings.

Parastandardized Assessments

One problem with published standardized bedside assessments is that they are essentially screening instruments. Screening instruments can indicate the severity of the disorder; typically very few items sample *within* severity levels, particularly at the very mild and very severe ranges. Thus, these assessments may need to be augmented to obtain a broader sampling within the patient's level of performance. For this reason, bedside screening instruments may not be adequate to monitor day-to-day change. If clinicians make frequent assessments to monitor changes daily or twice daily, it is useful to develop a routine of probe tasks customized to the patient's performance level that can be repeated at each visit. A clinician can fashion a *para*standardized assessment routine, whereby essentially the same procedures are followed at each visit. Obviously, if you are not using a published procedure or test you will not have a normative reference group, but "normed" comparisons may be unnecessary for your assessment purposes. One could argue that the very notion of "aphasic norms" is an oxymoron; however, norms for aphasic performance are useful when mild or subtle aphasia is being differentially examined.

The format for bedside, parastandardized assessment of changes in communicative behavior conforms well with the sort of research designs, such as single-case research, used in applied behavioral analyses. When clinicians sample across time (the independent variable) to see if the patient can or cannot perform a particular task or set of tasks (the dependent variable), they are conducting an experimental analysis. In such an analysis, the patient serves as his or her own control for day-to-day variation.

Daily Ward Visits

To sample and characterize responsivity, mood, affect, comprehension of others, verbal expression, and stimulability with the minimally responsive patient, the clinician might note a number of descriptors during daily ward visits (Table 4.1).

REPORTING FINDINGS

In addition to observations from bedside assessments, it is important to ask families as well as ward and rehabilitation personnel, "How is he doing with

TABLE 4.1   Descriptors to Note During Daily Ward Visits

Responsiveness
Asleep; not arousable?
Arousable to voice and touch?
Somnolent but arousable?
Awake?
Able to sit?
Sustains attention for how long? (seconds? minutes?)
Alert, communicative, but fatigues easily?
Alert, communicative, and able to attend to the examiner throughout this (duration) visit

Mood and affect
Cannot be assessed?
Demonstrates apathy? (in what way?)
Frustration? (in what way?)
Anger? (in what way?)
Pleasure? (in what way?)
Happiness? (in what way?)
Sadness? (in what way?)
Fear? (in what way?)
Shows emotional lability? (how?)
Shows little affect variability? (describe any lack of response to affect-eliciting stimuli—
    e.g., jokes, smiles, etc.)

Understanding others
Looks at the speaker?
Responds to his or her name?
Responds to inquiries—e.g., "Are you tired?" "Did you have lunch?"
Looks at objects, items, or individuals in the room when the names are spoken?
Follows simple oral directions?—e.g., "Close your eyes"; "Make a fist"; "Point to the TV";
    "Look at the door."
Responds appropriately (with surprise, smiles, etc.) when absurd or humorous remarks are
    made—e.g., "Did President Clinton stop in to see you today?"
Indicates yes or no reliably when asked biographical questions—e.g., "Are you married?";
    "Do you live in [city]?"; "Are you retired?"
Indicates yes or no reliably when asked orientation questions—e.g., "Is this a hotel?"; "Is it
    winter?"; " Are you Mr. [right name], Mr. [wrong name]?"
Looks at objects, items, or individuals in the room when shown the written name?
Points to his or her name in a list of three choices?
Follows simple written directions?

Expressing needs and wants to others
Uses facial expression and body language?
Nods yes or no reliably or uses words and gestures that indicate yes or no? (what words or
    gestures are used to indicate yes or no?)
Points with specificity to indicate wants?
Uses a picture (or alphabet) communication board?
Uses gestures to demonstrate requests?
Uses social greetings—e.g., "hello," "fine," etc.?
Uses some understandable and meaningful words? (what are they?)
Uses short phrases or sentences? (give some examples)

TABLE 4.1   *(continued)*

Ability to be stimulated

Can be stimulated to produce "automatic" expressions? (days of the week; counting; singing)

Repeats his or her name?

Repeats words and short phrases?

Imitates gestures? (give examples)

Understands questions or requests better if "key" words are written to cue him or her to the topic?

Understands questions or requests better if picture cues are presented?

Understands questions or requests better if augmented by gestures?

Understands questions or requests better if given in short phrases?

Responds to phonologic or descriptive cues when attempting to name?

Expresses himself or herself better when provided with writing materials?

Expresses himself or herself better when provided with a communication board (alphabet, pictures)?

---

communication?"; "Do you understand what she wants?"; "Can she follow directions?"; "How does he tell you what he wants?"; and so forth. The family and the other professionals involved in patient care and rehabilitation are sources of information about daily, functional communication, and what they reveal about everyday communication can substantiate or challenge the speech-language assessment findings. The speech and language findings, along with the observations of other staff provided in ward conferences and medical progress notes, collectively are considered when writing the initial evaluation report or preparing for the initial conference with the family. Likewise, it is also important to know how both the staff and the family or significant others describe what the aphasic person is capable and incapable of doing.

These descriptions can become the starting point for the speech-language pathologist's contribution to family and staff conferences. In conferences with the family or at staff meetings, the speech-language pathologist should begin with what the staff or family think are the aphasic person's problems, and acknowledge, amend, or elaborate on those observations. In preparation for the initial conference, clinicians need to have enough data to feel prepared to (1) describe the present communicative status in "functional" terms; (2) advise the staff and family regarding the nature of the problems and best avenues for communication; and (3) determine the suitability and justification for initiating or delaying therapy. The questions in Table 4.2 can aid in this assessment.

SOAP Format

Most medical chart notes and summaries are expected to be written in the so-called SOAP format. Each section of the note or report is headed by: "S"

TABLE 4.2   Questions Used to Prepare an Examiner for an Initial Conference with Family or Staff

Describing present status

What is the patient's level of alertness and responsiveness to others?

What are the characteristic features and severity of the communication problem?

What evidence suggests that the communication status reflects aphasia, motor speech deficits, general cognitive disturbances, or a combination of deficits?

Advising family members and ward staff

What advice seems appropriate for staff and family members to enhance communication with the patient at this time?

Will any environmental adjustments or assistive devices benefit this patient at this time?

What educational and counseling needs should be addressed immediately and in the near future with family members?

Determining a suitable, justifiable treatment plan

Even though this patient may be able to participate in physical and occupational therapies, can he or she be expected at this juncture to participate in cognitively demanding activities, such as standardized testing and language therapy?

What is the appropriate type and amount of involvement by the speech-language pathologist with this patient (e.g., daily bedside visits to continue assessment, daily visits to enhance a specific communication skill, counseling with family members, initiation of individual treatment, participation in discharge planning, etc.)?

---

for *subjective* comments, "O" for *objective* findings, "A" for your *assessment* or interpretation based on these findings; and "P," a statement of your *plan*. The SOAP format was initially applied in what are called *problem-oriented* medical records and in sequential medical records. Both the intake and subsequent progress notes can be written in SOAP format for easier access of information. Files kept in a problem-oriented or sequential record format allow all personnel involved in the patient's care to record their notes sequentially and in the same section of the medical file. Alternatively, the *source-oriented* medical record format segregates notes with separate sections for physicians, nurses, dietitians, social service personnel, rehabilitation personnel, and others. In practice, medical progress notes are brief, two- or three-sentence statements of the patient's present status. The physician may make remarks as brief as, "Afebrile, hemiparesis persists." Thus, the management plan may be gained from speaking with the physician and primary nurse, or gleaned from the section containing "doctor's orders." It is important to remember that *brief notes get read and long narratives do not*.

Balancing the need for accuracy and brevity can be difficult. The self-discipline to keep notes short and to the point is an important skill to acquire in medical speech-language pathology. It is best to limit notes to one's particular area of expertise, to avoid repeating information read in preceding notes from other staff, and to emphasize information that may have an impact on the diagnosis or direction of care. Similarly, initial evaluation summary reports should contain only the pertinent background to the problem and significant findings. Clinic forms or reports limited to one page are probably more likely to be read than reports that are continued on additional pages.

ANALYSIS OF APHASIA IN PREPARATION FOR TREATMENT: PREDICTING OUTCOME

Aphasia therapy begins at its end. That is, treatment should begin with a notion of an intended endpoint. You cannot begin treatment unless you have a general idea what to expect to accomplish with a patient and his or her family. You need to assess aphasia to determine what you think will be an acceptable endpoint, or goal, for treatment. To achieve this difficult aim, the speech-language pathologist needs to make a comprehensive standardized assessment of the patient.

The PICA (Porch, 1981) is well-recognized as a reliable, valid measure of the severity of communicative deficits across modalities. This index provides outcome predictions for the first 6 months after onset as a guideline for prognosis in patients receiving treatment and as a measure to compare the effects of therapy. Other standardized tests, such as the WAB (Kertesz, 1982), provide a severity score but have not been examined for predictive potential. There may be some predictive value to diagnosing the type of aphasia, based on the natural evolution of aphasic syndromes. For example, if a patient has an "irreversible" aphasia based on findings from the *Minnesota Test for Differential Diagnosis of Aphasia* (MTDDA) (Schuell, 1972), the prognosis is poor. Alternatively, using the predictions of the *Boston Diagnostic Aphasia Examination* (BDAE) (Goodglass & Kaplan, 1983) or the WAB, patients found to have milder forms of Wernicke's aphasia, for example, might be predicted to evolve to an anomic disorder, while patients with more severe forms of a particular type of aphasia generally continue to display those characteristics in the chronic state but in milder form (Goodglass & Kaplan, 1983).

Avenues for Treatment

The problem with standardized test batteries for aphasia is that they are designed to locate broad, general deficits (e.g., an impairment in "confrontation naming" or "auditory comprehension") and thus fail to provide a sufficiently fine-tuned analysis to allow an examiner to develop a plan of treatment. It does not take a great deal of testing to appreciate that a patient has a problem with auditory comprehension or verbal formulation or nonfluent oral expression. However, breaking apart the various components of these general deficits requires the judicious use of supplemental tests or customized assessment protocols.

In most rehabilitation settings (home health agencies, rehabilitation centers, outpatient clinics, and the like), the time that one can reasonably justify

TABLE 4.3   Steps Used to Determine Avenues for Treatment

Step 1. Background gathering
Determine medical and social history.
Determine family's observations, concerns, and expectations.
Determine current medical and neurologic status.
Determine the gradient of improvement from the acute through the present stage of recovery.

Step 2. Comprehensive, standardized testing
Identify severity of the overall communication deficits.
Identify relative deficit pattern (e.g., reading is relatively worse than auditory comprehension).
Determine whether the patient is sufficiently responsive to be a suitable candidate for treatment.

Step 3. Assessment of functional communication
Determine whether the patient communicates within his or her living environment at a level commensurate with tested abilities.
Determine whether treatment should focus on a particular deficit area (e.g., verbal fluency or reading) or should focus on expanding the patient's ability to use residual language abilities in his or her living environment. That is, decide if treatment should be deficit-oriented or function-oriented.

Step 4. Supplemental testing
Focus on the areas where the patient demonstrates particular or questionable deficits.
Design tasks that will further refine an analysis of specific processes.

to devote to testing is limited. Spending several weeks testing and analyzing aphasia is not practical. Nonetheless, an expanded analysis of a particular process or ability may help to identify the best avenues for therapy and save treatment time.

Determining avenues for treatment generally starts with a broad examination leading to progressively more detailed analysis (Table 4.3).

SUPPLEMENTAL ASSESSMENT OF AUDITORY AND GRAPHIC COMPREHENSION PROCESSES

Minimum standards for the quality of patient care in long-term care facilities and rehabilitation center speech-language pathology programs should stipulate that every patient who undergoes speech-language treatment is evaluated with at least one comprehensive, standardized aphasia test. Administration of an aphasia battery, such as the BDAE, WAB, or MTDDA, mentioned earlier, or the *Luria-Nebraska Neuropsychological Battery* (LNNB) (Cristensen, 1975) or *Neurosensory Center for Comprehensive Examination for Aphasia* (NCCEA) (Spreen & Benton, 1977) permits the clinician to examine many different aspects of the patient's communication. Lyon's (1986) review of standardized tests may aid clinicians in selecting the instrument best suited to their settings and populations. Simmons (1986) points out that comprehensive batteries provide a sample across input and output communicative processes and highlight areas where special or supplemental testing is indicated.

Deficits in auditory comprehension, oral expression, naming, reading, and so forth, can have different patterns of presentation. Evidence of a broad deficit is an indication to look for the source or sources of the problems. The following sections contain sample tasks that could augment testing by examining processes within input and output domains. One needs to remember, as was emphasized earlier, that an assessment task labeled as a test of auditory analysis or phonological output may tap several associated abilities. An auditory analysis task that requires the patient to understand a specific word within a sentence could reflect a problem with grammar or syntax, a short-term memory deficit, a problem with a particular lexical category, a problem with semantic processes, or a defect in selective attention—and not necessarily a problem with phonologic auditory analysis. The following discussion is meant to *illustrate* ways to approach an examination for and within specific deficits with standardized and supplemental tests.

Auditory Input

The *Token Test* (DeRenzi & Vignolo, 1962), the *Auditory Comprehension Test for Sentences* (ACTS) (Shewan, 1981), and the *Revised Token Test* (McNeil & Prescott, 1978) are widely used instruments for supplemental testing of auditory input processes. The advantage of the latter two is that they provide an analysis of factors contributing to the breakdown of sentence comprehension. In addition, subtests from the MTDDA, BDAE, and WAB provide a variety of tasks to examine processing contributing to auditory comprehension. Comprehension of functionally relevant words and sentences can be analyzed with the *Functional Auditory Comprehension Task* (FACT) (LaPointe & Horner, 1978). Particular features of auditory comprehension, such as auditory discrimination, auditory (word) analysis, and the assessment of the auditory input lexicon, can also be examined either by designing individualized assessment tasks in addition to using supplemental tests, or by selecting subtests from existing tests. As examples, one can examine auditory discrimination of similar word pairs with a subtest from the MTDDA or one can test discrimination of intonation and rhythm with items such as those found in the BDAE. The *Peabody Picture Vocabulary Test* (PPVT) (Dunn, 1965) has been used by speech pathologists and neuropsychologists, when applying the published age-appropriate norms, to assess the auditory input lexicon. An analysis of error patterns used to determine the presence of a category-specific deficit or a problem with one word type (e.g., nouns versus verbs) could elucidate relative strengths within the lexicon. It might be useful to preface an assessment of the auditory comprehension lexicon or sentence comprehension with an examination for deficits in auditory discrimination or word analysis (Table 4.4).

TABLE 4.4 Criteria for Examining for Deficits in Auditory Discrimination or Word Analysis

Auditory analysis ability
1. Discriminating word pairs separated by at least two phonemic features ("cake" versus "late").
2. Discriminating similar word pairs with only one phonemic feature ("late" versus "lake").
3. Identifying the number of syllables within a word.
4. Identifying specifically designated phonemes within words.
5. Identifying specific words within a sentence.
6. Identifying stress, intonation, and rhythm in words and phrases.

Auditory input lexicon
1. Comprehending single words from various categories (objects, body parts, or pictures).
2. Comprehending single words representing different parts of speech (nouns, adjectives, verbs, prepositions, etc.).
3. Comprehending words indicating location and direction (on, by, left, right, up, down, etc.).
4. Distinguishing real words from nonwords ("house" versus "hadge").
5. Understanding functional directives ("point," "draw," "write," "take," "give," etc.).
6. Comprehending abstract versus concrete words (abstract: "respected"; concrete: "document").
7. Comprehending low-frequency versus high-frequency vocabulary ("cup" versus "couplet").

Auditory memory
1. Pointing to pictures in a series.
2. Pointing to numbers or objects in a series.
3. Following simple directions ("open your mouth," "point to the book," etc.).
4. Following two-step directions ("turn over the book and give it to me").
5. Pointing to the pictures that correspond to short narratives read by the examiner.

Morphosyntactic features in auditory input
1. Deriving meaning from morphemes (indicates understanding of "shoe" versus "shoes" or "man" versus "men")
2. Deriving meaning from syntactic structure ("the empty bottle was full").
3. Deriving meaning from the morphology ("the girls' dog ran from them").

Graphic Input

The *Reading Comprehension Battery for Aphasia* (RCBA) (LaPointe & Horner, 1979) is a popular supplemental test of reading functions, with subtests sampling single-word, sentence, and paragraph reading, as well as providing performance comparisons for visual, auditory, and semantic confusions in error analysis. Research in reading processes also suggests that standardized reading tests, such as the *New Adult Reading Test* (NART) (Nelson, 1984) and the *Nelson Reading Test* (Nelson, 1962), may be useful in assessing reading in normal and brain-damaged persons. Such tests have supplemental utility

TABLE 4.5   Tasks Used to Assess Graphic and Reading Ability

Graphic analysis ability
1. Matching shapes and figures.
2. Matching letters (upper case to lower case, manuscript to cursive).
3. Matching numbers.
4. Scanning to identify target letters on a horizontal line.
5. Scanning to identify target letters presented on a vertical line.

Graphic-auditory associations
1. Matching letters to phonemes ("p" to /p/) and phonemes to letters.
2. Pointing to words read to the patient.
3. Pointing to the written form of nonwords read to the patient.
4. Identifying homophones from lists.
5. Identifying irregular real words read to the patient.

Graphic input lexicon
1. Matching number symbols (the number "2") to corresponding amounts (a picture of a pair).
2. Demonstrating comprehension of written words of common names from various categories of items (body parts, foods, clothing, etc.).
3. Indicating recognition of words versus nonwords read by the patient.
4. Demonstrating comprehension of words from different word categories (nouns, adjectives, etc.).
5. Demonstrating comprehension of words indicating attributes (adjectives, adverbs).
6. Demonstrating comprehension of irregular words ("guest," "island").

with aphasic persons (Nicholas & Brookshire, 1987). More comprehensive academic skills tests (Gates & MacGinitie, 1969) also lend themselves to reading assessment after neurologic disease. To augment an assessment of reading ability, clinicians might find it helpful to design tasks to assess the patient's graphic analysis ability, grapho-motoric associations, graphic input lexicon, and sentence or paragraph comprehension (Table 4.5).

SUPPLEMENTAL ASSESSMENT OF ORAL EXPRESSION AND VERBAL FORMULATION

Supplemental assessments of oral expression and verbal formulation include evaluations of oral-buccal and verbal apraxia (Dabul, 1979); tests of naming ability (Goodglass & Kaplan, 1983; Newcombe, Oldfield, Ratcliff, & Wingfield, 1971; Nicholas, Brookshire, MacLennan, & Porazza, 1989), sentence formulation (Wener & Duffy, 1983), and word fluency (Adamovich & Henderson, 1984; DeRenzi & Faglioni, 1978; Wertz, Dronkers, & Shubitowski, 1986); and assessments of expository speech and discourse (Goodglass & Kaplan, 1983; Kertesz, 1982; Ulatowska, North, & Macaluso-

TABLE 4.6 Tasks Used to Assess Verbal Expressive and Semantic Abilities

Auditory-to-verbal associations
1. Repeating phonemes.
2. Repeating automatic sequences (counting, days of the week, etc.).
3. Repeating familiar social expressions ("OK," "How are you?").
4. Repeating one- or two-syllable words.
5. Repeating phrase- and sentence-length material.

Phonologic output ability
1. Spontaneously using social greetings.
2. Expressing single-syllable word names from pictures or objects.
3. Expressing two- and three-syllable words.
4. Expressing multisyllabic words and words with consonant clusters.
5. Formulating compound words and short sentences when given their parts ("Put the word *house* and the word *boat* together into one word"; "Put the words *football*, *church*, and *window* into a sentence.").

Semantic associations
1. Categorizing pictures.
2. Identifying objects, pictures, or words from a description of their use or attributes (*shoe* "find the one you wear on your foot").
3. Naming within categories (animals, foods).
4. Describing or demonstrating knowledge of the purpose, use, or attributes of a picture.
5. Describing or demonstrating knowledge of how objects are similar or different.
6. Understanding synonyms, antonyms, and definitions.
7. Understanding verbal analogies.

Haynes, 1981; and see Simmons' review, 1986). To analyze oral expression and verbal formulation in preparation for therapy, it may be helpful to focus clinical assessment on different aspects of expressive abilities, including auditory-to-verbal associations, phonologic output ability, and lexico-semantic ability. These processes can be examined with nonstandardized assessment tasks (Table 4.6).

Grapho-Motor Abilities and Written Language

Of all of the standardized tests used with aphasic persons, the PICA provides one of the best analyses of graphic abilities. The PICA bases scores on the two measures of writing—motoric (letter size, line execution, orientation of words on a horizontal plane) and linguistic (spelling, grammar, syntax, semantic errors, and so forth) (Golper, Fisher, Gordon, & Marshall, 1984). Analysis of graphic abilities might also include evaluating the ability to reproduce drawings or to draw to communicate a message (Elman, Roberts, & Wertz, 1988; Lyon & Sims, 1989). Along with published tests and assessment methods, an analysis of grapho-motor abilities for writing and drawing could include tasks listed in Table 4.7.

**TABLE 4.7   Tasks Designed to Evaluate Motoric
and Lexical Features of Writing and Drawing**

Grapho-motor associations
1. Copying symbols, letters, and numbers.
2. Copying a patient's first and last name.
3. Copying the names of pictures.
4. Copying sentences.
5. Reproducing or producing drawings.

Graphic output lexicon
1. Writing the patient's first and last name.
2. Writing a relative's name.
3. Writing location names.
4. Writing names of pictures or common objects.
5. Writing names within categories, such as "fruits."
6. Writing the names of items from the naming tests or other vocabulary tests.

TABLE 4.8   Tasks for Evaluating Gestural Input Lexicon and Expression

1. Demonstrating recognition and use of hand or finger gestures for number and amounts.
2. Demonstrating recognition and use of gestures that represent a single word or concept ("OK," "Come," "Go," "Stop").
3. Demonstrating recognition and use of gestures that refer to attributes ("fat," "sleepy," "hungry," "noisy," "smelly").
4. Demonstrating recognition and use of gestures referring to actions ("Drive," "Eat," "Play cards," "Sweep the floor").
5. Demonstrating recognition and use of gestures that express a short story ("I played cards at my house yesterday").

Gestural Input and Gestural Expression

Gestural comprehension and expression can be examined with the *Assessment of Nonverbal Communication/New England Pantomime Tests* (Duffy & Duffy, 1985), a standardized test appropriate for use with aphasic persons. Clinicians can also apply portions of the *Communicative Activities of Daily Living* (CADL) (Holland, 1980), which provides photographs to test comprehension of gestures and facial expression, or they might pay special notice to gestural abilities as demonstrated during the administration of the BASA or the PICA. In assessing gestural understanding and use of gestures, one might design tasks that evaluate several areas (Table 4.8).

Related Neuropsychological Deficits

Some comprehensive assessment batteries for aphasia include sections or subtests for related neuropsychological deficits (Cristensen, 1975; Goodglass

& Kaplan, 1983; Kertesz, 1982; Porch, 1981; Spreen & Benton, 1977). Identification of related deficits ought to be an integral part of the diagnosis, supplemental testing, and treatment planning of aphasia management. Neuropsychological evaluations will help determine the presence of such conditions as hemispatial neglect, dyspraxia, visuoperceptual deficits, visuo-construction deficits, agnosias, problems with executive processes, and, at least in milder cases of aphasia, contributory memory dysfunction. To provide an illustrative reference, a list of commonly used tests and tasks for evaluating related neuropsychological deficits is provided in the appendix to this chapter. Some of the published tests listed here should be administered or interpreted by clinicians with special training in neuropsychology.

Appendix

Related Neuropsychologic Tests and Assessments*

ORIENTATION AND ATTENTION

Mental status screening tests (Folstein, Folstein, & McHugh, 1975; Mattis, 1978; Pfeiffer, 1975)

Confabulation (Mercer, Wapner, Gardner, & Benson, 1977)

Place and time orientation (Benton, Van Allen, & Fogel, 1964; Milner, 1971)

Space and body orientation (Goodglass & Kaplan, 1983; Hecaen & Angelergues, 1963; Semmes, Weinstein, Ghent, & Teuber, 1963; Wepman & Turaids, 1975)

Route-finding and direction (Gooddy & Reinhold, 1963; Weinstein, Semmes, Ghent, & Teuber, 1963)

Vigilance and mental tracking (Bender, 1938; Lewis & Kupke, 1977; Smith, 1967; Talland, 1961)

Symbol-digit and digit-symbol tests (Smith, 1973; Wechsler, 1955)

Hemispatial neglect and visual inattention line bisection tests (Albert,1973; Diller, Ben-Yishay, Gerstman, Goodkin, Gordon & Weinberg, 1974; Kinsbourne, 1974; Schenkenbert, Bradford, & Ajax, 1980)

Neglect in picture description tasks (Battersby, Bender, Pollack, & Kahn, 1956; Bisiach & Luzzatti, 1978; Deutsch, Tweedy, & Lorinstein, 1980; Goodglass & Kaplan, 1983)

VISUAL RECOGNITION: FAMILIAR AND UNFAMILIAR

Faces tests (Benton, Hamsher, Varney, & Spreen, 1983; Milner, 1968; Warrington & James, 1967)

Recognition of facial emotion (DeKovsky, Heilman, Bowers, & Valenstein, 1980)

Design and figure recognition (Cristensen, 1975; Ekstrom, French, Harman, & Dermen, 1976; Wechsler, 1955)

Figure-ground tests (Ayres, 1966; Cristensen, 1979; Kirk, McCarthy, & Kirk, 1968)

VISUAL SCANNING AND TRACKING

Letter cancellation tasks (Talland, 1961)

Visual search tasks (Goldstein, Welch, Rennick, & Shelly, 1973)

---

*Also see Lezak's (1983) review of neuropsychological tests and batteries.

VISUAL ORGANIZATION

Visual organization and forms tests (Hooper, 1958; Likert & Quasha, 1970; Wechsler, 1955)

AUDITORY PERCEPTION

Speech sounds perception and discrimination tests, and audiologic speech perception test battery (Halstead, 1947; Schuell, 1972)
Nonlinguistic auditory perception (Halstead, 1947; Seashore, Lewis, & Saetweit, 1960)

AUDITORY RECOGNITION

Emotional tone recognition (Bender, Fink, & Green, 1951)

TACTILE INATTENTION

Tactile extinction tasks (Bender, Fink, & Green, 1951; Weinstein, 1978)

TACTILE PERCEPTION, DISCRIMINATION, AND RECOGNITION

Stereognosis tasks (Hutt & Gibby, 1970)
Skin writing and fingertip writing tasks (Hutt & Gibby, 1970)

CONSTRUCTIONAL PRAXIS

Copying (Borad, Goodglass, & Kaplan, 1983; Butters & Barton, 1970; Taylor, 1959; Taylor, 1979)
Free drawing (Benton & Fogel, 1962; Butters & Barton, 1970; Rey, 1964)
Object assembly, stick designs and block design (Botwinick & Storandt, 1974; Graham & Kendall, 1960; Rapaport, Gill, & Schafer, 1968; Spreen & Benton, 1977; Wechsler, 1955)

VERBAL MEMORY

Immediate retention, retrieval, and recognition (Cristensen, 1975; Graham & Kendall, 1960; Schuell, 1972; Spreen & Benton, 1977; Terman & Merrill, 1973; Wechsler, 1955)

VISUAL MEMORY

Immediate retention, retrieval, and recognition (Botwinick & Storandt, 1974; Graham & Kendall, 1960; Kirk, McCarthy, & Kirk 1968; Milner, 1968; Milner, 1971; Rey, 1964; Terman & Merrill, 1973; Wechsler, 1945)

GLOBAL AMNESIA

Amnesia tests and ratings (Artiola, Fortuny, Briggs, Newcombe, Ratcliff, & Thomas, 1980; Levin, O'Donnell, & Grossman, 1979)

EXECUTIVE FUNCTIONS

Limb apraxias (Hecaen, 1981; Heilman, 1979)
Manual dexterity (Porteus, 1959; Purdue Research Foundation, 1948)
Planning and purposeful behavior (Jones-Gotman & Milner, 1977; Porteus, 1959; Wechsler, 1955)
Cognitive flexibility (Stroop, 1935)
Motor impersistence and perseveration (Benton, 1977; Joynt, Benton, & Fogel, 1962)

CONCEPT FORMULATION

Visual analogies (Raven, 1965; Terman & Merrill, 1973; Wechsler, 1955)
Block-counting tasks and picture problems (Tow, 1955)
Proverbs interpretation (Wechsler, 1955)
Abstract words, similarities and differences (Wechsler, 1955)
Sorting tests (Berg, 1948; Cain, Egbert, & Weingartner, 1977)

PSYCHIATRIC AND PERSONALITY TRAITS

Ratings of psychiatric symptoms (Beck, Ward, Mendelson, Mock, & Erbaugh, 1961; Heaton & Pendleton, 1981; Lubin, 1965; Neugarten, Havighurst & Tobin, 1961; Overall, Gorham, 1962)
Projection tests (Murray, 1938; Rorshach, 1942)
Personality inventories (Hathaway & McKinley, 1951)

REFERENCES

Adamovich B.L., & Henderson J.A. (1984). Can we learn more from word fluency measures with aphasic, right brain injured and closed head trauma patients? *Clinical Aphasiology Conference Proceedings* (pp. 124–131). Minneapolis: BRK Publishers.

Albert, M.L. (1973). A simple test of visual neglect. *Neurology 23*, 658–664.

Artiola, I., Fortuny, L., Briggs, M., Newcombe, F., Ratcliff, G., & Thomas, C. (1980). Measuring the duration of post traumatic amnesia. *Journal of Neurology, Neurosurgery, and Psychiatry 43*, 377–379.

Ayres, A.J. (1966). *Southern California figure-ground visual perception test* [manual]. Los Angeles: Western Psychological Services.

Battersby, W.S., Bender, M.B., Pollack, M., & Kahn, R.L. (1956). Unilateral "spatial agnosia" ("inattention") in patients with cortical lesions. *Brain, 79*, 68–93.

Beck, W.T., Ward, C.H., Mendelson, M., Mock, J., & Erbaugh, J.K. (1961). An inventory for measuring depression. *Archives of General Psychiatry, 4*, 561–571.

Bender, L.A. (1938, 1979). A visual motor gestalt test and its clinical use. *American Orthopsychia Association Research Monographs* (No 3).

Bender, M.B., Fink, M., & Green, M. (1951). Patterns in perception on simultaneous tests of face and hand. *AMA Archives of Neurology and Psychiatry, 66*, 355–362.

Benton, A.L. (1977). Interactive effects of age and brain disease on reaction time. *Archives of Neurology, 34*, 369–370

Benton, A.L., & Fogel, M.L. (1962). The assumption that a common disability underlies failure in copying drawings and copying two-and three-dimensional block patterns is not justified. *Archives of Neurology 7*, 347–358.

Benton, A.L., & Hamsher, K. (1978). *Multilingual aphasia examination*. Iowa City: Benton Laboratory of Neuropsychology.

Benton, A.L., Hamsher, K., Varney, N.R., & Spreen, O. (1983). *Contributions of neuropsychological assessment*. New York: Oxford University Press.

Benton, A.L., Van Allen, M.W., & Fogel, M.L. (1964). Temporal orientation in cerebral disease. *Journal of Nervous and Mental Disorders, 139*, 110–119.

Berg, E.A. (1948). A simple objective test for measuring flexibility of thinking. *Journal of General Psychiatry, 39*, 15–22.

Bisiach, E., & Luzzatti, C. (1978). Unilateral neglect of representational space. *Cortex, 14*, 129–133.

Borad, J.C., Goodglass, H., & Kaplan, E. (1983). Normative data on the Boston diagnostic aphasia examination parietal lobe battery and the Boston naming test. *Journal of Clinical Neuropsychology, 2*, 209–216.

Botwinick, J., & Storandt, M. (1974). *Memory, related functions and age*. Springfield, IL: Charles C Thomas.

Butters, N., & Barton, M. (1970). Effect of parietal lobe damage on the performance of reversible operations in space. *Neuropsychology, 8*, 205–214.

Caine, E.D., Ebert, M.H., & Weingartner, H. (1977). An outline for the analysis of dementia. *Neurology, 23*, 1087–1092.

Carmines, E.G., & Zeller, R.A. (1981). Reliability and validity assessment. In J.L. Sullivan (Ed.), *Quantitative applications for the social sciences*. Beverly Hills: Sage Publications.

Cristensen, A.L. (1975). *Luria's neuropsychological investigation*. New York: Spectrum Publication.

Cristensen, A.L. (1979). *Luria's neuropsychological investigation text* (2nd ed.). Copenhagen: Munksgaard.

Dabul, B. (1979). *Apraxia battery for adults.* Tigard, OR: C.C. Publications.

Darley, F. (1982). *Aphasia.* Philadelphia: W.B. Saunders.

DeKovsky, S.T., Heilman, K.M., Bowers, D., & Valenstein, E. (1980). Recognition and discrimination of emotional faces and pictures. *Brain & Language 9*, 206–214.

DeRenzi, E., & Faglioni, P. (1978). Normative data and screening power for a shortened version of the Token test. *Cortex, 14*, 41–49.

DeRenzi, E., & Vignolo, L.A. (1962). The Token test: A sensitive test to detect receptive disturbances in aphasia. *Brain, 85*, 665–678.

Deutsch, G., Tweedy, J.R., & Lorinstein, I.B. (1980, February). *Some temporal and spatial factors affecting visual neglect.* Paper presented at the eighth annual meeting of the International Neuropsychological Society, San Francisco.

Diller, L., Ben-Yishay, Y., Gerstman, L.J., Goodkin, R., Gordon, W., & Weinberg, J. (1974). *Studies in cognition and rehabilitation in hemiplegia.* New York: New York University Institute of Rehabilitation Medicine.

Duffy, R.J., & Duffy, J.R. (1985). *Assessment of nonverbal communication/New England pantomime tests.* Austin, TX: PRO-ED.

Dunn, L.M. (1965). *Expanded manual for the Peabody picture vocabulary test.* Minneapolis: American Guidance Service.

Ekstrom, R.B., French, J.W., Harman, H.H. & Dermen, D. (1976). *Manual for kit of factor-referenced cognitive tests.* Princeton, NJ: Educational Testing Service.

Elman, R.J., Roberts, J., & Wertz, R.T. (1988). Reliability and classification of writing and drawing performance in mildly aphasic patients and normal individuals. In T.E. Prescott (Ed.), *Clinical Aphasiology: Vol 17.* (pp. 95). Boston: College-Hill Press.

Folstein, M.F., Folstein, S.E., McHugh, P.R. (1975). Mini mental state. *Journal of Psychiatric Research, 12*, 189–198.

Frattali, C.M., Thompson, C.M., Holland, A.L., Wohl, C.B., & Ferketic, M.M. ASHA FACS—a functional outcome measure for adults. (1995). *ASHA 37*, 40–46.

Gates, A.I., & MacGinitie, W.H. (1969). *Gates-MacGinitie reading tests.* New York: College Press, Teachers College, Columbia University.

Goldstein, G., Welch, R.B., Rennick, P.M., & Shelly C.H. (1973). The validity of a visual searching task as an indication of general brain disease. *Journal of Consulting and Clinical Psychiatry, 41*, 434–437.

Golper, L.A., Fisher B., Gordon, M., & Marshall, R. (1984). *Motoric and linguistic features in aphasic writing.* Presented at the American Speech-Language-Hearing Association Annual Convention, San Francisco.

Gooddy, W., & Reinhold, M. (1963). The sense of direction and the arrow-form. In E. Halpern (Ed.), *Problems of Dynamic Neurology.* Jerusalem: Hebrew University Hadassah Medical School.

Goodglass, H., & Kaplan, E. (1983). *Boston diagnostic aphasia examination.* Philadelphia: Lea & Febiger.

Gordon, M. (1990). *The other side.* New York: Penguin Books.

Graham, F.K., & Kendall, B.S. (1960). Memory-for-designs-test: Revised general manual. *Perceptual & Motor Skills Monograph Supplement* (No 2-VIII, 1), 147–188.

Granger, C., & Hamilton, B. (1985). *Functional index measure (FIM).* Buffalo, NY: The Task Force for Development of a Uniform Data System for Medical Rehabilitation, Project Office, Department of Rehabilitation Medicine, Buffalo General Hospital.

Hall, K.M., Hamilton, B., Gordon, W.A., Zasler, M.D., & Johnston, M.V.F. (1988). *Functional assessment measure (FAM)*. Santa Clara Valley Medical Center for Rehabilitation Research.

Halstead, W.C. (1947). *Brain and intelligence*. Chicago: University of Chicago Press.

Hathaway, S.R., & McKinley, J.C. (1951). *The Minnesota multiphasic personality inventory manual* (revised). New York: Psychological Corporation.

Heaton, R.K., & Pendleton, M.G. (1981). Use of neuropsychological tests to predict adult patients' everyday functioning. *Journal of Consulting and Clinical Psychiatry, 49*, 807–821.

Hecaen, H. (1981). Apraxia. In S.B. Bilskov & T.J. Boll (Eds.), *Handbook of clinical neuropsychology*. New York: Wiley-Interscience.

Hecaen, H. & Angelergues, R. (1963). *La cetite psychique*. Paris: Masson et Cie.

Heilman, K.M. (1979). Apraxia. In K.M. Heilman & K. Valenstein (Eds.), *Clinical neuropsychology*. New York: Oxford University Press.

Helm-Estabrooks, N., Ramsberger, G., Morgan, A.R., & Nicholas, M. (1989). *Boston assessment of severe aphasia*. San Antonio, TX: Special Press.

Holland, A.L. (1980). *Communicative abilities in daily living*. Austin, TX: PRO-ED.

Hooper, H.E. (1958). *The Hooper visual organization test* [manual]. Los Angeles: Western Psychological Services.

Hutt, M.L., & Gibby, R.G. (1970). *An atlas for the Hutt adaptation of the Bender-Gestalt test*. New York: Grune & Stratton.

Jones-Gotman, M., & Milner, B. (1977). Design fluency: The invention of nonsense drawings after focal cortical lesions. *Neuropsychology 15*, 653–674.

Joynt, R.J., Benton, A.L., & Fogel, M.L. (1962). Behavioral and pathological correlates of motor impersistence. *Neurology, 12*, 876–881.

Kaplan, E., Goodglass, H., & Weintraub, S. (1983). *The Boston naming test*. Philadelphia: Lea & Febiger.

Keenan, J.S., & Brassel, E.G. (1975). *Aphasia language performance scales*. Murfreesboro, TN: Pinnacle Press.

Kertesz, A. (1982). *The Western aphasia battery*. New York: Grune & Stratton.

Kinsbourne, M. (1974). Lateral interactions in the brain. In M. Kinsbourne & W.L. Smith (Eds.), *Hemispheric disconnection and cerebral function*. Springfield, IL: Charles C Thomas.

Kirk, S.A., McCarthy, J.J., & Kirk, W.D. (1968). *Illinois test of psycholinguistic abilities* [examiner's manual] (rev. ed.). Urbana, IL: University of Illinois Press.

LaPointe, L. & Horner, J. (1978, Spring). The functional auditory comprehension test (FACT): Protocol and test format. *FLASHA Journal*, 27–33.

LaPointe, L.L., & Horner, J. (1979). *Reading comprehension battery for aphasia*. Austin, TX: PRO-ED.

Levin, H.S., O'Donnell, V.M., & Grossman, R.G. (1979). The Galveston orientation and amnesia test: A practical scale to assess cognition after head injury. *Journal of Nervous and Mental Disorders, 167*, 675–684.

Lewis, R., & Kupke, T. (1977, May). *The Lafayette Clinic repeatable neuropsychological test battery: Its development and research applications*. Paper presented at the Annual Meeting of the Southeastern Psychological Association, Florida.

Lezak, M.D. (1983). *Neuropsychological assessment* (2nd ed.). New York: Oxford University Press.

Likert, R. & Quasha, W.H. (1970). *The revised Minnesota paper form board test* [manual]. New York: Psychological Corporation.

Lubin, B. (1965). Adjective check lists for measurement of depression. *Archives of General Psychiatry, 12*, 57–62.

Lyon, J. (1986). Standardized test batteries: Advances in aphasia testing. In L.L. LaPointe (Ed.), *Seminars in speech and language: Aphasia: Nature and assessment, 7*, 159. New York: Thieme.

Lyon, J. & Sims, E. (1989). Drawing: Its use as a communicative aid the aphasic and normal adults. In T.E. Prescott (Ed.), *Clinical Aphasiology* (Vol 18, p. 339). Boston: College-Hill Press.

Mattis, S. (1978). Mental status examination for organic mental syndrome in the elderly patient. In L.A. Bellak & T.B. Karasu (Eds.), *Geriatric Psychiatry*. New York: Grune & Stratton.

McNeil, M. & Prescott, T. (1978). *Revised token test*. Austin, TX: PRO-ED.

Mercer, B., Wapner, W., Gardner, H., & Benson, D.F, (1977). A study of confabulation. *Archives of Neurology, 34*, 429–433.

Milner, B. (1968). Visual recognition and recall after right-temporal lobe excision in man. *Neuropsychology 6*, 191–209.

Milner, B. (1971). Interhemispheric differences in the localization process in man. *British Medical Bulletin, 27*, 272–277.

Murray, H.A. (1938). *Explorations in personality*. New York: Oxford University Press.

Nelson, H.E. (1984). *New adult reading test (NART) test manual*. Windsor, England: NFER-Nelson.

Nelson, M.J. (1962). *The Nelson reading test*. Boston: Houghton-Mifflin.

Neugarten, B.L., Havighurst, R.J., & Tobin, S.S. (1961). The measurement of life satisfaction. *Journal of Gerontology, 16*, 134–343.

Newcombe, F., Oldfield, R.C., Ratcliff, G.G., & Wingfield, A. (1971). Recognition and naming of object-drawings by men with focal brain wounds. *Journal of Neurology Neurosurgery & Psychiatry 34*, 329–340.

Nicholas, L.E., & Brookshire, R.H. (1987). Error analysis and passage dependency of test items from a standardized test of multiple sentence reading comprehension for aphasic and non brain damaged adults. *Journal of Speech and Hearing Disorders, 52*, 358–366.

Nicholas, L.E., Brookshire, R.H., MacLennan, D.L, & Porazza, S.A. (1989). Revised administration and scoring procedures for the Boston naming test and norms for non brain damaged adults. *Aphasiology, 3*, 569–580.

Overall, J.E., & Gorham, D.R. (1962). The brief psychiatric rating scale. *Psychiatric Reports, 10*, 799–812.

Pfeiffer, E. (1975). SPMSQ: Short portable mental status questionnaire. *Journal of the American Geriatric Society, 23*, 433–441.

Porch, B.E. (1981). *The Porch index of communicative ability*. Palo Alto, CA: Consulting Psychologists Press, 1981.

Porteus, S.D. (1959). *Porteus maze test and clinical psychology*. Palo Alto, CA: Pacific Books.

Purdue Research Foundation (1948). *Examiner's manual for the Purdue pegboard*. Chicago: Science Research Associates.

Rapaport, D., Gill, M.M., & Schafer, R. (1968). *Diagnostic psychological testing* (rev. ed.). New York: International Universities Press.

Raven, J.C. (1965). *Guide to using the coloured progressive matrices*. London: H.K. Lewis.

Rey, A. (1964). *L'examen clinique en psychologie*. [The clinical examination in psychology.] Paris: Presses Universitaires de France.

Rorshach, H. (1942). *Psychodiagnostic: A diagnostic test based on perception* (P. Lemkau & B. Kronenburg, Trans.). New York: Grune & Stratton.

Schenkenbert, T., Bradford, D.C., & Ajax, E.T. (1980). Line bisection and unilateral visual neglect in patients with neurologic impairment. *Neurology 30*, 509–517.

Schuell, H. (1972). *The Minnesota test for differential diagnosis of aphasia*. New York: The Psychological Corp.

Seashore, C.E., Lewis, D., & Saetweit, D.L. (1960). *Seashore measure of musical talents* (rev. ed.). New York: Psychological Corporation.

Semmes, J., Weinstein, S., Ghent, L., & Teuber H.L. (1963). Correlates of impaired orientation in personal and extrapersonal space. *Brain, 86*, 747–772.

Shewan, C. (1981). *The auditory comprehension test for sentences*. Chicago: Biolinguistic Clinical Institute.

Simmons, N.N. (1986). Beyond standardized measures: Special tests, language in context and discourse analysis in aphasia. In L.L. LaPointe (Ed.) *Seminars in speech and language: Aphasia: Nature and assessment, 7*, 181. New York: Thieme, 1986.

Skenes, L., & McCauley, R. (1985). Psychometric review of nine aphasia tests. *Journal of Communication Disorders, 18*, 461–474.

Smith, A. (1973). *Symbol digit modalities test* [manual]. Los Angles: Western Psychological Services.

Smith, S. (1967). Serial sevens subtraction test. *Archives of Neurology 17*, 78–80.

Spreen, O., & Benton, A.L. (1977). *Neurosensory center comprehensive examination for aphasia*. Victoria, BC: University of Victoria.

Stroop, J.R. (1935). Studies of interference in serial verbal reactions. *Journal of Experimental Psychology, 18*, 643–662.

Talland, G.A. (1961). Effect of aging on the formation of sequential and spatial concepts. *Percepual & Motor Skills, 13*, 210–217.

Taylor, E.M. (1959). *The appraisal of children with cerebral deficits*. Cambridge, MA: University Press.

Taylor, L.B. (1979). Psychological assessment of neurosurgical patients. In T. Rasmussen & R. Marino (Eds.), *Functional neurosurgery*. New York: Raven Press.

Terman, L.M., & Merrill, M.A. (1973). *Standford-Binet intelligence scale* [manual for the 3rd rev., form L-M]. Boston: Houghton Mifflin.

Tow, P.M. (1955). *Personality changes following frontal leucotomy*. London: Oxford University Press.

Tyler, L.E. (1971). *Tests and measurements* (2nd ed). Englewood Cliffs, NJ: Prentice-Hall.

Ulatowska, H.K., North, A.J., & Macaluso-Haynes, S. (1981). Production of narrative and procedural discourse in aphasia. *Brain and Language, 13*, 345–371.

Warrington, E. & James, M. (1967). An experimental investigation of facial recognition in patients with unilateral cerebral lesions. *Cortex, 3*, 317–326.

Wechsler, D. (1945). A standardized memory scale for clinical use. *Journal of Psychiatry, 19*, 87–95.

Wechsler, D. (1955). *Wechsler adult intelligence scale* [manual]. New York: Psychological Corporation.

Weinstein, S. (1978). Functional cerebral hemispheric asymmetry. In M. Kinsbourne (Ed.), *Asymmetrical function of the brain*. Cambridge, England: Cambridge University Press.

Weinstein, S., Semmes, J., Ghent, L., & Teuber, H.L. (1963). Spatial orientation in man after cerebral injury: II. Analysis according to concomitant defects. *Journal of Psychiatry, 42*, 249–263.

Wener, D.L., & Duffy, J.R. (1983). An investigation of the sensitivity of the reporter's test to expressive language disturbances. *Clinical Aphasiology Conferences Proceedings* (abstract). *83*, 15. Minneapolis: BRK Publishers.

Wepman, J.M., & Turaids, D. (1975). *Spatial orientation memory test* [manual of directions]. Palm Springs, CA: Language Research Associates.

Wertz, R.T., Dronkers, N.F., & Shubitowski, Y. (1986). Discriminant function analysis of performance of normals and left hemisphere, right hemisphere, and bilaterally brain damaged patients on a word fluency measure. *Clinical Aphasiology Conference Proceedings 86*, 257–266. Minneapolis: BRK Publishers.

West, J.F. & Sands, E. (1987). *Bedside evaluation and screening test for aphasia.* Frederick, MD: Aspen.

Chapter 5

Basic Hearing Assessment

Ronald C. Jones

Most clinicians agree that aphasia is such a complex disability that, for the purpose of providing treatment, it is difficult to classify individuals with aphasia into specific diagnostic groups. This is particularly true for the aphasic patient suspected of also having a hearing loss. Even the patient with a mild aphasia tends to confuse the simplest of auditory signals and give the appearance of having poor ability to discriminate speech. Patients with more severe aphasia often need the simplest of words to be repeated several times in order to respond. So the presence of a significant hearing loss serves only to confound an already difficult situation. It is very important, therefore, that the speech-language clinician test a patient's hearing, or interpret test results, before administering speech and language assessments. Otherwise, the clinician is at a clear disadvantage from not knowing whether a patient's poor auditory responses are the result of aphasia or hearing loss.

The purpose of this chapter is to provide the speech and language clinician with guidelines for conducting basic hearing assessments with patients who are aphasic. This chapter should help clinicians differentiate between hearing loss and loss of auditory function due to aphasia.

PRIMARY AUDITORY DISORDERS ASSOCIATED WITH APHASIA

When individuals with aphasia have difficulty recognizing common speech signals, the condition is known by various terms, but generally it is known as *acoustic agnosia* (Darley, 1982; Luria, 1966). A primary characteristic of this condition is that the patient's errors for speech-sound discrimination increase as differences between sounds decrease. Thus, more

87

errors are likely to occur with discriminations made between sounds such as /t/ and /p/, or /t/ and /d/, than between /s/ and /m/, or /k/ and /r/. Understandably, the effects of this condition can be easily confused with the speech-sound recognition errors commonly seen among persons with even mild hearing loss.

When an auditory perception disturbance resulting from aphasia involves more than just simple speech-sound discrimination and includes disturbances with nonsymbolic (nonlanguage) sounds (e.g., mechanical or animal noises) or human nonlinguistic sounds (coughing, sneezing, hand clapping, etc.), the condition is known as an auditory agnosia (Eisenson, 1971). Severe forms of auditory agnosia are termed *pure word deafness* or *cortical deafness*. The condition is characterized by an inability to comprehend or discriminate spoken language, although the ability to read, write, and speak is relatively intact (Eisenson, 1973). Pure word deafness is thought to be the rarest of conditions because it would take precisely placed lesions within the auditory cortex and corpus callosum to generate such a condition and at the same time not affect areas surrounding these regions. From a purely audiologic perspective, though, auditory agnosia would be quite demonstrable and would resemble a profound sensorineural hearing loss.

Differentiating between the various auditory disturbances caused by aphasia, and those produced by hearing loss, becomes an important matter for the speech and language clinician to consider.

ROLE OF THE AUDIOLOGIST

The speech-language clinician assumes the lead role in managing the communication of patients with aphasia, but he or she occasionally may need the consultative assistance of the audiologist. In such a case, the audiologist assumes responsibility for conducting hearing tests, making necessary medical referrals (to an ear-nose-throat specialist), and providing any necessary follow-up rehabilitative services (e.g., hearing aids, counseling, auditory training, etc.). These activities should be conducted in concert with the speech-language clinician's treatment plan. The audiologist might also serve as a member of the multidisciplinary assessment and rehabilitation team assigned to provide comprehensive patient management.

When an audiologist is not readily available to consult with the speech-language clinician, or where such services are available but would be inordinately delayed because of scheduling problems, the speech-language clinician is obligated to conduct the preliminary audiometric tests. It is assumed here, of course, that the clinician is familiar with the use of an audiometer and with the basic pure-tone hearing test. If this is not the case, then the clinician is advised to consult again with an audiologist for reference materials or formal training.

AUDIOMETRIC EVALUATION OF PATIENTS WITH
APHASIA BY SPEECH-LANGUAGE CLINICIANS

Instrumentation and Equipment

The audiologist has one other important role to play: to consult with the speech-language clinician about the type of equipment needed to conduct basic audiometric tests and to provide assistance if testing reveals a hearing loss. Essentially, the equipment includes a calibrated portable pure-tone audiometer, an otoscope, and a personal sound amplification system. (These instruments are discussed later in the chapter.)

Test Considerations

The speech-language clinician should consider at least two elements of the hearing assessment. These are (1) determining which test stimuli should be used (either a speech or nonspeech signal) and (2) determining the most suitable method of test presentation for a specific patient in a particular situation.

Test Signal

Investigations (Chandler & Sedge, 1982; Miller, 1960; Street, 1957) have repeatedly shown that for testing the hearing of patients with aphasia, the best stimuli to use are nonspeech signals. This is because the auditory processing of simple sound signals, such as pure tones, occurs principally within the cochlea and lower brainstem. These areas are anatomically remote from the damaging effects of a stroke and other survivable head injuries (Mencher, 1967). However, the processing of speech requires mediation by the cortex, where the effects of a stroke can be considerable (Bard & Rioch, 1937; Goldberg & Neff, 1962; Lorente de Nó, 1933; Magoun, 1952; Mueller & Beck, 1982; Rubens, 1979).

Conventional audiometric tests call for the use of sound frequencies that range from 250 Hertz (Hz) to 8000 Hz. These frequencies represent the important speech signals. For test convenience, the frequency range is divided into even octave intervals. The pure tones that represent these octaves are 250 Hz, 500 Hz, 1000 Hz, 2000 Hz, 4000 Hz, and 8000 Hz. Sometimes mid-octave tones (15000 Hz, 3000 Hz, and 6000 Hz) are also used. Because these test frequencies represent important components of speech (vowels and consonants), the response by an individual with aphasia to these stimuli provides an excellent approximation of auditory sensitivity for detecting common speech sounds.

Signal Intensity.   The normal hearing level for a pure-tone signal is zero decibels (dB). This "0 dB" level does not denote the absence of sound intensity. Rather, it is the lowest level at which the average normal hearing person responds to pure-tone test signals. The fact is, an individual with normal hearing may well have a hearing threshold that is below zero, or even just slightly above. Normal hearing, therefore, is best described as a range of intensities occurring somewhere between −10 dB and +20 dB, with the average being 0 dB.

The speech-language clinician is cautioned not to assume that an aphasic patient's normal responses to pure-tone audiometry will yield normal ability to recognize speech. As indicated previously, speech recognition involves cortical function and is therefore subject to the effects of aphasia. The real value of pure-tone audiometry with patients who are aphasic is that it helps to identify possible peripheral (outer, middle, inner ear) hearing deficits, which can usually be minimized through medical treatment (for outer and middle-ear disease), or with hearing aids and other assistive listening devices (for cochlear disturbances).

The Audiogram.   The audiogram represents an array of important information, and should be carefully reviewed. With reference to the audiogram shown in Figure 5.1, the scale for sound frequency (Hertz) is located along the top axis of the graph, and the scale for sound intensity (decibels) is located along the side axis. Conventionally, an "O" is used to represent the right ear's threshold response, and an "X" is used for the left ear.

Test Presentation

A number of researchers have examined various methods for conducting pure-tone audiometry with patients who are aphasic (Carhart & Jerger, 1959; Ludlow & Swisher, 1971; Wilson, Fowler, & Shanks, 1981). In general, they have found that the less severely impaired an aphasic patient is, the more likely he or she can respond to a routine audiometric threshold procedure (Carhart & Jerger, 1959). However, for patients with more severe aphasia, specific modifications of the procedure are often required. Such variations in patients' responses should be considered by the clinician before testing is attempted.

Threshold Testing Technique.   The audiometric threshold technique used by audiologists is reviewed here to familiarize the speech-language clinician with conventional test procedures. The method routinely used to measure hearing threshold is called the *ascending-descending* technique (Carhart & Jerger, 1959). Quite simply, a sound signal (pure tone) is presented through earphones using a calibrated audiometer. The intensity of the signal should start somewhere near the patient's presumed normal hearing threshold (around 10–20 dB). If the patient fails to respond (with a positive gesture, verbal response, etc.), the signal is repeated, but increased by 5 dB. The process continues until there is a response. When the patient responds, the signal intensity is reduced by

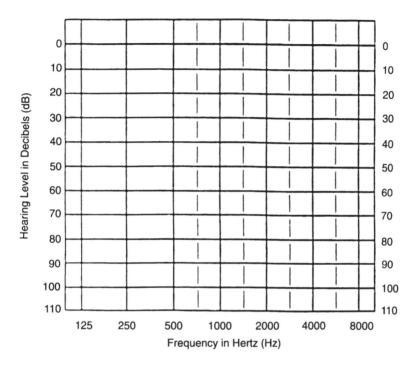

Figure 5.1 *A conventional pure-tone audiogram.*

10 dB, presumably dropping below the patient's hearing threshold. Again the signal intensity is increased in 5-dB increments, repeating the process at least two or three times for each test signal. The threshold is recorded on an audiogram as the lowest sound level at which the patient responded at least 50% of the time.

Threshold Test Modification.　Many individuals with severe aphasia have considerable difficulty understanding directions and following routine or patterned procedures. For these patients, it is often necessary to alter the procedure for the basic hearing test. For patients who can respond to simple directions but are either slow to respond or may be confused by the ascending-descending technique, the sound signal should be presented at an intensity level well above the patient's presumed threshold. A good starting point is the level of average conversational speech—60 decibels (or higher if necessary). If the patient responds, the signal intensity should be reduced in 10-dB increments until he or she fails to respond. This descending procedure should be repeated at each test frequency two or three times. Hearing threshold is recorded on an audiogram at the lowest sound level at which the patient consistently responded. This procedure, appropriately called the *descending technique*, has been found effective with most aphasic patients without adversely affecting test validity or reliability (Wilson et al., 1981).

Another test modification for patients with severe aphasia is behavioral observation audiometry (BOA), a technique audiologists use routinely with infants and small children. The clinician relies on visual observation of the patient, looking for responses to common environmental sounds (telephone ring, doorbells, television, etc.). The patient's eye or head rotation in the direction of a sudden sound, or physical reaction (startle, reflex, etc.) to a loud sound, if present, should be observed. This approach is obviously neither as quantifiable nor as accurate as pure-tone audiometry but is acceptable under certain extreme circumstances. With the BOA method, test results should not be recorded on an audiogram. Instead, the speech-language clinician should issue a written narrative report of the types of sounds that the patient responded to, and the nature of the responses. This report should be incorporated with other data from communication tests.

In cases where conventional audiometric techniques cannot be used with a patient who is aphasic, an audiologist should be consulted. The audiologist may retest the patient's hearing using more objective and quantifiable methods. These tests might include acoustic immittance measures (to rule out middle-ear problems); or brain stem response audiometry (ABR) (to rule out a retrocochlear problem). Again, these and other audiologic procedures should be conducted in concert with the speech-language clinician's treatment plan.

Audiometric Profiles.   Figure 5.2 illustrates four profiles of threshold responses from pure-tone thresholds tests. These represent (1) normal hearing; (2) mild hearing loss; (3) moderate to severe hearing loss; and (4) profound hearing loss. (Note that only air conduction thresholds are shown.)

Although the pure-tone signals used in audiometry represent the important speech sounds, the relationship between the signals and a person's actual speech discrimination ability is a difficult association to establish. In general, however, it is reasonable to assume that an increasing amount of hearing loss corresponds to increasing difficulty in understanding speech (Table 5.1).

Effects of Aging on Hearing Sensitivity.   Researchers who have studied the effects of aging on hearing have documented the steady progression of hearing loss with advancing age (Bunch, 1929; Hinchcliffe, 1962). Typical pure-tone audiometry gives the best evidence of this effect, particularly at frequencies beyond 1000 Hz. Figure 5.3 demonstrates the dramatic effects of aging on hearing, and shows, as well, similarities between aging males and females.

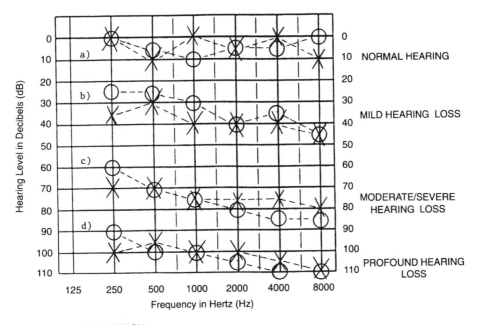

AIR CONDUCTION
O RIGHT EAR
X LEFT EAR

Figure 5.2   *Pure-tone audiogram illustrating profiles for: (a) normal hearing; (b) mild hearing loss; (c) moderate to severe hearing loss; and (d) profound hearing loss.*

TABLE 5.1   Classification of Hearing Loss: Illustration of the Relationship Between Hearing Level Taken from Audiometric Data and the Ability to Understand Speech

Average Hearing Threshold Level 1000–4000 Hz

Hearing Level dB (HTL)	Degree of Loss	More Than	Not More Than	Ability to Understand Speech
0	None	—	25	No significant difficulty with faint speech
25	Mild	25	40	Difficulty only with faint speech
40	Moderate	40	55	Frequent difficulty with normal speech
55	Moderately severe	55	70	Frequent difficulty with loud speech
70	Severe	70	90	Can understand shouted and amplified speech
90	Profound	90	—	Usually cannot understand even amplified speech

Source: Modified from H. Davis, S.R. Silverman. (1970). Hearing and Deafness. New York: Rinehart & Winston.

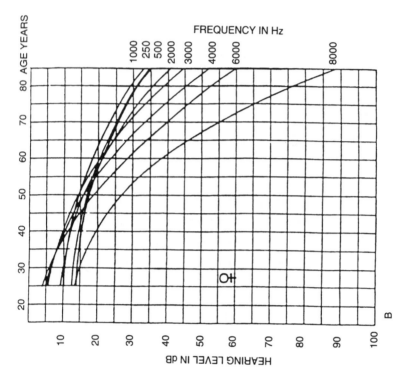

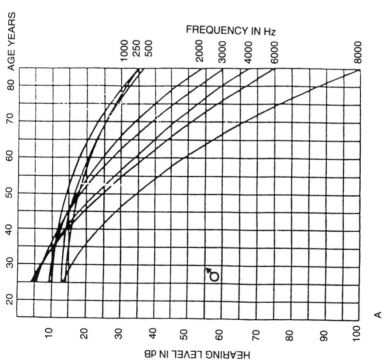

Figure 5.3   *Composite male (A) and female (B) presbycusic curves. (Modified from C.P. Lebom & R.C. Reddell. (1972). The Presbycusis Component in Occupational Hearing Tests. Laryngoscope, 82, 1399–1409.)*

Related research shows that by 40–50 years of age, hearing thresholds beyond 1000 Hz begin to decrease noticeably, and by 60–80 years, the lower frequencies become involved (Corso, 1963; Glorig & Roberts, 1965; Harford & Dodds, 1982; Hinchcliffe, 1962; Lebo & Reddell, 1972; Robinson & Sutton, 1979). This information should alert clinicians who work with elderly aphasic patients to anticipate the presence of measurable hearing loss, particularly for higher-frequency sounds.

Basic Procedure for Auditory Assessment

The assessment procedure presented here is multifaceted by design. The intent is to avoid relying on any one source of data for determining the auditory condition of a patient, particularly when more than one source is important. The procedure described below includes: (1) case history, (2) auditory comprehension testing, (3) otoscopic inspection, and (4) identification audiometry.

Case History

Much of the information needed to determine the patient's preexisting auditory capabilities can be obtained through a case history. Family members, friends, and other persons acquainted with the aphasic patient, as well as some patients themselves, can provide a fairly comprehensive picture of prestroke auditory skills. Questions about how well the patient heard conversations in quiet and in noisy settings, or how well the patient used or enjoyed television, radios, and the telephone, can be important in discerning how normal or abnormal the patient's hearing performance was before the stroke. In addition, if the patient wore a hearing aid, knowing the type of aid, its vintage, which ear (if not both), and how often it was used, can illuminate the extent to which the patient's hearing was previously affected and managed. Of course, copies of any previous audiograms are invaluable. Clinicians should consider constructing a questionnaire encompassing these and other pertinent questions.

Informal Auditory Comprehension Tests

In addition to the case history, experienced speech-language clinicians have long used methods for assessing auditory comprehension without the use of conventional audiometric instruments and formal test procedures (Schuell, 1966). This approach is particularly important when comprehensive audiologic services are unavailable or when information about the aphasic patient's auditory abilities is urgently needed.

Although not intended to be a measure of hearing, the information obtained from informal auditory comprehension tests can alert the clinician and other caregivers of the possible presence of an auditory communication problem. Tests might include the following tasks:

1. Identifying objects named in a picture
2. Following simple directions
3. Answering simple questions
4. Completing sentences
5. Paraphrasing what was heard
6. Writing answers to what was heard

Test items and materials should be culturally sensitive to the patient. A patient's familiarity or social comfort with test items and materials may prompt a more spontaneous and accurate response.

Otoscopic Inspection

Several physical and pathologic conditions can involve the ear and affect hearing. Therefore, it is important to examine the outer ear before conducting a hearing evaluation. Speech-language clinicians who conduct routine oral-peripheral examinations should find it relatively simple to also conduct a peripheral examination of the ear (Table 5.2). (If a physical examination of the patient has already included an ear examination, that information should be reviewed and integrated into the audiologic assessment report.)

In performing the otoscopic inspection, a well-lighted otoscope must be used. There are five procedures:

1. Select a speculum (funnel-shaped tip) large enough to give a clear view of the ear canal walls and the tympanic membrane (TM).
2. Turn on the otoscope.
3. Gently pull the auricle upward, backward, and outward.
4. When inserting the speculum, use the side of the little finger or fingertip to anchor the hand holding the otoscope against the patient's cheekbone or mastoid bone. This is to ensure that a sudden head or hand movement will not cause ear discomfort from the scope or speculum.
5. Rotation of the head or the tip of the speculum will probably be necessary. Use the light from the scope like a beacon to view the entire TM.

An otologic referral is warranted if the inspection reveals any abnormalities or pathologic conditions, or if information from the case history reveals a history of unresolved ear disease.

Identification Audiometry Hearing Screening

Hearing threshold testing (previously described) is unquestionably superior to hearing screening tests. This is because threshold tests serve to quantify absolute (or near-absolute) hearing sensitivity, even with modified approaches, while screening tests yield a general impression of sensitivity. One criterion for threshold testing, however, is that it must be

TABLE 5.2   Structures to be Examined in Otoscopic Inspection

A. Auricle
   1. Positioning of the ear
   2. Deformity or injury
   3. Preauricular tags, dimples, or pits
   4. Growths or skin conditions
   5. Deformity from frostbite
   6. Cauliflower ear
   7. Other unusual conditions
B. External ear canal
   1. Partial or complete closure (atresia)
   2. Abnormal narrowing (stenosis)
   3. Excessive buildup of cerumen or debris
   4. Growths
   5. Active infection
   6. Odor
   7. Postoperative scarring or alterations
   8. Blood in the canal
   9. Dislodged pressure equalization tube
  10. Other irregularities
C. Tympanic membrane (TM)
   1. Perforation
   2. Bulging or retraction
   3. Fluid or bubbles behind the TM
   4. Abnormal color
   5. Tube in the TM
   6. Evidence of trauma
   7. Other irregularities

conducted in a low-noise setting, preferably a sound suite, an acoustically treated test site. Unfortunately, such settings are rarely available to speech-language clinicians, whose work environments vary from home health care to nursing homes, hospital clinics, and other less rarified settings. Therefore, if a patient needs a hearing assessment, and there is neither a readily available audiologist nor a suitable test environment for threshold testing, a hearing screening should be conducted. Again, threshold testing is preferable.

Screening Frequencies.   Only four of the eight pure-tone test frequencies need to be used for a hearing screening. Traditionally, these signals represent the frequencies at the low, middle, and high end of the range of speech frequency (e.g., 500 Hz, 1000 Hz, 2000 Hz, and 4000 Hz). I suggest, however, that 500 Hz be eliminated, and that 3000 Hz be included. The 500-Hz signal can be easily confused with environmental sounds or body noises and be missed on a screening test. The 3000-Hz signal strengthens the high-frequency representation on the test and aids in recognizing any adverse effects of high-frequency hearing loss.

For hearing screening, setting the level of the screening tone (1000 Hz, 2000 Hz, 3000 Hz, and 4000 Hz) at 20 dB, and getting a patient to respond consistently at this level, signifies that the person can hear within the normal hearing range. Failure to respond at this level, at any one of the test frequencies, signifies a screening-test failure. This warrants a more thorough audiometric evaluation.

Audiometer Calibration.   Before conducting the hearing evaluation, the speech-language clinician must ensure that the audiometer is calibrated—that the intensity levels and frequencies selected are accurate.

Audiometers can be calibrated in two ways. One way is to have the audiometer manufacturer or distributor perform an annual electrical/acoustical calibration (in accordance with the American National Standards Institute [ANSI], 1969). This is time-consuming and can be costly, but it is necessary to certify the accuracy of the test results. For convenience, the procedure might be scheduled to coincide with the calibrations that a consulting audiologist must also obtain for his or her test equipment.

The other method is for the clinician to perform a *biological calibration*. The biological calibration is a simple check of the audiometer's signals performed each day the audiometer is used. The clinician tests his or her own *normal* hearing to ensure that the audiometer signals (frequency and intensity) are operational, and to determine whether the test room is adequately quiet with no noises to interfere with the test signals. A biological calibration should be part of the testing routine. However, it does not substitute for the annual electrical/acoustical calibration.

The following is a generic hearing screening procedure that can be modified to suit clinicians' particular needs. This procedure has been adapted from the procedure recommended by the American Speech-Language-Hearing Association (ASHA, 1985, 1990).

1. The patient should be advised that his or her hearing is going to be tested. The patient should respond in some appropriate fashion when he or she hears a sound coming from each earphone.
2. The earphones should be placed comfortably over the patient's ears.
3. The audiometer should be set to 1000 Hz tone at 60 dB (average level of conversational speech). The signal is then introduced. The right ear should be routinely tested first. The patient's response should be observed.
4. If the patient responds, the signal should be reduced to 20 dB (upper limit of the normal hearing range) and presented again. If the patient responds, normal hearing for that frequency should be recorded on the audiogram. If the patient fails to respond, an "NR" (no response) should be written on the audiogram.

5. The procedure should be repeated for 2000 Hz, 3000 Hz, and 4000 Hz. If the patient fails to respond to any one of the four signals at 20 dB, then a screening failure should be recorded. The patient should then be rescreened, later, before an audiologic referral is made.
6. Repeat the entire procedure for the other ear.

Follow-up Reporting. When a patient completes the entire auditory assessment procedure, the clinician should be able to identify (1) any history of prior hearing problems; (2) a performance level for auditory comprehension of language, based upon informal or formal language tests; (3) the physical status of the ear; and (4) the level of hearing determined from either a pure-tone threshold test or a pure-tone hearing screening. From these data, the clinician should be able to categorize the patient's auditory status as follows:

1. Patients with normal pure-tone results (passed screening) but who demonstrate poor auditory/speech reception or discrimination ability should be assumed to have an auditory disturbance associated with aphasia.
2. Patients with measurable hearing loss (failed screening) and no active ear disease should be seen by an audiologist for auditory rehabilitation therapy. These patients will likely need a personal amplification system.
3. Patients with no previous history of hearing loss but who fail a hearing screening should be retested as soon as possible. Their diagnostic profile is incomplete without a clear determination of their hearing status.
4. Patients with a history of hearing problems who also fail the hearing screening should be seen for a medical and audiologic evaluation. The audiologist should probably administer more detailed diagnostic tests and follow-up with auditory rehabilitation therapy (hearing aid[s], auditory training, etc.). Use of a personal amplification system may be warranted.

Personal Amplification Systems. A personal amplification system may constitute a privately purchased personal hearing aid of any number of types (e.g., ITE, BTE, Eyeglass, Body Level) or a personal amplifier provided by the speech-language clinician.

The personal amplifier is a small tabletop or body-worn device that consists of earphones, a battery-operated amplifier, and an extension microphone. Speech-language clinicians have long used them to assist patients during therapy sessions. These units have traditionally been referred to as *auditory training units* but today are identified by their trade names. Personal amplifying units continue to be an essential component of the speech-language clinician's diagnostic and rehabilitative instrumentation and should be made available if a patient needs one. The audiologist can be consulted regarding which type of personal amplification system is most suitable.

SUMMARY

Few would argue with the statement that the sense of hearing is fundamental to the development and promotion of normal speech and language. It would follow, therefore, that hearing assessment of an individual with aphasia is an essential component of overall communication management and should be conducted prior to the initiation of clinical treatment. Without such an assessment, there would be constant doubt about the patient's true auditory status and full communication capabilities.

Pure-tone audiometry, conducted either as a threshold procedure or as a screening measure, is the recommended test for speech-language clinicians to use with their patients who have aphasia. The results of pure-tone testing identify common hearing loss, and by inference, differentiate it from a loss of auditory function resulting from the aphasia.

REFERENCES

American National Standards Institute Specifications for Audiometers. ANSI S3.6-1969. New York American National Standards Institute, Inc., 1970.

American Speech-Language-Hearing Association. (1985). Guidelines for identification audiometry. *ASHA, 27*, 49–52.

American Speech-Language-Hearing Association. (1990). Guidelines for screening for hearing impairments and middle ear disorders. *ASHA, 32*, (Suppl. 2), 17–24.

Bard, P., & Rioch, D.M.C.K. (1937). A study of four cats deprived of neocortex and additional portions of the forebrain. *Bulletin Hopkins Hospital, 60*, 73–125.

Bunch, C.C. (1929). Age variations in auditory acuity. *Archives of Otolaryngology 9*, 625–626.

Carhart, R., & Jerger, J.F. (1959). Preferred method for clinical determination of pure tone thresholds. *Journal of Speech and Hearing Disorders, 24*(11), 330–345.

Chandler, D., & Sedge, R.D. (1982). Pure tone sensitivity and speech recognition findings following head injury. *Seminars in Hearing, 8*(3), 241–251.

Corso, J.F. (1963). Age and sex differences in puretone thresholds. *Archives of Otolaryngology 77*, 53–73.

Darley, F.L. (1982). *Aphasia* (p. 75). Philadelphia, PA: W.B. Saunders.

Davis, H., & Silverman, S.R. (1970). *Hearing and deafness*. New York: Rinehart & Winston.

Eisenson, J. (1971). Aphasia in adults: Basic considerations. In L.E. Travis (Ed.), *Handbook of speech pathology and audiology* (p. 1226). New York: Appleton-Century-Crofts.

Eisenson, J. (1973). *Adult aphasia* (pp. 11–12). Englewood Cliffs, NJ: Prentice Hall.

Glorig, A., & Roberts, J. (1965). Hearing levels of adults by age and sex. United States 1960–1962. *National Center for Hearing Statistics Series, II*, No. 11. Washington, DC: U.S. Department of Health, Education, and Welfare, Public Hearing Service.

Goldberg, J.M., & Neff, W.D. (1962). Frequency discrimination after bilateral ablation of cortical auditory areas. *Journal of Neurophysiology, 24*, 119–128.

Harford, E.R., & Dodds, E. (1982). Hearing status of ambulatory senior citizens. *Ear Hear, 3*, 105–109.

Hinchcliffe, R. (1962). Aging and sensory thresholds. *Journal of Gerontology, 17,* 45–50.

Lebo, C.P., & Reddell, R.C. (1972). The presbycusis component in occupational hearing tests. *Laryngoscope, 82,* 1399–1409.

Lorente de Nó, R. (1933). The anatomy of the eighth nerve. *Laryngoscope, 43,* 1–38.

Ludlow, C.L., & Swisher, L.P. (1971). The audiometric evaluation of adult aphasics. *Journal of Speech and Hearing Research, 14,* 535–543.

Luria, A. (1966). *Human brain and psychological processes.* New York: Harper & Row.

Magoun, H.W. (1952). The ascending reticular activating system. *Research Publications - Association for Research in Nervous and Mental Disease, 30,* 480–492.

Mencher, G.T. (1967). The reliability of electrodermal audiometry with aphasic adults. *Journal of Speech and Hearing Research, 10,* 328–332.

Miller, M.H. (1960). Audiologic evaluation of aphasic patients. *Journal of Speech and Hearing Disorders, 25,* 333.

Mueller, H.G., & Beck, W.G. (1982). Brainstem level test results following head injury. *Seminars in Hearing, 8*(3), 253.

Robinson, D.W., & Sutton, G.J. (1979). Age effect in hearing—a comparative analysis of published threshold data. *Audiology, 18,* 320–334.

Rubens, A.B. (1979). Agnosia. In K. Heilman and B.E. Valenstein (Eds.), *Clinical neuropsychology* (pp. 233–267). New York: Oxford University Press.

Schuell, H. (1966). A re-evaluation of the short examination for aphasia. *Journal of Speech and Hearing Disorders, 31,* 137–147.

Street, B.S. (1957). Hearing loss in aphasia. *Journal of Speech and Hearing Disorders, 22,* 60.

Wilson, R.H., Fowler, C.G., & Shanks, J.E. (1981). Audiological assessment of the aphasic patient. In R.T. Wertz (Ed.), *Aphasia: Interdisciplinary approach. Seminars in speech, language, and hearing* (pp. 229–314). New York: Thieme-Stratton.

Chapter 6

Management of Aphasic Individuals from Culturally and Linguistically Diverse Populations

Gloriajean L. Wallace

PREVALENCE OF STROKE IN MINORITY POPULATIONS

Stroke, the third leading killer after cancer and heart disease (American Heart Association, 1994), can affect anyone, regardless of ethnicity. Available evidence, however, indicates a disproportionately high incidence of stroke among racial and ethnic minorities. Particularly, there is a disproportionately high incidence of stroke among blacks (Council on Scientific Affairs, American Medical Association, 1991; Kurtzke, 1985; Saunders, 1991; U.S. Department of Health and Human Services, 1985; Wallace, 1993a; Yano, Reed, & Kagan, 1985; Yatsu, 1991), who represent the largest minority group in the United States (12% of the overall population). Blacks also comprise approximately 9% of the population age 45 years and above (National Center for Health Statistics, 1994, Table 1) but comprise 11% of the stroke deaths among individuals age 45 years and above (National Center for Health Statistics, 1994, Table 34).

Comparisons of overall population representation and stroke death incidence is not as disparate for other minority groups when they are viewed as a whole. For instance, for the population of individuals age 45 and above, Hispanics comprise 4% of the population, yet only 2% of all stroke deaths; Asian/Pacific Islanders comprise 2% of the population, yet only 1% of all stroke deaths; and American Indians comprise less than 1% of the population, and less than 1% of all stroke deaths (National Center for Health Statistics, 1994, Table 34). While such overall group statistics make it appear that these and other minority groups are not at as great a risk for stroke as are blacks, specific subgroups of these populations have, in fact, been identified to be at very high risk. For instance, the risk for stroke has been reported to be higher among Puerto Ricans than for other Hispanic populations and higher than for the population at large. Likewise, the risk for stroke among Hawaiians and Samoans is higher than for other Asian/Pacific Islander groups and higher than for the population at large (American Heart Association, 1994; U.S. Department of Health and Human Services, Public Health Service, 1990; Wallace, 1993b).

RISK FACTORS FOR STROKE IN MINORITY POPULATIONS

The major risk factors for stroke in minority populations include uncontrolled hypertension, elevated serum cholesterol levels, and arteriosclerosis (Moss, 1993; Singleton & Johnson, 1993). All of these risk factors are exacerbated because of dietary habits that include the use of excessive amounts of salt and polyunsaturated fat during food preparation and seasoning (Wallace, 1992). This is particularly true for blacks, many of whom incorporate traditional Southern dietary practices into their lifestyles and other minority groups who have shifted to more Americanized cholesterol-laden diets.

Diabetes, a condition that results in vascular changes, is another risk factor for stroke that is pervasive within minority communities. African-Americans are 1.6 times more likely to incur diabetes as the population at large; more than 2 million African-Americans are affected by this disease. Nearly 6% of African-American males and 8% of African-American females have diabetes. Hispanics are over 55% more likely to incur diabetes than is the population at large (American Diabetes Association, 1992). An estimated 2.5 million Hispanics, or one in every 10 individuals, has this disease, which affects almost 10% of the Cuban population, 13% of the Mexican-American population, and more than 13% of the Puerto Rican population. The incidence of diabetes is also high among American Indians, who are 10 times more likely to incur diabetes than is the general population (American Diabetes Association, 1992). Members of one tribe, the Pimas of Arizona, are 300% more likely to incur diabetes than is the population at large (American Diabetes Association, 1992). Compared to Americans as a whole, diabetes among minority groups goes undetected for longer periods of time, which accounts for the higher death rate and higher rate of complications. The incidence of diabetes among minority communities discussed above may be attributed to hereditary factors as well as to dietary practices that promote the heavy consumption of carbohydrates.

Sickle cell anemia, a risk factor for stroke, disproportionately affects those of African and Mediterranean ancestry and others (who unknowingly may have traces of this ancestry) (Barnhart, Henry, & Lusher, 1974; Johnson & El-Hazmi, 1984; Platt et al., 1994; Prohovnik, Pavlakis, & Piomelli, 1989). This disease causes red blood cells, which are normally round, to assume a curved or sickled shape. This abnormal shape makes it difficult for them to pass through the small blood vessels. As a result, areas of the brain that are supplied by small blood vessels do not receive oxygen, which can result in stroke.

Cocaine poses a risk for stroke because of its vasoconstricting properties (Brust, 1993; Das, 1993; Holden, 1989; Killam, 1993; Kokkinos & Levine, 1993; Levine, Brust, Futrell, et al., 1990; Levine, Washington, Jefferson, et al., 1987; Mody, Miller, McIntyre, Cobb, & Goldberg, 1988; Wallach, 1989). The use of cocaine is a problem of disproportionate magnitude in inner cities, which are often densely populated by minorities.

Many public health efforts have been initiated to reduce stroke risk factors (for example, programs emphasizing stroke education and blood pressure and cholesterol screening). While these efforts have resulted in a significant stroke reduction within the general population, the rate of reduction for stroke and stroke risk factors among those from the minority community has proceeded at a much slower pace (American Heart Association, 1994).

CHANGING DEMOGRAPHICS AND STROKE IN THE COMMUNITY

The U.S. Bureau of the Census reports a more rapid than anticipated increase in the number of persons immigrating to the United States—a trend that may have an impact on the prevalence of stroke. This increase includes a great influx of individuals from countries south of the continental borders, and from Asia and the Pacific Rim nations. If current trends in immigration and birth rates persist, the Hispanic population will further increase by an estimated 21%, the Asian presence by 22%, blacks almost 12%, and whites a little more than 2% by the end of the twentieth century (U.S. Bureau of the Census, 1990). By 2010, one-third of all Americans will be people of color and by 2056, European-Americans will be a minority group (Taylor, 1992). The slow decline in stroke risk factors together with the rise in overall population figures suggest that the problem of stroke and the need for stroke rehabilitation within the multicultural community will only increase over time.

Given the high risk for stroke and likely resulting communication impairment among individuals from this fast-growing segment of our community, there is a need for greater attention to issues relating to cultural and linguistic variables that may impinge on rehabilitation. Aside from the numbers, attention to multicultural issues is important to ensure the very best delivery of personalized rehabilitation management for all patients, regardless of their ethnicity.

PERSONALIZING TREATMENT FOR DIVERSE POPULATIONS

In aphasia, speech-language pathologists have always individualized clinical management, because of our awareness of the impact of content relevancy on communication performance (Brookshire, 1978, p. 25; Holland, 1977; Schuell, 1953, p. 197; Schlanger & Schlanger, 1970; Wallace & Canter, 1985). This concept is not new. Efforts in this area have focused on using astute observation and accumulating a detailed social history, including information about the individual's pre-stroke lifestyle, interests, skills, and attitudes. They have also entailed acquainting ourselves with information about family structure, level of support, and family history to maximize the participation of significant others in treatment. However, cultural and linguistic issues pertaining to populations outside of a speech-language pathologist's own experience are often not well understood. It is difficult, therefore, to factor them into the clinical planning process. As a result, cultural variables may only be considered from an ethnocentric perspective, where it is assumed that assessment and treatment should proceed from a framework fashioned for middle-class European-Americans (Pederson, 1987), and issues relating to second language use and rehabilitation of the bilingual patient may receive little attention. Given that all communication (normal and pathologic) emerges from a cultural context, as our population becomes increasingly diverse, speech-language pathologists will need to broaden their knowledge about cultural issues, to adapt their clinical style(s) of interaction, and to sharpen their sensitivities for cultures that are different from their own. These changes will be important to maximize speech-language pathologists' ability to help all patients reintegrate into the community and participate fully in life, based on what is relevant and practical.

THE ROLE OF THE SPEECH-LANGUAGE PATHOLOGIST IN MANAGING DIVERSE POPULATIONS

The American Speech-Language-Hearing Association (ASHA) has taken the stance that it is important to infuse multicultural information into the framework of clinical management. Furthermore, ASHA has asserted that professional certification of university programs by the ASHA Educational Standards Board (ESB) is contingent on the demonstration of programmatic infusion of multicultural information into the academic curricula (including neurogenics coursework) (ASHA, 1992a). While this position has advanced the cause of multiculturalism within our professions, ASHA has, to date, not provided *specific* guidance concerning the role that speech-language pathologists should play in the management of diverse populations, nor about the scope of information needed to fulfill the role. In the absence of definitive guidance by ASHA, it is reasonable to expect that, at minimum, clinicians should have at their fingertips the necessary resources for developing culturally and linguistically appropriate rehabilitation strategies. Toward this end, the reader is asked to consider three questions:

1. Will you assume a direct role or an indirect role in the rehabilitation of patients from culturally and linguistically diverse populations?
2. Do you have in place a set of strategies and procedures that can be implemented when fulfilling a direct or indirect role as rehabilitation team member?
3. Are you familiar with variables, including cultural and communication variables, that may affect the design and use of rehabilitation services by individuals from the minority community?

WHO WILL PROVIDE THE SERVICE

If it were possible to match patients with clinicians from similar cultural and linguistic backgrounds, the decision about whether to implement a direct or indirect model of service delivery would clearly be less complex. However, given the paucity of minorities within the professions, it is unlikely that such a match is possible. Only 4% of the ASHA-certified speech-language pathology membership is of non-European ancestry (ASHA, 1992b).

An alternative consideration might be to match patients with clinicians who have attained bicultural and bilingual/bidialectal competency as a result of specific academic and clinical training. However, the paucity of such professionals also prohibits significant matching. Campbell (1986; Campbell, Brennan, & Steckol, 1992; Campbell & Taylor, 1992) surveyed 713 speech-language pathologists regarding their level of preparedness to work with diverse populations. Survey respondents for this study were not identified by area of specialty. Sixty-six percent of the survey respondents reported that they did not feel competent to evaluate or treat communication disorders in culturally and linguistically diverse populations. This finding was consistent with others (Committee on the Status of Racial Minorities, 1985, 1987; Snope, 1982). Furthermore, 91% of the 713 speech-language pathologists surveyed by Campbell indicated that they had received no coursework and no clinical training relevant to the management of diverse populations during their professional education. These results coincide with earlier findings by Shewan and Malm (1989). Thus, the bulk of clinical management will, by necessity, be undertaken by nonminority speech-language pathologists, most of whom are monolingual and monocultural. This will necessitate training about cultural issues pertaining to the diverse patients that speech-language pathologists see (Wallace & Bridges-Freeman, 1991) and will necessitate the use of trained

TABLE 6.1   Schemata of Service Delivery Options Based on Clinician Competencies and Patient Characteristics

Patient Profile	*Clinician Profile*			
	Monolingual (English) Monocultural (Mainstream U.S.)	*Monolingual (English) Bicultural*	*Bilingual Bicultural*	*Bilingual Monocultural (Mainstream U.S.)*
Monolingual (English) Monocultural (mainstream U.S.)	D-S	D-S	D-S	D-S
Bilingual Bicultural	ID-S CC	ID-S	D-S	D-S CC
Bilingual Monocultural (other than mainstream U.S.)	ID-S CC	ID-S	D-S	D-S CC
Monolingual (other than standard English) Mono-cultural (other than mainstream U.S.)	ID-S CC	ID-S	D-S	D-S CC

D-S = clinician will provide direct service to patient; ID-S = clinician will provide indirect service to patient; this will occur with the assistance of an interpreter, preferably a paid trained assistant from the patient's community; CC = the clinician is advised to learn about the patient's culture prior to service provision.

interpreter assistants when there is a language mismatch between clinician and patient (ASHA, 1995).

IMPLEMENTATION OF DIRECT OR INDIRECT SERVICES

As delineated above and shown in Table 6.1, speech-language pathologists will assume either a direct or an indirect role based on their level of competency for interweaving cultural and linguistic characteristics of the patient into the management plan.

The Bilingual Speech-Language Pathologist

The bilingual speech-language pathologist will have language skills necessary to provide direct services to both bilingual and monolingual patients.

TABLE 6.2 Summary of Important Information to Obtain about the Person with Aphasia Prior to Clinical Contact

1. Overview of ethnic group, including prominent cultural mores
2. Cultural history and history of immigration to the United States
3. Generational status
4. Communication patterns (verbal and nonverbal)
5. Social organization
6. Time concept
7. Predominant religion(s)
8. Health practices
9. Food preferences
10. Risk factors for communication impairment

In instances when the bilingual clinician is unfamiliar with the patient's specific culture, care should be taken to obtain this information prior to the initiation of clinical management. During the "S" or subjective portion of our "SOAP" (subjective, objective, assessment, and plan) clinical information-gathering process, we generally obtain a host of information about the patient's background. However, this typically does not include relevant information about the patient's culture. A suggestion of the type of additional information that one may choose to obtain prior to service delivery is summarized in Table 6.2 and discussed below. (For more information about SOAP, see Chapter 4.)

While general information about cultural mores is valuable, one should keep in mind that just as diversity can be found across groups, diversity can also be found within groups. This is particularly important to remember when comparisons are made across socioeconomic categories and levels of education. Generally, the higher the socioeconomic status and level of educational attainment, the more acculturated the individual (Milroy, 1987). For this reason, it may be best to think in terms of ranges of culture, rather than absolutes, and to use information as a general rather than absolute barometer. Attempts should be made to validate interpretations of observed behavior with the patient and/or the patient's family. Useful information may include:

1. *An overview of the ethnic group, including general information about prominent cultural mores and general characteristics of the population.* This will provide the clinician with a general flavor of the culture. One should keep in mind that the individual may differ markedly from the group description. Although all individuals from the multicultural community do not fit a low socioeconomic, low educational attainment profile, many do. This is especially true when one considers older individuals. The lack of money to pay for rehabilitation services, and a patient's inability to obtain transportation to treatment (particularly if treatment

takes place outside of the patient's community) may hinder service delivery. For this reason, impediments to service delivery need to be explored. Information pertaining to highest educational level attained and pre-stroke literacy skills needs to be determined prior to language assessment and selection of treatment goals. An additional important point to note is that minority patients may not receive rehabilitation even when they can afford it and it is geographically accessible, because of the challenges associated with the provision of services to patients whose language or customs may differ from those of the professionals assigned to work with them.

2. *Cultural history and history of immigration to the United States.* Conditions surrounding immigration to the United States may range from relatively pleasant to harsh; motives can range from voluntary pursuit of a more prosperous lifestyle, to involuntary flight to avoid political persecution. Understanding the conditions under which the patient or the patient's ancestors immigrated to the United States may provide greater insight into the personal profile of the patient. Particular attention should be given to obtaining information about the history of accessibility of and satisfaction with the U.S. health care system. Many ethnic groups have a long history of discrimination and inaccessibility to health care services, and for this reason may have developed a pattern of visiting a medical professional only when they are faced with a potentially life-threatening condition.

   A sensitivity to historical issues that influence health-seeking behavior may provide insight into ways in which the clinician can increase the patient's trust and comfort with health and rehabilitation services. Insight in this area may also facilitate the establishment and maintenance of clear patient-clinician channels of communication.

   Because many minority populations have had limited access to health care in the United States (Kenton, 1991), ancillary health services such as speech pathology are virtually unknown professions within these communities. Patients who are not familiar with what rehabilitation services have to offer may be reluctant to follow through for appointments. For this reason, greater marketing of speech-language pathology rehabilitation services in the multicultural community is sorely needed.

3. *Generational status.* This will provide valuable information about the patient's level of acculturation, based on length of residency within the United States from a personal and an ancestral perspective.

4. *Communication patterns.* The clinician will need to obtain detailed information about the linguistic, nonverbal pragmatic, and cognitive style characteristics of the ethnic group. Information pertaining to specific dialect of a language should also be obtained. In-depth inquiry pertaining to the patient's premorbid auditory comprehension, speaking, and literacy skills as compared to the ethnic group is important. Comparisons of the patient's pre-stroke skills to those of a spouse, sib-

ling, or other close family member in the same generation as the patient may also prove helpful (Payne-Johnson, 1983). When preparing to determine the language(s) and dialect(s) to target during assessment, and when deciding on the most productive language to target for treatment, the following information will undoubtedly be of use:

- Information pertaining to the context of acquisition for the first and second language
- Level of comprehension and expressive language proficiency for the first and second languages (in both written and spoken modalities) prior to the stroke
- Context of use for the first and second language prior to the stroke (for example, English usage at work, and use of another language within the home when conversing with family and friends)
- Extent of code switching used prior to the stroke (a complete discussion of code switching and implications for assessment and treatment of the bilingual speaker is presented by Reyes (1995).

With the exception of the bilingual aphasia test (Paradis, 1987), there are very few assessments available in languages other than standard English. Therefore, it will likely be necessary for the clinician to design criterion-referenced assessments and/or alternative scoring procedures when evaluating the patient's competency in languages other than standard English. This will minimize bias (Holland, 1983). A final comment in the area of communication is the important reminder that a solid understanding of culturally appropriate nonverbal aspects of communication will go a long way to promote healthy interaction among patient, family, and clinician.

5. *Social organization.* Many members of minority communities are group-oriented, as compared to members of mainstream American culture who emphasize the independent functioning of the individual separate from the family and extended family unit (Reyes, 1994). Because of the importance of family and extended family among many minority cultures, it will be important for the clinician to delineate and include all "significant others" in the clinical management process, with the understanding that the "significant other" category may extend far beyond the mainstream American nuclear family of mother, father, and immediate children.

Because the extended family may be extremely involved with the patient, the clinician may find it disconcerting to provide treatment in a setting where many individuals besides the patient and the immediate family are present in the hospital room. Rather than feeling disconcerted in this situation, we should seize the opportunity to engage additional sources for treatment assistance. We may need to examine our concepts of the importance of extended family so that we are more tolerant of the presence of family and extended family members during assessment and treatment.

Furthermore, the clinician needs to be sensitive to the patient's point of view on the acceptability of having family and extended family members observe assessment and treatment. For some patients, particularly those of Asian ancestry, it may be difficult to have family and extended family observe as they are presented with and required to respond to simple activities of daily living that they may no longer be able to do without assistance. Having family and extended family members witness the patient's post-stroke difficulty with such tasks may be a source of shame for the patient. For some patients it is a matter of pride; for others it is a matter of a fear of becoming too dependent on others, or a fear of what family members will think of them.

6. *Time concept.* Hall (1959) in his classic book *Silent Language* delineates two major types of interactional styles based on emphasis or de-emphasis on time. According to Hall, individuals with *monochronic style* view time linearly, and tend to focus on interactions and activities one at a time. Individuals with monochronic orientation can segment their activities according to the element of time. They emphasize promptness and are able to terminate an activity when the clock indicates that it is time to do so. Punctuality is a major characteristic of this group. Other individuals have a *polychronic* time orientation. These individuals can handle several interactions and activities at the same time and are able to go back and forth between tasks with great ease. The emphasis is on the involvement of people and the completion of transactions rather than adherence to schedules. Mainstream American culture is monochronic (Lingenfelter & Mayers, 1986). Many minority cultures, on the other hand, are polychronic. Differences in time orientation across patients have implications for how treatment sessions should be structured, and for the development of more appropriate models of service delivery. Home-based, rather than clinically based models of service delivery, may be more likely to promote regular attendance and prompt arrival for appointments for individuals with polychronic orientation (Reyes, 1994; Reyes, 1995; Wallace, 1992).

7. *Predominant religion(s).* While the majority of individuals in the United States are Christians or Jews, all U.S. citizens do not ascribe to these beliefs. It is also important to note that religion often influences one's belief of why an illness occurred, and whether it is proper to cure an illness or to leave it untreated (as might occur when a patient feels that the illness or disability was deserved) (Wallace, 1992). Reyes refers to this factor as *locus of control* (1994). Individuals with an external locus of control believe that events are independent of their actions, and more a result of external forces imposed by God or fate. Individuals with an internal locus of control believe that events are contingent upon their actions and that they can influence their own destiny. An internal versus an external locus of control may influence one's approach to treatment tasks, especially those in which judgment of accuracy are cogni-

tively based. Reyes notes that the locus of control may also influence whether one seeks the services of the speech pathologist and may influence one's motivation and thus one's progress in therapy.

8. *Health practices.* It is important to understand the patient's and family's understanding of health and illness, and the relevancy of rehabilitation services (Green, 1982; Kraut, 1990; McCaslin & Calvert, 1975; Rakowski, Hickey, & Dengiz, 1987; Snow, 1984; Spector, 1985). These concepts may vary across ethnic groups. Some cultures prefer to let a health condition run its course without Western medical or rehabilitative intervention because of a belief that the person experiencing the difficulty needs to experience the challenges associated with the illness rather than receive treatment to overcome the illness. In some cultures, efforts to provide rehabilitation and independence are not readily accepted because of a tradition of caring for ill persons rather than rehabilitating them back to independence. In such instances, requiring the patient to attend rehabilitation services to learn to function independently would be considered disrespectful and would cause great shame to the family.

Patient and family acceptance of traditional versus orthodox forms of healing (rehabilitation) vary across the ethnic groups. Some non-Western groups believe in non-Western traditional healing techniques to the exclusion of Western orthodox methods. Herbal medicine, massage, prayer, meditation, visualization, and other forms of healing may be preferred over Western modes of treatment. A respectful understanding of these factors is necessary before one can address this issue with the patient. A clinician who can see the issue from the patient's point of view stands a better chance of obtaining patient cooperation for orthodox treatment when traditional healing has failed, and of obtaining patient cooperation for treatment with non-Western traditional and Western methods simultaneously.

9. *Food preferences.* Since many stroke patients also have concomitant motor speech impairments and dysphagia, it is helpful to determine food preferences so that those considerations can be incorporated into the feeding plan when necessary. Alexander, Riquelme, Trent, & Williams (1994), for example, have reported success with the use of pureed plantains for Hispanic dysphagic patients in comparison to other pureed foods such as potatoes.

10. *Risk factors for communication impairment.* Obtaining information in this area will assist with health promotion efforts, so that the clinician can facilitate the prevention of future strokes (Marge, 1984). An extensive discussion of health promotion and stroke prevention is provided in Chapter 19.

Linguistic competency and information about culture provide a minimum knowledge base for providing services to linguistically and culturally diverse patients. The clinician providing services to this population will likely need exceptional clinical skills to be able to select, gather, synthesize, and make judgments about relevant information (including criterion-referenced behavioral data), in the absence of *specific* guidelines, norms, and materials for use with minority populations.

While specific guidelines and training standards for the bilingual speech-language pathologist have not yet been delineated by ASHA, the ASHA Committee on the Status of Racial Minorities has provided *general* skills that a bilingual speech-language pathologist should possess (ASHA, 1988). These include:

1. Ability to describe the process of normal speech and language acquisition for both bilingual and monolingual individuals and how those processes are manifested in oral (or manually coded) and written language.
2. Ability to administer and interpret formal and informal assessment procedures to distinguish between communication differences and communication disorders in oral (or manually coded) and written language.
3. Ability to apply intervention strategies for treatment of communicative disorders in the patient's language.
4. Ability to recognize cultural factors that affect the delivery of speech-language pathology and audiology services to the patient's language community.

The Monolingual Speech-Language Pathologist

The monolingual speech-language pathologist will, of course, provide direct services to the English-speaking patient from mainstream American culture and to individuals who differ from the clinician in culture but not language. The latter instance will, however, require that clinicians take time to learn about pertinent aspects of a patient's culture with which they may not be familiar (see Table 6.2).

For the patient who speaks a language other than standard English, the monolingual speech-language pathologist will need to provide indirect consultative services. This will entail the use of an interpreter (preferably a paid, trained bilingual/bicultural assistant). Kayser (1993) notes that the role of interpreter is not to be taken lightly. According to Kayser, the role of interpreter is complex and should not be filled by family members. Kayser (1995) provides a list of skills that the interpreter should possess. These include:

1. A fluid command of the language such that the interpreter can communicate the same concept in different ways.
2. An ability to shift pragmatic and linguistic styles depending on the dialect being spoken.
3. Some speech pathology training to enable the interpreter to understand the rationale, procedures, and information that is obtained during assessment.

4. A good command of medical, educational, and professional terminology.
5. Good memory skills to enable the interpreter to retain chunks of information during the interpretation process.

A detailed discussion of procedures relating to the management of bilingual patients by the monolingual speech-language pathologist is beyond the scope of this chapter. The reader should refer to Kayser (1995) and Wallace (1996) for this information. Case studies relating to the management of diverse adult neurogenics patients by bilingual and monolingual speech-language pathologists can also be found in Wallace (1996, in press). General steps that the monolingual speech-language pathologist may wish to consider when providing indirect service with the bilingual patient are listed below.

1. Obtain information about the patient's culture and language system.
2. Become familiar with a few simple words in the patient's native language and be able to pronounce them correctly.
3. Obtain a good working knowledge of nonverbal communication skills appropriate for the patient's culture, and for interaction with individuals in the patient's generation.
4. Locate, train, and work with an interpreter in preparation for the assessment process.
5. Select culturally and linguistically appropriate criterion-referenced tasks to obtain comparative information across languages.
6. Determine the most productive language to target in treatment.
7. Develop culturally appropriate treatment goals and strategies.
8. Develop culturally sensitive methods for incorporating the family into the treatment process.
9. Locate, train, and work closely with an interpreter (in conjunction with the family and extended family unit) who will provide the direct rehabilitation service. Jon Lyon's Communication Partners concept, discussed in Chapter 8, is particularly well-suited for incorporating community members into the treatment process.
10. Determine whether treatment is efficacious and make ongoing adjustments to treatment goals and strategies as necessary.

SUMMARY AND CONCLUSIONS

The interest in diversity and its impact on the rehabilitation process is newly emerging. Much research is needed, including studies to:

1. Investigate cultural and linguistic variables that may influence the rehabilitation process.
2. Develop valid and reliable assessment instruments, with standardization information that is appropriate for application to diverse populations.

3.   Determine the most efficient way of determining the language of choice to treat bilingual aphasic individuals.
4.   Delineate best practices when incorporating interpreters into the aphasia management process.

In addition, research is needed to explore efficacious, and perhaps alternative, models of service delivery for diverse populations by a profession of individuals who for the most part are monolingual and monocultural.

I have shared information gleaned from my work with diverse populations with the hope that this chapter will serve as a springboard to stimulate clinical and research interest in this area. Issues pertaining to cultural and linguistic diversity must receive greater attention if we are to provide quality, individualized rehabilitation services to all patients with aphasia, including those from cultural and linguistic backgrounds that may differ from our own.

REFERENCES

Alexander, K.N., Riquelme, L., Trent, D., & Williams, B. (1994). Diversity in caseload management of patients with motor speech disorders and dysphagia. Miniseminar presented at the 1994 ASHA convention, New Orleans.

American Diabetes Association. (1992). *Diabetes facts*. Alexandria, VA: Author, National Office.

American Heart Association. (1994). *Heart and stroke facts: 1994 statistical supplement*. Dallas, TX: Author, National Center.

American Speech-Language-Hearing Association. (1988). *Bilingual speech-language pathologists and audiologists. Definition prepared by the Committee on the Status of Racial Minorities*. Rockville, MD: Author.

American Speech-Language-Hearing Association. (1992a). Multicultural action agenda 2000. *ASHA, 34*, 38–66.

American Speech-Language-Hearing Association. (1992b). *Omnibus Survey*. Rockville, MD: Author.

American Speech-Language-Hearing Association. (1995). Position statement and guidelines for the training, credentialing, use, and supervision of support personnel in speech-language pathology. *ASHA, 37*(Suppl 14), 21.

Barnhart, M.I., Henry, R.L., & Lusher, J. (1974). *Sickle cell*. Kalamazoo, MI: Upjohn.

Brookshire, R. (1978). Auditory comprehension and aphasia. In D. Johns (Ed.), *Clinical management of neurogenic communicative disorders*. Boston: Little, Brown.

Brust, J.C. (1993). Clinical, radiological and pathological aspects of cerebral vascular disease associated with drug abuse. *Stroke, 24*(12 suppl.), 1129–1133.

Campbell, L. (1986). A study of the comparability of master's level training and certification and needs of speech-language pathologists (Doctoral dissertation, Howard University, Washington, DC, 1985). *Dissertation Abstracts International, 46*, 10B. (University Microfilms No. 85–28, 727)

Campbell, L., Brennan, D., & Steckol, K. (1992). Preservice training to meet the needs of people from diverse cultural backgrounds. *ASHA, 34*, 29–32.

Campbell, L., & Taylor, O. (1992). ASHA-certified speech-language pathologists: Perceived competency levels with selected skills. *Howard Journal of Communications, 3* (Winter-Spring), 163–176.

Committee on the Status of Racial Minorities. (1985). Clinical management of communicatively handicapped minority language populations. *ASHA, 27,* 29–32.

Committee on the Status of Racial Minorities. (1987). *Multicultural professional education in communicative disorders: Curriculum approaches.* Rockville, MD: American Speech-Language-Hearing Association.

Council on Scientific Affairs, American Medical Association. (1991). Hispanic health in the U.S. *Journal of the American Medical Association, 265,* 248–252.

Das, G. (1993). Cardiovascular effects of cocaine abuse. *International Journal of Clinical Pharmacology and Therapeutic Toxicology, 31,* 11, 521–528.

Green, J. (1982). *Cultural awareness in human services.* Englewood Cliffs, New Jersey: Prentice-Hall.

Hall, E.T. (1959). *The silent language.* Garden City, NY: Doubleday.

Holden, C. (1989). Street wise crack research. *Science, 246,* 1376–1381.

Holland, A. (1977). Comment on "spouses understanding of the communication disabilities of aphasic patients." *Journal of Speech and Hearing Disorders, 42,* 307–311.

Holland, A. (1983). Nonbiased assessment and treatment of adults who have neurologic speech and language problems. *Topics in Language Disorders, 3,* 67–75.

Johnson, M., & El-Hazmi, M. (1984). *The world and the sickle cell gene.* New York: Trade-Medic Books.

Kayser, H. (1993). Hispanic cultures. In D. Battle (Ed.), *Communication disorders in multicultural populations* (pp. 144–147). Boston: Butterworth-Heinemann.

Kayser, H. (1995). Interpreters. In H. Kayser (Ed.), *Bilingual speech-language pathology: an Hispanic focus* (pp. 207–221). San Diego: Singular Publishing.

Kenton, E. (1991). Access to neurological care for minorities. *Archives of Neurology 48,* 480–483.

Killam, A.L. (1993). Cardiovascular and thrombosis pathology associated with cocaine use. *Hematology and Oncology Clinics of North America, 7,* 1143–1151.

Kokkinos, J., & Levine, R.R. (1993). Stroke. *Neurology Clinics 11,* 577–590.

Kraut, A. (1990). Healers and strangers: Immigrant attitudes toward the physician in America—a relationship in historical perspective. *Journal of the American Medical Association, 263,* 1807–1811.

Kurtzke, J. (1985). Epidemiology of cerebrovascular disease. In F.H. McDowell & L.R. Caplan (Eds.), *Cerebrovascular disease survey report* (revised). Bethesda, MD: National Institute of Neurological and Communication Disorders and Stroke.

Levine, S., Brust, J., Futrell, N., et al. (1990). Cerebrovascular complications of the use of the "crack" form of alkaloidal cocaine. *New England Journal of Medicine, 323,* 699–703.

Levine, S., Washington, J., Jefferson, M., et al. (1987). "Crack" cocaine-associated stroke. *Neurology, 37,* 1849–1853.

Lingenfelter, S.G., & Mayers, M.K. (1986). Ministering cross-culturally. Grand Rapids, MI: Baker Book House.

Marge, M. (1984). Prevention: A Challenge for the profession. *ASHA, 26,* 35–37.

McCaslin, R., & Calvert, W. (1975). Social indicators in black and white: Some ethnic considerations in delivery of service to the elderly. *Journal of Gerontology 30,* 60–66.

Milroy, L. (1987). *Language and social networks*. Oxford: Basil Blackwell.

Mody, C., Miller, B., McIntyre, H., Cobb, S., & Goldberg, M. (1988). Neurologic complications of cocaine abuse. *Neurology, 38*, 1189–1193.

Moss, S. (1993). Neurogenic communication disorders resulting from stroke. *ASHA, 35*, 61-62.

National Center for Health Statistics. (1994). *Healthy, United States 1993*. Hyattsville, MD: Public Health Service.

Paradis, M. (1987). *The assessment of bilingual aphasia*. Hillsdale, NJ: Lawrence Erlbaum.

Payne-Johnson, J. C. (1983). Treatment of dialectal differences of sociolinguistic origin. In W. Perkins (Ed.), *Language handicaps in adults* (pp. 137–145). New York: Thieme-Stratton.

Pederson, P. (1987). Ten frequent assumptions of cultural bias in counseling. *Journal of Multicultural Counseling and Development, 15*, 16–24.

Platt, U.S., Brambilla, D.J., Rosse, W.F., Milner, D.F., Castro, O., Steinberg, M.H., & Klug, P.P. (1994). Mortality in sickle cell disease: Life expectancy and risk factors for early death. *New England Journal of Medicine, 330*, 1639–1644.

Prohovnik, I., Pavlakis, S.G., Piomelli, S., et al. (1989). Cerebral hyperemia, stroke and transfusion in sickle cell disease. *Neurology, 39*, 344–348.

Rakowski, W., Hickey, T., & Dengiz, A. (1987). Congruence of health and treatment perceptions among older patients and providers of primary care. *International Journal of Aging and Human Development, 25*, 63–77.

Reyes, B. (1994). Management of adult neurogenic patients: A multicultural perspective. *Seminars in Speech and Language, 15*, 165–173.

Reyes, B. (1995). Considerations in the assessment and treatment of neurogenic disorders in bilingual adults. In H. Kayser (Ed.), *Bilingual speech-language pathology: an Hispanic focus* (pp. 153–182). San Diego: Singular Publishing Group.

Saunders, E. (1991). *Cardiovascular diseases in blacks*. Philadelphia: F.A. Davis.

Schlanger, P., & Schlanger, B. (1970). Adapting role-playing activities with aphasic patients. *Journal of Speech and Hearing Disorders, 35*, 229–243.

Schuell, H. (1953). Auditory impairment in aphasia: Significance and retraining techniques. *Journal of Speech and Hearing Disorders, 18*, 14–21.

Shewan, C.M., & Malm, K.E. (1989). The status of multilingual/multicultural service issues among ASHA members. *ASHA, 31*, 78.

Singleton, L., & Johnson, K. (1993). *The black health library guide to stroke*. New York: Henry Holt.

Snope, T. (1982). *Master report of surveys and discrepancies. Professional self-study project*. Rockville, MD: American Speech-Language-Hearing Association.

Snow, L.F. (1984). Folk medical beliefs and their implications for care of patients. *Annals of Internal Medicine 81*, 82–96.

Spector, R. (1985).*Cultural diversity in health and illness* (2nd ed.). Norwalk, CT: Appleton-Century-Crofts.

Taylor, O. (1992). Opening statement. In O. Taylor, H. Kayser, S. Fujikawa, F. Herzon, & G. Wallace (Eds.), *Research and research training needs of minority persons and minority health issues* (pp. 1–11). Bethesda, MD: National Institute on Deafness and Other Communication Disorders, Published Working Group Report.

United States Bureau of the Census. (1990). *Statistical abstract of the United States: 1990* (110th ed.). Washington, DC: U.S. Government Printing Office.

United States Department of Health and Human Services. (1985). *Report of the secretary's task force on black and minority health.* Bethesda, MD: Author.

United States Department of Health and Human Services, Public Health Service. (1990). *Healthy people 2000.* DHHS Publication No. (PHS) 91-50212. Washington, DC: U.S. Government Printing Office.

Wallace, G. (1992). Adult neurogenic disorders. In D. Battle (Ed.), *Multicultural issues and speech-language pathology* (pp. 239–255). Boston: Butterworth-Heinemann.

Wallace, G. (1993a). Neurological impairment among elderly African-American nursing home residents. *Journal of Health Care for the Poor and Underserved, 4,* 40–50.

Wallace, G. (1993b). Stroke and traumatic brain injury (Ma'i Ulu) in America Samoa. *Hawaii Medical Journal, 52,* 234–250.

Wallace, G. (1996, in press). *Multicultural neurogenics: A clinical resource for speech-language pathologists providing services to neurologically-impaired adults from culturally and linguistically diverse backgrounds.* Tucson, AZ: Communication Skill Builders.

Wallace, G., & Bridges-Freeman, S. (1991). Adults with neurological impairments from the multicultural populations. *ASHA, 33,* 58–60.

Wallace, G., & Canter, J. (1985). Effects of personally relevant language materials on the performance of severely aphasic individuals. *Journal of Speech and Hearing Disorders 50,* 385–390.

Wallach, S. (1989). Medical complications of the use of cocaine. *Hawaii Medical Journal, 48,* 461–462.

Yano, K., Reed, D.M., & Kagan, A. (1985). Coronary heart disease, hypertension, and stroke among Chinese-American men in Hawaii: The Honolulu heart program. *Hawaii Medical Journal, 44,* 297–300.

Yatsu, F.M. (1991). Strokes in Asians and Pacific-Islanders, Hispanics and Native Americans. *Circulation, 83,* 1471–1472.

Chapter 7

Can-Do Therapy: A Positive Approach for Maximizing Recovery During Rehabilitation

Martha S. Burns

In the mid- and late 1970s, Norman Cousins (1979) popularized the notion that stress and mental attitude play a significant role in determining the course of illness. In 1989, Cousins expanded this view, suggesting that hope, humor, and the power of the mind might augment medical treatment and maximize recovery. His impetus, along with that of Ader (1981), Locke and colleagues (Locke, 1986; Locke, Ader, Besedovsky, Hall, Solomon, Strom, & Spector, 1985), and many others, was instrumental in launching the new field of psychoneuroimmunology and a body of scientific research based on the relationship between mental attitude, illness, and recovery. Similarly, trend-spotters John Naisbitt and Patricia Aburdene (1990) characterized the 1990s as a new age of self-determination and individualism. The "I can do it" era is upon us.

In aphasia rehabilitation, clinical scientists and practitioners have been perhaps somewhat slower to embrace the power of positive mental attitude and individual determinism. However, one finds in recent clinical literature a discernible trend toward basing aphasia treatment on mutual goals set by the patient and his or her family as well as by the functional outcome needs of the individual and the family nucleus (Andrews & Andrews, 1990; Davis & Wilcox, 1985). In fact, one need only review the emphasis of many of the chapters of the present text to note the changing emphasis on the role of the individual and family in the rehabilitation process.

This chapter is designed to help clinicians harness the power of the individual and family in aphasia recovery. The chapter includes three sections that contain practical clinical suggestions and treatment techniques designed to maximize the recovery of aphasic individuals. Treatment approaches outlined in this chapter have been designed to be consistent with current knowledge about mechanisms of neurological recovery and language processing (Burns & Halper, 1988; Ojemann, 1991). They are discussed in terms of three clinical principles:

1. *Emphasize the positive.* Use personal, communicative, and linguistic strengths in goal-setting and treatment methods.
2. *Focus on functional outcome.* Adapt treatment content to personal interests, background, and goals.
3. *Respond to patient and family feedback.* Change treatment goals and methods through continual reappraisal of patient responsiveness.

Brief case studies of individuals are presented where appropriate to illustrate methodology and their effects on recovery.

EMPHASIZE THE POSITIVE

In their seminal book on brain-recovery mechanisms, Stanley Finger and Donald G. Stein (1982) state that "there are many situations and instances in which [professionals] have been entirely too pessimistic about the possibility of restitution, and it is not difficult to argue that these attitudes and beliefs can affect how patients actually perform in the period after brain injury." They conclude that individually designed treatment programs are probably most effective when "they focus on providing a supportive environment that emphasizes the *skills that the patient can employ at the time of therapy*" (p. 332, emphasis added).

Although few aphasia clinicians would argue with this basic viewpoint, it is all too easy to fall into the trap of emphasizing deficits and limitations to prepare the patient and family for the ultimate realities of a disability. Further, none of us wishes to deceive the aphasic individual or provide false hopes of an unobtainable future. However, Cousins (1979, 1989) and others (Ader, 1981; Locke, 1986; Locke et al., 1985; Finger & Stein, 1982) persuasively argue that emphasis on the bad news of an illness can actually accelerate a negative outcome. Conversely, Cousins (1989) argues that emphasizing "specific evidence that recovery is possible acts like a tonic and actually enhances the prospects for effective medical treatment" (p. 87).

The rationale underlying aphasia treatment oriented toward an individual's strengths and a positive recovery outlook is not designed to foster denial but to inspire the person to muster all available personal resources to fight the hard battle of aphasia rehabilitation that lies ahead. It is from this perspective that the following therapeutic suggestions have been developed.

Make a Modular Map of Linguistic and Communication Strengths and Weaknesses

There is recent evidence that language processing in the brain involves several separate and localizable systems (modules) that process language in parallel rather than in sequence (Damasio, 1990; Ojemann, 1983; Ojemann, 1991; Raichle, 1990). This new model of language processing expands on the sequential model of language processing first hypothesized by Carl Wernicke over a century ago and reinterpreted in recent years by Norman Geshwind (1965). Connectionistic theory, and the behavioral classifications of aphasia type derived from it (i.e., Broca's, conduction, and Wernicke's aphasia), are based on this sequential cerebral processing model.

The recent data accumulated from positron emission tomography (PET) scanning (Damasio, 1990; Raichle, 1990), isotopic techniques, interoperative electrical stimulation (Ojemann, 1983; Ojemann, 1991), as well as microelectrode recordings during surgery (Ojemann, 1983; Ojemann, 1991), and lesion studies suggest that the classic connectionistic model needs to be revised. First, there is tremendous variability in brain organization for language from one individual to another. Second, there are many cognitive modules, independent from language but augmentative or supportive of language systems, which may include logical/mathematical, musical, intra- and interpersonal, spatial, and bodily intelligences (Gazzaniga, 1985; Geshwind, 1965). These modules may be used therapeutically to circumvent damaged language systems, as in the use of gestures and mimes to communicate, or they may be used to augment damaged systems, such as by applying musical rhythms and melodies to decrease apraxic struggle and improve prosodic inflection. Finally, modular theory posits that auditory comprehension need not necessarily precede oral expression in language processing. Rather, the two occur simultaneously and can be treated therapeutically through any language-performance tasks. Thus, to be effective, aphasia therapy does not necessarily have to follow an "auditory comprehension first, oral expression second" process. For some patients, treatment goals that stress multiple language modalities through functional tasks may be just as effective as more traditional modality-specific tasks.

Based on the above discussion, it would appear that an effective method of targeting language and communication goals for any patient would be to use as much information as possible from the patient's individual cognitive (linguistic and nonlinguistic) profile. So, after completing an initial diagnostic assessment, the clinician could compile a list of communication or language skills that testing reveals have been impaired, as well as those that testing, informal probes, and family input indicate the individual has maintained. By plotting the patient's relative strengths and weaknesses on a graph, linguistic behaviors may be selected for therapeutic intervention. The patient's cognitive strengths can be used as assets to design treatment tasks and strategies for facilitative cues.

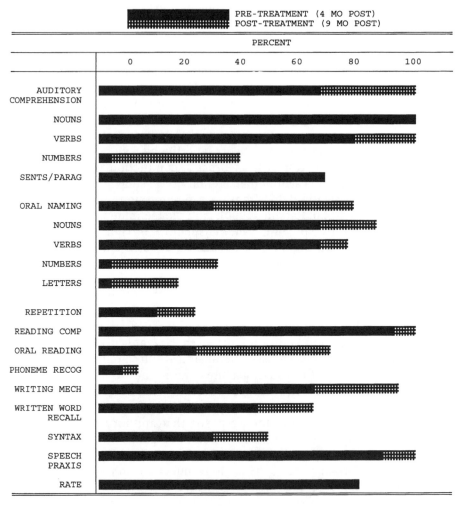

Figure 7.1 *Modular aphasia profile of M.D., an acute aphasic. Treatment was targeted to the 20–50% performance range.*

Target a Midrange Ability Level for Treatment Goals

Once the modular map has been developed for a patient, the clinician can share the information with the patient and the family and use the map to target treatment goals and select treatment stimuli.

Figure 7.1 illustrates such a map for one patient, M.D. One can see that by targeting linguistic behaviors of oral naming (especially verbs), reading comprehension, oral reading, written-word recall, and syntax—all behaviors that fell into a midlevel range after pretreatment testing—the patient showed substantial improvement in these and other nontargeted modules after 5 months of therapy.

Use the Patient's Strengths to Select Materials and Facilitative Cues

For each individual, retained strengths can be used as facilitators, augmentative techniques, or adaptive communicative mechanisms. With M.D., one strength, mathematics, was preserved after the stroke. This strength was used to foster syntactical understanding and usage as mathematical-like formulas to aid comprehension and expression of specific grammatical constructions. After 5 months of treatment, M.D.'s written-word recall became a relative strength, which he used to augment oral expression through written self-cuing. Another patient, M.C., who was a ballerina before her stroke, retained outstanding bodily intelligence. She found the use of gestures and mime to be a valuable communicative strength to augment oral expression, which, for several months poststroke, was limited to the single-word level and only 50% intelligibility.

Use Communication Skills If Linguistic Skills Are Severely Limited

For a person with severe aphasia, the modular map may include only such abilities as responsiveness to his or her name, the pragmatic ability to glean information from gestures and prosody, the ability to use content and shared information to comprehend simple conversations of familiar persons in highly familiar situations, or the ability to recognize questions and the willingness to try to respond.

Although speech-language pathologists have been trained to carefully distinguish actual linguistic competence from a person's use of prosody and gesture to augment comprehension, therapeutic intervention that stresses these intact communication abilities and pragmatic skills has been advocated by many professionals in recent years (Davis & Wilcox, 1985; Collins, 1986, 1990).

Use the Patient's Strengths to Aim for Communicative Success

By setting communication goals and using procedures that incorporate intact abilities, the aphasic person can begin the treatment process by succeeding. For example, if gesture and exaggerated facial or prosodic cues assist comprehension of yes/no questions, treatment can initially use these cues and draw attention to the ways these cues are used. Gradually, the clinician can fade the use of these cues as the person learns how to focus on linguistic content by using natural prosody as an aid.

Many published treatment programs for very severe patients by Nancy Helm-Estabrooks and colleagues (Helm & Barresi, 1980; Helm & Benson, 1978; Helm-Estabrooks & Morgan, 1987), such as visual action therapy (VAT), voluntary control of involuntary utterances (VCIU), and the use of drawing, use intact nonverbal and limited verbal skills to untap or augment residual receptive and expressive linguistic abilities.

Emphasize the Patient's Strengths to Empower the Family and Patient

Andrews and Andrews (1990) discuss how emphasizing abilities can be used to set mutually defined treatment goals when sharing information about the aphasia evaluation with the aphasic patient and his or her family. As both the patient and family are informed about intact communication skills, they can be encouraged to use them in communicating with the individual. Family members can also be advised that "speech therapy" occurs each time the aphasic individual communicates effectively with others, and to the extent family members learn how to achieve that communication, they are helping the person through an important phase of language rehabilitation. Often the clinician can in turn learn new pragmatic cuing devices from the family as they discover for themselves what seems to foster communication with the aphasic person.

In some cases, emphasizing retained linguistic skills helps the patient and family better understand aphasia itself. They can see that language skills have not been irrevocably lost, and that effective treatment involves improving the person's ability to gain access to preserved linguistic knowledge. This in turn helps family members resist the temptation to reteach words or talk for the person. It constructively redirects a loved one's natural desire to help by guiding him or her toward creative experimentation with facilitatory techniques that assist the communicative interchange. It also helps the patient to begin to become his or her own therapist by trying new techniques himself or herself.

Burns, Dong, and Oehring (1995) have case study data from a cost-benefit study comparing conventional aphasia therapy with family-based therapy. They found that for individuals with chronic aphasia, family-based treatment shows promise as a cost-effective adjunct or alternative to traditional treatment. Judgments of effectiveness in this study were based in part on family members' perceptions of improved communication during the family interactions.

Give the Patient and Family Positive Prognostic Statements

The vast majority of people with aphasia recover some language ability. Families and patients need to know this. Unlike many diseases and degenerative neurological processes, the good news is that aphasia improves with time. The first thing a clinician can tell patients who are medically and neurologically stable is, "You will most likely get better. No one can say for certain how much better you will get, but most people who have strokes continue to improve for many months."

Many aphasia clinicians and doctors feel compelled to stress the negative outcome with patients and their families by using statements such as, "You may never be able to work again," or "You should prepare for the possibility that your life will be significantly changed." Whose life has not been significantly changed by naturally occurring events such as divorce, a death in the family, an economic recession, a war? Why do clinicians feel obligated to prepare the person with aphasia for the worst possible outcome? Is the aim to protect the patient and family from false hope, or to protect the clinician in the event that treatment is not successful?

There is no reason to put prognostic statements and outcome projections in negative terms. Even when the patient or family member asks such pointed questions as, "Will I ever work again?" or "Will he ever be able to talk?", there are positive yet accurate ways to respond. For example, an excellent reply to the first question emphasizes the range of options open to persons with aphasia. "I have worked with some individuals with aphasia who have been able to work again. Some with mild aphasia have returned to their original position without much difficulty. Others decided to change to a new job or position with fewer language demands. Some persons with aphasia have been able to modify their old job with the help of their superiors or others they work with, so that they could perform satisfactorily. And some have decided to retire or work as volunteers. As you get closer to the termination of treatment, we can discuss options and perhaps consult with a vocational counselor."

Many family members of patients with little or no verbal output ask whether their loved one will ever be able to speak again. The clinician often interprets this question as, "Will the person speak normally?" The answer is often guarded, such as, "Aphasia almost always reduces a person's ability to talk effectively," or "He may speak a little, but the chances are not very good that he will talk the way he did before."

Many times, the family member simply wants to be reassured that the clinician will try to work on speech and has not given up on their family member. An equally correct but positive reply that is sensitive to this need might be, "Right now, as you can see, speech is very difficult and not useful. But even though he cannot use words to express himself, he can (gesture, indicate yes and no, understand what you say, use his facial expression and pointing to communicate, etc.). My goal for the next few weeks is to build on these abilities and help the two of you use these to communicate with each other. In time, some useful speech may recover. I will certainly do everything I can to stimulate this." By emphasizing what the person can do as well as providing realistic short-term goals, the clinician can guide the family member toward realistic short-term expectations and reassure them that the aim is to reach the highest attainable goals.

Use Other Aphasics with Similar Symptoms As Examples

Stroke clubs and aphasia groups provide an excellent opportunity for persons with aphasia to share success stories. Although few actors with aphasia successfully return to the stage, many patients with aphasia find gratification from new hobbies or modified work settings. One former actress found gratification in helping with an acting workshop for children. Another woman who had been a librarian before her stroke found her skills were useful in a local nursing home library. One university professor with an apraxia of speech but no dyslexia or agraphia was able to teach a limited schedule of basic courses by writing out his lectures ahead of time. His greatest satisfaction came from his ability to edit and critique manuscripts his colleagues planned to submit for publication. A clinical psychiatrist with mild Broca's aphasia found his reduced rate of speech actually improved his ability to listen to his clients, and he has developed a subspecialty of working with language-impaired clients and their families.

FOCUS ON FUNCTIONAL OUTCOME

In 1956, Martha Sarno (cited in Sarno, 1969) published the *Functional Communication Profile,* a behavioral scale listing 45 communicative behaviors that was designed to be completed largely through conversation. Since then, many aphasiologists have stressed the importance of using functional assessment and treatment strategies to maximize the patient's performance in real-life situations.

Yet despite this emphasis on functional assessment and treatment, the vast majority of speech-language clinicians still rely heavily on standard published workbooks and programmed materials. This in part may be due to large caseloads and heavy demands on time, which preclude developing personalized treatment stimuli for clients. However, highly individualized approaches need not take excessive preparation time if family members are included in the treatment team and are encouraged to select and adapt materials that respect the patient's vocational or avocational interests. Even when preparation time is needed to develop appropriate materials, the time spent is usually well worth the energy and enthusiasm that such an approach fosters. When developing functional outcome goals and treatment stimuli to reach these goals, three issues need to be considered:

1. Active intervention in the environment
2. Gainful employment or avocational interests
3. Social contact/interactive stimulation

Active Intervention in the Environment

Before initiating the treatment program, a clinician should identify the interactive routines and needs of the family. These might include family dinners, intimate social gatherings with friends or grown children, religious celebrations or weekly attendance at church or synagogue, and eating out. These events can then be staged and practiced through one of three treatment vehicles: group sessions and trips, actual in-home treatments with family members present, and role playing.

Each interactive session should be planned in advance and the client informed of expectations. Planning involves determining who the participants will be, where the interaction might take place, and the goals. The client and family can determine these parameters before practice, or they can be systematically varied during the session. In earlier writings (Burns & Halper, 1988; Halper & Burns, 1989), Burns and colleagues provide sample conversational routines to practice, including planning with colleagues a farewell party for retiring employees, planning a picnic with friends, discussing a family reunion with other family members, and conversing with other passengers on a plane trip.

For many clients with aphasia, real events in family life make the best material for practice. For example, a client expressed frustration with trying to follow a conversation with passengers in a car, so he, his wife, and the clinician practiced typical conversations sitting with their backs to each other. Another client became concerned when he attended a gala banquet and had difficulty following the conversation at a large table. To prepare for the next similar event, his wife and two of her friends joined him to practice conversing across their dining room table. As he experienced difficulties, he and his wife tried to determine which aspects of the situation posed the greatest problems. They then worked together to find a solution. The client learned from the experience that he was very dependent on lip reading and eye contact to aid comprehension. Consequently, he learned to make a conscious effort to directly attend to each new speaker. After practicing this a few times at home, he attended the next event and that found his comprehension had improved markedly.

Employment or Avocational Background

One of the best sources of clinical material comes from the patient's own vocational or avocational background. Not only are materials related to previous job or interests more motivating because of their familiarity, often they present a means for easily tapping into the individual's premorbid strengths and interests. As long as the clinician is careful to adapt the activities to the person's competence level, these types of activities provide incentive and optimism that at least some level of prestroke functioning can be reattained. By experimenting with these types of adapted materials, clients can also see how goals can be achieved through the use of creative adaptations. Finally, vocational materials provide a clinical opportunity for the aphasiologist to help the person with aphasia deal with some of the realities of his or her language impairment in a positive, constructive way. Case studies are used to illustrate how such stimuli can be developed.

W.A. was a 62-year-old female former secretary with a severe Broca's aphasia. She had been an avid bridge player before her stroke but all therapeutic attempts to rekindle this skill had been unsuccessful because her symbolic memory was too poor to remember previous hands played during a game. She was very upset that she could not again play bridge, but since card playing was such an important avocational interest, her husband decided to try similar games. Soon, with a few adaptations, she was able to play "hearts" and canasta and in time the two of them resumed card parties with friends.

A.D. was a 56-year-old former political science professor with an anomic aphasia. He was less interested in returning to lecturing than in resuming his career as a writer of college textbooks. His written expression, although within normal limits for adults, was now enough of a struggle that a textbook seemed beyond the range of possibility. After trying several page-length essays on political science topics of interest, he found the technical language and abstract concepts too difficult to express clearly through writing. He decided to give up his goal to again write books until the clinician suggested he try a less demanding topic. After experimenting with several lighter subjects, which he felt were either too mundane or of limited interest to him, he came upon the idea of writing about his aphasia rehabilitation experience. He spent the next 3 months working on this project; from that experience, he went on to revise and republish a previous text.

W.M. was a 35-year-old owner and manager of a commercial muffler franchise. Several months after his stroke, the corporation discontinued the franchise. His expressive language skills were reduced to such an extent that attempting to procure a new franchise to manage seemed out of the question. Shortly after this incident, his wife filed for divorce. The client was despondent and ready to quit therapy. In an effort to find some treatment avenue for him, the speech-language therapist showed him the technical manual for her car. After looking through it, he realized that he could comprehend many of the diagrams and felt his mechanical skills were still excellent. His treatment goal then became improving reading comprehension for technical manuals so that he could return to mechanical work. Initially, the therapist simplified the technical descriptions and limited written material to one or two sentences. Soon, the clinician realized that she was inadvertently making technical mistakes through her edits, and he began to correct her adaptations. After several months of work, they gradually increased the complexity of the material, moving on to current automo-

bile manuals. He began working on his own car and eventually found employment in a friend's automobile repair garage.

M.D. is a 42-year-old tax lawyer and executive vice president of a large telecommunications corporation who has a moderate subcortical aphasia. By only 4 months post-onset, he had made significant gains in auditory comprehension as an inpatient at a local rehabilitation hospital. However, he was very depressed by the severity of his language impairment. Of particular concern were his reduced reading comprehension and poor calculation skills. Since he had been a math major in college, the therapist began experimenting with various levels of mathematics. At first, he was frustrated by anything more complex than two-digit addition. However, within 1 month, by working with his wife (a former teacher) to break down complex problems into smaller subproblems, he was able to master two-by-three-digit multiplication, two-by-four-digit division, percentile conversions, addition and multiplication of fractions, and multiplication of decimals.

To work on reading comprehension, therapist and client experimented with various adaptations of business articles from the newspaper. First, they discovered that he could comprehend virtually any article when he read it aloud chorally with another person. The therapist then made a tape recording of herself reading aloud and asked the patient to listen to the tape as he silently read the same material. The patient practiced this activity for 1 week. Although it proved helpful, he still struggled to comprehend the grammatical phrasing on the tape and became frustrated that the tape did not allow him enough time to ponder difficult sentence constructions. He then spent 2 weeks reading articles that the therapist had rewritten into simple sentences. At first these were prerecorded, but he soon discovered that he could comprehend these adapted articles without the taped assistance. The next step was to pair the adapted summaries with the real news articles, first reading the summary, then going to the original. After 4 weeks, M.D. found he could comprehend the actual articles if important content words and key phrases were first highlighted with a marker. This freed him from being frustrated by complex grammatical constructions that carry little meaning but are very difficult to decode.

Social Contact and Interactive Stimulation

A final important aspect of treatment geared toward functional outcome is to permit actual clinical manipulation and practice of pragmatic devices and nonverbal aids to augment communication. Although these communication goals can be addressed through group sessions and role-playing discussed above, they can also be practiced directly as part of a standard treatment session. Methodologies such as Promoting Aphasics' Communicative Effectiveness (PACE) (Davis & Wilcox, 1985) provide carefully designed procedures for developing these interactive skills in a structured way. (See especially Chapter 9 by Audrey L. Holland.)

RESPOND TO PATIENT AND FAMILY FEEDBACK

The person with aphasia is most often the best judge of whether techniques, procedures, and goals are appropriate and effective. It is wise to solicit opinions of the treatment often from both client and family. When the client seems frustrated or progress is minimal, the speech-language specialist should change treatment goals and methods and continually reappraise the patient's responsiveness. Patient and family feedback are a powerful source of information and fresh ideas. Two principles that are useful in this regard are:

1.   Change goals when clinician, client, or a family member discovers new areas of interest or need.
2.   Continually experiment with new methods for reaching long-term goals more quickly.

Change Goals When Clinician, Client, or Family Member Discovers New Areas of Interest or Need

Perhaps the best aphasia treatment uses the client and his or her family as a primary force in the treatment process. Often clients have the best insight into their processing systems; family members are also an excellent source of information about prestroke cognitive patterns and strategies. Two case studies illustrate this point.

J.R. was a 72-year-old homemaker who had raised seven children and three grandchildren. She was first seen several days after a severe left-sided stroke and treated initially for a dysphagia from which she recovered quite quickly. She also presented with a global aphasia. Approximately 2 weeks after the severe stroke, treatment for global aphasia began. The woman was unresponsive on all language tasks, although family members repeatedly stated that she spoke to them and seemed to comprehend some of their conversations. Several clinicians tried to work with her during the next few weeks, but she failed to point to pictures, follow commands, answer yes/no questions, or attempt verbalizations. Characteristically, she would look away from the clinician or close her eyes.

The staff had decided to discharge her temporarily, pending a change in her responsiveness, when one of her granddaughters happened to visit during a treatment session. She told the clinician that her grandmother was slow to warm up to strangers; she often did not speak to new people until she had carefully sized them up. She also distrusted professional women, because she believed strongly that well-intentioned women should stay home to raise a family. The granddaughter also related that her grandmother's first child had died as an infant in a small southern hospital with a female doctor attending.

After conferring, the staff and family decided that the change of clinicians that had been made earlier had actually been counterproductive. A family member suggested that the first clinician, a young graduate student of the same cultural background as the aphasic woman, return for aphasia assessment. The staff realized that she was the only speech-language pathologist who had not worn a lab coat during treatment sessions. After one or two nonconfrontational meetings, the student was able to elicit enough responses to develop a solid treatment program. The patient returned to her hometown shortly thereafter and worked successfully with a young male speech-language pathologist for several more months.

A.D. was a 62-year-old teacher who, when first seen 5 months after a left-side stroke, exhibited a severe nonfluent aphasia with moderate comprehension impairment and a recurrent utterance of "no soap." He had shown little progress in oral or written expressive language during his previous inpatient rehabilitation program. Attempts to teach an augmentative gestural system had failed and he was unable to break his use of the involuntary utterance.

When treatment began on an outpatient basis, his wife was present for all sessions. She noted that he had been a math teacher for 40 years and believed that he thought mathematically. She noted also that he could count aloud. She wondered whether he might learn language through some type of mathematical model. The clinician had noticed that he used gestures, prosody, and facial expression to communicate reasonably well, despite the use of his recurrent utterance. PACE (Davis & Wilcox, 1985) was a new procedure at the time, but the clinician and wife decided to try it by using number concepts to describe complex action pictures. The gentleman quickly learned the technique and after a few sessions described a picture as follows: "1-2-3-4 (points to himself to indicate men or people) . . . bbrbrbr (automobile sound) . . . outside (gestures out the window)." This represented the first time that he was able to inhibit his recurrent utterance and utter a real word spontaneously. He eventually used mathematical formulas to work on comprehension and expression of some grammatical concepts such as verb tense and pronouns, and continued to use counting in a very creative conversational way to denote days of the week, time concepts, and to take telephone messages for his wife.

Continually Experiment with New Methods for Reaching Long-Term Goals Quicker

Even when existing goals and procedures seem to be working well for the individual with aphasia, it is always interesting and often fruitful to experiment with new techniques and approaches to meet goals. Often, procedures and stimuli become quite boring for clients, especially when they are working on one area for a long time. An individual who has been working on paragraph comprehension for several weeks might enjoy changing to anecdotes from *Reader's Digest*, humorous newspaper columns or short gossip columns about people of interest to him or her.

Sometimes patients can grasp a concept but finding a new representation will speed their ability to use or apply it. An agrammatical client, for example, who is struggling to understand and use Wh-pronouns might find an algebraic equation in which x stands for the unknown person or place a useful key to rewriting sentences or finding the appropriate referent.

Finally, experimentation with new methods might lead to a representation that readily facilitates processing for that particular person. A businessman with severe anomia, for example, after experimenting with numerous self-facilitatory naming techniques, found that an organizational chart and floor plan solved his problem of recalling names of colleagues at work.

SUMMARY

Language rehabilitation in aphasia can be one of the most dynamic and successful processes in all of clinical practice because of the wealth of material and ideas generated by the individual and available within the family. When the clinician focuses on harnessing the power of the individual and works to generate a positive energetic treatment environment, miracles can, and do, happen.

REFERENCES

Ader, R. (Ed.). (1981). *Psychoneuroimmunology.* New York: Academic Press.

Andrews, J., & Andrews, M. (1990). *Family based treatment in communicative disorders: A systemic approach.* Sandwich, IL: Janelle Publications.

Burns, M., & Halper, A. (1988). *A comprehensive approach to treatment of the aphasias.* Rockville, MD: Aspen.

Burns, M., Dong, K.Y., & Oehring, A. (1995). Family involvement in the treatment of aphasia. *Topics in Stroke Rehabilitation, 2,* 68.

Collins, M. (1986). *Diagnosis and treatment of global aphasia.* San Diego: College-Hill Press.

Collins, M. (1990). Global aphasia. In L.L. LaPointe (Ed.), *Aphasia and related neurogenic language disorders (pp. 113-129).* New York: Thieme Medical Publishers.

Cousins, N. (1979). *Anatomy of an illness.* New York: W.W. Norton.

Cousins, N. (1989). *Head first: The biology of hope.* New York: E.P. Dutton.

Damasio, A. (1990). Synchronous activation in multiple cortical regions: A mechanism for recall. *Seminars in Neuroscience, 2,* 287–296.

Davis, G.A., & Wilcox, M.J. (1985). *Adult aphasia rehabilitation: Applied pragmatics.* San Diego: College-Hill Press.

Finger, S., & Stein, D.G. (1982). *Brain damage and recovery: Research and clinical perspectives.* New York: Academic Press.

Gazzaniga, M.S. (1985). *The social brain: Discovering the networks of the mind.* New York: Basic Books.

Geshwind, N. (1965). Disconnection syndromes in animals and man. *Brain, 88,* 237–294.

Halper, A., & Burns, M. (1989). *Speech/language treatment of the aphasias: Treatment materials for oral expression and written expression.* Rockville, MD: Aspen.

Helm, N., & Barresi, B. (1980). Voluntary control of involuntary utterances: A treatment approach for severe aphasia. In R. Brookshire (Ed.), *Proceedings of the conference on clinical aphasiology.* Minneapolis: BRK Publishers.

Helm, N., & Benson, F. (1978). *Visual action therapy for global aphasia.* Paper presented at the Academy of Aphasia, Chicago, IL.

Helm-Estabrooks, N., & Morgan, A. (1987). Back to the drawing board: A treatment program for non-verbal aphasia patients. In R. Brookshire (Ed.), *Proceedings of the conference on clinical aphasiology.* Minneapolis: BRK Publishers.

Locke, S. (Ed.). (1986). *Psychological and behavioral treatments for disorders associated with the immune system: An annotated bibliography.* New York: Institute for the Advancement of Health.

Locke, S.E., Ader, R., Besedovsky, H., Hall, N., Solomon, G., Strom, T., & Spector, N.A. (Eds.). (1985). *Foundations of psychoneuroimmunology.* New York: Aldine.

Naisbitt, J., & Aburdene, P. (1990). *Megatrends 2000.* New York: William Morrow.

Ojemann, G.A. (1983). Brain organization for language from the perspective of electrical stimulation mapping. *Behavioral and Brain Sciences, 6,* 189–230.

Ojemann, G.A. (1991). Cortical organization of language. *Journal of Neuroscience, 11*(8), 2281–2287.

Raichle, M. (1990). Exploring the mind with dynamic imaging. *Seminars in Neuroscience, 2,* 307–315.

Sarno, M.T. (1969). The functional communication profile. *Rehabilitation Monograph 42,* New York University Medical Center.

Chapter 8

Optimizing Communication and Participation in Life for Aphasic Adults and Their Prime Caregivers in Natural Settings: A Use Model for Treatment

Jon G. Lyon

Treatment of aphasia is aimed at returning patients to residential settings with optimal use of linguistic and communicative functions. In doing so, it is hoped that the consequences of becoming aphasic might be lessened and that lives may become more normalized. With a return to established routines, the fundamental structure for ensuring quality of life might also be enhanced. Yet today, most rehabilitative effort and time are directed toward repair or circumvention of disordered linguistic and communicative dysfunctions within clinical domains. Behaviorally based stimulation drills constitute the core of aphasia treatment in hospital and rehabilitative centers.

The rationale for stimulation-based treatment of aphasia is well-documented (Darley, 1982; Rosenbek, LaPointe, & Wertz, 1989; Schuell, Jenkins, & Jimenez-Pabon, 1964). However, the scientific worth of basic assumptions comprising current treatment practices remain largely unproven. One premise is that underlying disordered processes should be differentiated and systematically ordered and managed from the easiest to most difficult to repair. A second premise is that a sterile, clinical environment is preferable for isolating, controlling, and simplifying processes to be treated. Third, and most important, there is an unspoken assumption that treatment gains first established in clinical settings will transfer to natural settings. Yet to date, data and clinical experience regarding this last premise are sparse and inconclusive (Thompson, 1989). Indeed, it would appear that clinical gains with aphasic adults are not assured of transference or use in natural settings without further intervention (Kearns, 1989). However, the form of this additional remediation is equally controversial and unclear. One means toward achieving a resolution may be to isolate the causes of past shortcomings and to propose adjustments accordingly.

Recently, I identified three general sources of influence that may explain reduced communication as aphasic adults return to residential or community settings (Lyon, 1992). I divided these sources of influence into physiologic, linguistic-communicative, and psychosocial well-being causes. Physiologic causes address the reason for aphasia, linguistic-communicative causes speak to the aphasia itself, and psychosocial causes refer to the consequences of aphasia.

A physiologic cause refers to the influence of disrupted brain function on transference of treatment effects from clinical to natural settings. Processes needed for effective use, such as access and use of cognitive functions, may be impaired. This impairment results in either an insufficient or inefficient use of residual cognitive processing mechanisms (McNeil, 1991). Minimal transference of treatment effects from clinical to natural settings in other types of acquired adult neurogenic disorders of speech and language (e.g., certain dysarthrias and right-hemisphere damage) may suggest that this problem has a commonly shared physiologic basis.

As for linguistic-communicative causes, two types were identified (Lyon, 1992): (1) insufficient knowledge of underlying processes contributing to disordered language or communication (Byng, Kay, Edmundson, & Scotts, 1990; Caramazza, 1989; Lesser, 1987); or (2) failure to manage key communicative components from clinical to natural settings (Davis & Wilcox, 1985; Kearns, 1989; Kimbarow, 1989). To date, most of the clinical research in aphasia aims to ameliorate linguistic-communicative causes. Although such data may prove valuable in establishing a viable plan for communicative use in natural settings, I argued that management of a third possible cause, psychosocial well-being, may prove more influential.

The study of dysfunctional psychosocial well-being in aphasic adults is not new (Buck, 1968; Eisenson, 1984; Goldstein, 1942; Sarno & Hook, 1980). Yet the precise nature and influence of well-being on communication remains largely unspecified and unmanaged (Darley, 1991). The issue is not that psychosocial well-being is totally ignored or untreated (Herrmann & Wallesch, 1989, 1990; Muller & Code, 1983; Roblin, 1984; Wohrborg, 1989). Rather, it is the absence of an integrated treatment plan that simultaneously addresses dysfunctions of language, communication, and psychosocial well-being. I urged the adoption of a treatment plan that acknowledges and addresses the ongoing interrelationships and interdependencies among language, communication, and psychosocial well-being (Lyon, 1992). Also, I emphasized the need for a treatment model that ultimately permits and ensures remediation of disordered components within natural settings.

To achieve these ends, I proposed other conceptual adjustments to assessment and treatment in aphasia (Lyon, 1992). Disrupted processes from language and communication, the social use of communication, and psychosocial well-being must be sampled. The gestalt of perceived severity and motivation to enact change to disrupted processes, by clinician as well as patients and caregivers, determines the form and direction therapy should take. The fundamental aim of aphasia treatment is to restore "use" to disrupted processes, not separately, but in accordance with how they occur and interrelate in real life. A requisite is realizing that targeted goals in re-establishing use usually mean some form of functional sacrifice compared to normal usage. With this in mind, however, realistic goals can be established.

When balancing goals and the motivation to attain them, the cost most often extracted is increased time, effort, and persistence for the participants involved. Eventually, perceived return from treatment matches or exceeds the time and effort participants are willing to expend to realize further gains. When that occurs, treatment has reached a natural point of conclusion. Within my proposed framework, treatment is more an act of orchestration than of conscription. The prime objective is to restore use while still permitting a comfortable and sustainable means to daily life.

An in-depth review of a use model for aphasia treatment follows. After a descriptive accounting of this model's main components, an illustrative case study follows.

A USE MODEL FOR APHASIA TREATMENT

Rehabilitation of aphasia takes on a new form when viewed as a disruption to processes of language and communication, the social use of communication, and psychosocial well-being. Instead of attempting to simply fix or circumvent disordered parts of language (phrases, words, morphemes, and phonemes) or communication (verbal, written, pantomimed, or drawn) in aphasic adults, as is traditionally espoused, a use model for aphasia treatment strives to re-establish the viability and integrity of processes critical to communication and psychosocial well-being in natural settings.

DIFFERENCES AND SIMILARITIES WITH TRADITIONAL PRACTICES

The meaning of *use* in a use model needs to be differentiated from pragmatic applications of this term that abound in the literature (Davis & Wilcox, 1985; Holland, 1987; Kimbarow, 1989). Here *use* is *not* tied to how, when, or why particular linguistic or communicative forms should be employed in communicative exchanges. Instead, *use* refers to rejuvenating, actually "using," disrupted processes that permit an adult with aphasia to return to active participation communicatively and in chosen activities of daily life.

Emphasizing the restoration of use is not to assert that optimal linguistic or communicative functions, including pragmatic considerations, run counter to treatment objectives in a use model. In fact, at specific times in treatment, restoration of linguistic and communicative processes takes precedence over strategies to increase participation in communication or activities of daily living within natural settings. This is especially true during acute stages of aphasia. Initially, treatment in a use model is aimed at improving form and content as well as use of linguistic and communicative processes. However, even when therapy has this traditional flavor, a broader scope to treatment prevails. The immediate goal may be to restore optimal communicative use, but that function is embedded in the constant aim of restoring optimal control, direction, independence, and personal responsibility to the lives of patients and their families.

There is another important distinction between traditional practices and a use model for aphasia treatment. Once residual linguistic and communicative abilities are better defined, preciseness of form, content, or use in language or communication are intentionally de-emphasized. Typically, somewhere between 9 and 12 months post-onset, if not sooner, adults with aphasia and their prime caregivers begin to adjust to the altered linguistic and communicative systems. Also, these adults begin to recognize what their compromised mechanisms for communication will or will not tolerate within natural exchanges. Users may even begin to anticipate what the future may hold for them communicatively. It is within this window of recovery that establishing a more stable and comfortable mode of content exchange is critical. If aphasic adults are amenable to such changes, it is important to establish a communicative environment that rewards use, rather than form or content. Therapeutic success is contingent on the exchange of meaningful content, irrespective of its form, completeness, or efficiency. In this regard, it is the interaction that becomes the central focus of treatment. Active participation in the "doing" rather than "how it is done" becomes foremost.

THE VALUE OF COMMUNICATIVE USE

Participation in establishing and carrying out communicative exchanges fulfills three requisites to psychosocial well-being: (1) documentation that such activities are still possible, (2) increased comfort with an altered mode of exchange, and (3) proof that such activities are potentially valuable when properly supported. With repeated use, conversations often evolve to a point where execution becomes secondary to the anticipated reward. When this occurs, the participant, whether aphasic adult or prime caregiver, may tend to escape the constraints imposed by the aphasia. Instead of thinking that he or she "won't be able to" perform a task, the participant begins to savor the act of conversing or participating in life for its expected return or benefit alone. The dynamics of "forgetting" about being aphasic are also noted by Kagan and Gailey (1993). When "being aphasic" becomes secondary, the handicap from the disorder is significantly lessened. With less attention on being "unable" or "incomplete," or on being responsible for one who is aphasic, there is greater freedom to resume participation in activities of choice. Equally important, this renewed involvement is controlled not by the constraints of aphasia but instead by the functional worth of participating in communication and life despite the aphasia and its inherent drawbacks. Thus, rather than attempting to just restore form or efficiency to communication, as is traditionally espoused, the target of a use model is to rejuvenate and promote existing communication, its effective use, and with that, psychosocial well-being.

THE NATURE OF DISRUPTED PROCESSES IN A USE MODEL

The processes that support the use of communication and the presence of psychosocial well-being in adults with aphasia are well known to speech-language pathologists. Less is known, however, about their precise infrastructures and interrelationships between them. Nevertheless, a use model of treatment assumes a basic premise: that aphasia does *not* markedly alter the fundamental integrity of disrupted processes. That is, these processes are not lost, only altered. Use remains, but the form and content are different. Communicative functions normally derived effortlessly now require increased time and effort, and often constrained subject matter. Aphasic patients, and even more frequently, normal interactants commonly misinterpret this restricted use as a loss or an inability to participate. More important, misperceivers may never realize that alternative forms of communicative use are accessible and viable. Accordingly, demonstrated use of disrupted processes is an early treatment objective of a use model.

Resumption of use, though, is not dependent solely on demonstration of its viability, especially in moderate to severe aphasia. Optimal and ongoing functionality of disrupted processes requires more. Attention to variables that support participation in life, especially when substantial changes to well-being and lifestyles occur, is equally important. These include: what is perceived as possible, what is desirable, what is acceptable and tolerable (in terms of using altered processes), and what is sustainable (in terms of motivation and drive to alter these processes). Thus, clinicians may find that the precise formula for ensuring optimal use of disrupted processes is not readily at hand. Yet we know enough about the basic nature of these processes to structure an alternative and what is hoped to be a beneficial course.

THE ROLE OF THE SPEECH-LANGUAGE PATHOLOGIST

Before turning to the structure of therapy, the specific role of the speech-language pathologist needs clarification. To some degree, general procedural steps in a use model parallel those of traditional stimulation models for speech, language, and communication: careful observation and assessment, interaction, and demonstration of viable use; hierarchical ordering and behavioral management of disordered functions; and abundant care and reinforcement toward effecting a lasting change. Yet the approach to these steps in traditional models and a use model involves a key distinction. Speech-language pathologists in a use model strive to lead, and if desired, direct involved parties toward active participation in communication and daily life. Such a role contrasts with traditional practices of primarily targeting change of form, content, or use of language or communication. Ultimately, it is the recipients of treatment, adults with aphasia and prime caregivers, and not the treatment process or even the clinician, who determine the form and quantity of remediation. Treatment is not contingent on the type or degree of aphasia, or even on the clinical skills of the speech-language pathologist. Rather, necessity and feasibility of treatment is dependent on a sustained and focused drive of affected parties to accomplish change.

Valuing the opinions and desires of aphasic adults and caregivers in deciding the course of treatment does not diminish the importance of the role of the speech-language pathologist. The more able speech-language pathologists are to demonstrate and nurture the use of disrupted processes, the more likely recipients of therapy will be to choose to participate in remediation. However, speech-language pathologists should not be judged solely on efforts to reestablish linguistic and communicative constructs. Instead, therapeutic worth should be assessed according to a clinician's ability to guide patients and loved ones toward a comfortable, acceptable, and chosen equilibrium of communicative use. As emphasized earlier, our role is one of orchestration, not conscription. The prime challenge in this pursuit is to calm any natural fears of aphasic adults that they might be unable to adopt effective, alternative forms of use and to ensure that potential uses are not limited by the clinician's inability to demonstrate their communicative value. Our comfort level with gestures, drawing, or pantomime is a case in point.

TREATMENT

How does one set into motion a use model for aphasia treatment? Table 8.1 gives a general framework for establishing such a program.

Assessment

To begin with, the clinician assesses the prime components of language and communication, social use of communication, and psychosocial well-being.

TABLE 8.1   General Treatment Objectives in a Use Model for Aphasia Treatment

1. Assessment of disrupted processes within domains of communication and language, the social use of communication, and psychosocial well-being
2. Demonstration of viable use of select disrupted processes
3. Ranking of disrupted processes according to perceived importance
4. Facilitation of selected disrupted processes
5. Revisions to treatment plans
6. Termination of treatment

Table 8.2 lists the components by processing domain and communication participant. Aphasic adults (when able) and their prime caregivers evaluate all processing components. Prime caregivers are asked to evaluate separately their own use of communication with aphasic partners and their own psychosocial well-being. Processing components are judged from three temporal perspectives: what were they like before the aphasia, what are they like currently, and what might they be like in the future. Such time-based estimations aid in defining the scope of treatment. In this respect, expected gains from treatment should not exceed preinjury levels of function, nor should they surpass anticipated levels of re-establishment, although estimated projections of return may vary over time and with treatment.

Demonstration

Demonstration of how disrupted processes might be re-established is the next step. The therapeutic intent of this step is threefold: to verify that communicative or linguistic use is possible; to forge a working relationship for further intervention; and to provide a mutually agreed on reference point from which treatment commences. Through demonstration, aphasic adults and caregivers can select the form and content of therapy to come. Some of the selecting is volitional; some is automatic. The target, though, is to define a common ground on which to commence therapy.

Selection of processes for demonstration depends on a number of variables: time post-onset; severity of aphasia; perceived need of repair; commitment, motivation, and available time for repair; and setting(s) and condition(s) in which use is sought. Underlying this selection process is the previously stated objective to return optimal control, direction, independence, and responsibility to the lives of adults with aphasia and their prime caregivers. Processes that might be appropriately singled out for demonstration during the acute periods of rehabilitation are not appropriate at 6 or 18 months post-onset. Proper selection relies on a close, ongoing, therapeutic dialogue between patient and clinician. But it is important to realize that demonstration does not imply that users should or must adopt a suggested course. Demonstration is solely a departure point.

Demonstration is not without risk. While providing aphasic adults and prime caregivers with an opportunity to observe firsthand that communica-

TABLE 8.2 General Overview of Processes by Domain and Participant

1. Domain: Communication and Language

Aphasic adult
  Receptively (ability to comprehend)
    Speech
    Print
    Gestures
    Sketches
  Expressively (ability to make use of)
    Speech
    Writing
    Gestures
    Drawing

Prime caregiver
  Receptively (ability to comprehend the output of the aphasic adult)
    Speech
    Writing
    Gestures
    Drawings
  Expressively (ability to effectively convey content via)
    Speech
    Print
    Gestures
    Sketches

2. Domain: Social Use of Communication

Aphasic adult
  Comfort (comfort in being able to communicate)
    With family and friends
    With strangers
  Confidence (confidence in being able to communicate)
    With family and friends
    With strangers
  Interactant competence (ability of interactant to know how to extract content from the
      communicative exchange)
    With family or friends
    With strangers
  Conveyance (ability to convey desired content)
    With family or friends
    With strangers
  Initiation (ability to start a conversation)
    With family or friends
    With strangers
  Maintenance (ability to maintain a conversation)
    With family or friends
    With strangers

Prime Caregiver
  Same processes are examined as with aphasic adult; however, caregivers are asked to
      evaluate processes two different ways:

TABLE 8.2   *(continued)*

a. For themselves when communicating with their aphasic spouse/companion

b. For their aphasic spouse/companion in general

3. Domain: Psychosocial Well-Being

Aphasic adult

Purpose and direction to life—i.e., presence of a cause or reason for going ahead with life; something to look forward to

Contentment—i.e., satisfaction or comfort with life

Personal freedom—i.e., ability to do what you want on a daily basis

Initiation—i.e., ability and willingness to "start" activities of choice

Use of time—i.e., ability to stay busy throughout the day

Public image—i.e., ability and willlingness to go out in public

Self-image—i.e., ability to value self

Image of others—i.e., ability to value others

Comfort being alone—i.e., ability to be alone

Comfort with family and friends—i.e., ability to share space and time with family and friends

Comfort with strangers—i.e., ability to share space and time with strangers

Prime caregiver

Again, the same processes are examined. Also, caregivers are asked to evaluate themselves as well as their aphasic spouses/companions.

tion is still viable, demonstration simultaneously can define the severity of the existing communicative problem. If communicative use relies largely on nonstandard forms, as judged by its users, demonstration may impede rather than promote therapeutic progress. Readiness for demonstration is a prime consideration before proceeding with its implementation. The aforementioned importance of establishing a close, informal, ongoing dialogue concerning treatment should aid in determining the appropriateness of demonstration. If an adult with aphasia is fixated on the return of his speech, even when a clinician's knowledge and expertise would suggest otherwise, it is not appropriate to begin with demonstrations of how gestures or drawing might aid a functional return of expression. At best, it is appropriate to recommend the consideration of such means as interim alternatives while pursuing a functional restoration of speech. If these terms are agreeable to the patient, demonstration of gestures or drawing can proceed. But if a potential user views such a plan negatively, treatment should be confined to the demonstration and restoration of speech. With time and an improved sense of the limited viability of verbal expression, the patient may come to seek alternative modes of use. At that time, demonstration of the potential benefits of gestures and drawing can be reintroduced.

Prioritization

The third step in treatment is to establish a hierarchy of those processes to be treated. Because participants (adults with aphasia, prime caregivers, and speech-language pathologists) may view current needs and objectives of treatment differently, hierarchies for treatment need to be elicited separately. When the orderings show marked differences (which is not uncommon), resolution is the first requisite to effective treatment. It is important to rule out that such differences were due to faulty, misperceived, or insufficient information. For this reason, targeted processes are reviewed a second time. The speech-language pathologist clarifies the rationale for proceeding along the recommended course. When comprehension of proposed targets for therapy is not an issue, adjustments to the proposed treatment plan must follow. Compromise or acquiescence by the clinician are the more likely routes. The latter choice, acquiescence, may stand in contrast to traditional treatment methods. An example may help to clarify this latter point.

Not long ago, I evaluated and treated an adult with conduction aphasia. After assessing his language and communication, it was apparent that his verbal strength rested in his relatively well-preserved spontaneous speech. Accordingly, I attempted to demonstrate how free recall from pictured stimuli with a distinctive theme (e.g., action pictures from *Life* magazine) resulted in a host of new words without apparent strain. I contrasted the ease of his spontaneous speech with his labored efforts during verbal confrontation drills. But to this gentleman, simply chatting about pictures was not treatment. To him, this seemed like a casual task, unrelated to the "real" problem. The deficit, in his mind, was not an inability to talk. It was an inability to recall and say specific words when he wanted them. Despite my assessment, experience, and what I thought to be a sound rationale for treatment, he insisted that we work specifically on verbal repetition, the most difficult verbal task in his repertoire. I acquiesced. We settled on a revised verbal repetition drill. With cuing from printed and pictured stimuli, verbal repetition was possible, although still labored. The struggle, to some degree, served to verify to this man that he was truly working on the problem. In the long run, this gentleman regained some purposeful spontaneous speech, although not in the manner I would have chosen, nor in the easiest way, in my judgment.

Thus when treated parties, whether adults with aphasia or prime caregivers, understand treatment options yet still desire a different course, the speech-language pathologist is obligated to respect their wishes.

Facilitation

Facilitation is not a new concept to speech-language pathologists. It remains a prime justification for many types of linguistic/communication stimulation therapy. However, within the use model, facilitation refers to the promotion of treated processes in their natural settings. This contrasts with traditional practices of repairing linguistic and communicative components solely within clinical realms. As commonly acknowledged, stimulation of language and communication in clinical settings may bear little resemblance to conversational demands in daily life (Darley, 1991; Davis, 1986; Holland, 1987;

Kimbarow, 1989). In fact, clinical gains may prove regressive under certain circumstances if clinically acquired strategies fail or are only partially successful at home. Aphasic adults may conceivably deduce that communication simply is not viable in natural settings. Even worse, the adult with aphasia may come to feel that the problem rests with himself or herself.

Comparable dynamics may underlie psychosocial well-being as well. Aphasic adults may realize improvement in self-image and self-confidence from communicative gains achieved in clinical settings. Yet subsequent erosion of performance and support in natural settings may stand to counteract, even worsen, these short-lived clinical benefits. Thus, the focus on facilitation in a use model is to set into motion a process for returning communication and well-being to natural settings.

Communication Partners represents a treatment model for facilitating use in natural settings (Lyon, 1989, 1992). Normal community volunteers are recruited to serve as liaisons in moving treatment from clinical to natural settings. These volunteers—communication partners—are paired with aphasic adults and their prime caregivers. Initially, treatment sessions are conducted in clinical settings to teach communication partners how to communicate effectively with their aphasic peers. Once proficient in exchanging basic content, planned outings into the community are arranged.

The activities chosen within the community depend completely on the interests of the aphasic adult. One patient might choose to visit old friends not seen since her stroke; another may prefer to find community settings where card games are played; still another may want a three-wheeled bicycle to help him deliver newspapers on a paper route; and one more may desire garden plants for a backyard patio. Whatever the preference of the adult with aphasia, plans are mapped accordingly. Logistics are carefully reviewed. All participating parties must feel comfortable that the task ahead is realistic, achievable, and, above all, safely laid out. Thereafter, communication and aphasic partners set out on weekly outings.

Over time, Communication Partners serves as a facilitating agent, and aphasic adults begin to assume greater responsibility and control of their lives. Such personal gains do not emanate solely from the presence of a supportive therapeutic climate. They evolve as well from the personal gratification of knowing such activities are still possible and, more important, within the patient's capabilities. Prime caregivers benefit, too. Prime caregivers often assume full responsibility for the care of aphasic adults in the home. As a result, the caregiver can feel entrapped as well as overprotective. Communication partners permit caregivers to have a brief respite from such responsibilities and often allow the opportunity to re-evaluate what the patient is able to do independently.

This facilitation involves more than simply boosting speech, language, and communication within controlled, clinical settings. To be fully effective, it requires that we provide an effective means of integrating clinical gains into natural settings.

Revision

Continuous revision of a use model for aphasia treatment is essential for optimal improvement. As one targeted process is set into motion, results that are achieved are weighed against what was expected. When the two are widely divergent, when expectations far exceed results, this discrepancy can affect motivation. Immediate revisions are required to realign these critical reference points. Perhaps the difference is simply one of overestimation. Of greater concern, however, is when the difference seems to suggest the "inability" to resume a use. Generally, this is not the case. Use is rarely impossible; it may be, however, that the degree of effort, time, and consumption of resources to make processes work simply does not justify the end product. As long as affected parties realize this equation and knowingly choose their respective levels of involvement, treatment can be a success.

Termination

Treatment involves the inching forward of all parties toward an agreeable point of termination. Treated parties must measure what they want against the degree to which they, and others who must sustain these processes, are committed to achieving. When the compromise point arrives, therapy has reached its natural conclusion. Whether outwardly stated or inwardly confirmed, when treated parties would prefer to do without an end product rather than endure the costs of attaining it, it is time to quit. Sometimes accepting this reality can be problematic for patient, family, and, quite often, the clinician.

A CASE STUDY OF A USE MODEL IN APHASIA TREATMENT

N.S. is a 53-year-old adult with severe Broca's aphasia who experienced a left hemispheric, thromboembolic infarction to his middle cerebral artery 4 years ago. His acute and intermediate care occurred in a variety of clinical settings and in accordance with traditional practices of speech-language remediation. Basic processes for establishing control, independence, and direction to life were still absent when he was re-evaluated approximately 2 years ago. What was not absent, though, was N.S.'s desire. As previously stated, it is this factor more than any other—i.e., a burning passion to move ahead with life—that determines what can be accomplished with treatment. N.S.'s prime caregiver is his wife, a woman equally dedicated to her husband's optimal recovery, yet, at the time, uncertain about how to achieve this end. So, at 21 months post-onset, we began a journey together.

Assessment

The process began with an assessment of processing domains as seen by N.S. and his wife (Table 8.3). N.S.'s inability to convey information effectively and efficiently to his wife constituted the prime disruption to processes within the language and communication domain. His use of speech, writing, and gestures was highly restricted and largely nonfunctional; he had never been exposed to drawing for communicative purposes. His auditory comprehension of simple, everyday exchanges was functional, if presented somewhat slowly. Even so, frequent frustration and occasional anger were not uncommon in communicative exchanges between N.S. and his wife. In the domain of social use of communication, N.S. appeared comfortable only when addressing basic needs with his wife. He answered common yes/no questions, but many daily needs were addressed by simply following prior, pre-stroke daily habits. More complex topics or interactions with strangers were not considered comfortable, or likely to succeed. N.S. required the full support of the other interactant in a communique to achieve a successful exchange of content. As for the domain of psychosocial well-being, both N.S. and his wife reported marked difficulties. For N.S., purpose or direction in life, contentment with life, personal freedom, ability and willingness to initiate familiar or new activities, public image, and self-image were significantly restricted or diminished. His wife's lifestyle was restricted and demands on her life were far greater than before the onset of N.S.'s aphasia. While N.S.'s unmet needs were in the forefront of his wife's concerns, not far behind in importance were her own needs for more personal freedom and time.

Demonstration

Of all of N.S. and his wife's concerns, establishing an effective and efficient means of exchanging content was viewed as most essential. This need was apparent in both the domains of language and communication, and the social use of communication, in which an ability to exchange content was highly restricted. In addition, the form of exchange needed to fulfill two prime objectives: (1) to broaden the scope of contextual topics available (i.e., not be confined to just an exchange of basic needs or wants), and (2) to expand usage to interactants other than N.S.'s wife. Finally, personal and social involvement outside the home needed to be addressed as well.

Drawing was selected as a potential mode for re-establishing communicative exchange. It was hoped that its use, along with existing gestures and N.S.'s functional yes/no response, might expand the number of topics and interactants. N.S. and his wife were advised of this recommendation.They were informed that drawing was not necessarily a permanent substitute for speaking or writing, but rather a means of restoring viability to a part of communication that was nonfunctional. Drawing was merely a mode to get infor-

TABLE 8.3   Pretreatment Assessment of Disrupted Processes for N.S. and His Wife

1. Communication and Language

N.S. receptively

    Speech: functional comprehension of everyday conversation; inconsistent with complex formulations or two-step commands, questions, and statements

    Print: 60–70% accuracy with comprehension of single-word (noun/verb) and short functional phrases; poor full-sentence and paragraph comprehension

    Gestures: functional recognition of common gestures

    Sketches: excellent recognition of sketched objects and events

N.S. expressively

    Speech: spontaneous speech confined to the use of short, automatic, stereotypical utterances ("O.K.," "maybe," "all right"); no purposeful volitional speech or naming; verbal repetition confined to short, monosyllabic words

    Writing: able to write his name spontaneously; must copy otherwise

    Gestures: limited use in spontaneous exchange; occasionally could add gestures when requested; additions were often not differentiated enough to be useful; had been trained in AMERIND use; could gesture basic concepts (house, chair, toothbrush)

    Drawing: able to draw common objects and actions upon command; would commonly mix perspectives (e.g., part of drawing was from the side while part was from above)

N.S.'s wife receptively

    Speech: nonfunctional

    Writing: nonfunctional

    Gestures: largely unsuccessful; would try to make out undifferentiated attempts by N.S.

    Drawing: had not been attempted communicatively

N.S.'s wife expressively

    Speech: able to fully convey basic meaning via this modality

    Print: no need to use

    Gestures: no need to use

    Sketches: no need to use

2. Social Use of Communication

N.S.

    Comfort: comfortable with wife/family; not comfortable around strangers

    Confidence: 50% or better confident with wife although frequent, protracted periods necessary; 20% or less with strangers

    Interactant Competence: functional abilities for wife; poor abilities for all others

    Conveyance: highly limited

    Initiation: occasionally with wife; not present with others

    Maintenance: pursues intent with wife but unable to maintain without her support; not able to sustain with others

N.S.'s wife

    (HERS refers to wife's assessment of her own abilities when conversing with N.S.; N.S. refers to wife's assessment of N.S.'s abilities to converse with her and others.)

    Comfort:

        HERS: functional but occasional periods of frustration; some avoidance of exchanges with N.S.

TABLE 8.3   *(continued)*

N.S.: comfort with her alone; becomes angry when she can't understand intent.; N.S. is more patient with others although not comfortable

Confidence:

HERS: functional for basic needs and wants; not confident with content beyond that

N.S.: same as her assessment; limited confidence with others

Interactant Competence:

HERS: limited; only knows to ask questions until she figures out what's being conveyed

N.S.: not sure; probably views wife's ability as marginal; others are even worse

Conveyance:

HERS: basic needs known, other content is a struggle

N.S.: same as her assessment; worse for others

Initiation:

HERS: willing to start exchange, especially when something is on his mind

N.S.: same as her assessment; doesn't initiate with others

Maintenance:

HERS: N.S. wants to continue exchange but relies entirely on her to keep it going

N.S.: same as her assessment; requires others to maintain exchange

3. Psychosocial Well-Being

N.S.

Purpose: motivated to try to talk; not with a set direction or purpose to life

Contentment: not sad or depressed but certainly not content with life

Personal freedom: highly restricted; confined to the home daily while wife works

Initiation: willing to participate but minimal initiation when unaided

Use of time: sits and watches TV; no other activities

Public image: self conscious when in public but willing to go out with wife

Self-image: significantly reduced although proud of who he was before stroke

Image of others: favorable; perhaps slightly inflated now that he is so restricted

Comfort alone: functional; looks forward to wife's return at end of work day

Comfort with family: functional

Comfort with strangers: nil to minimal

N.S.'s wife

(HERS refers to wife's assessment of herself; N.S. refers to wife's assessment of N.S.)

Purpose:

HERS: aided by job that gives her direction; struggling to keep a healthy balance within relationship

N.S.: marginal

Contentment:

HERS: satisfactory; wished there was more that could be done for N.S.

N.S.: minimal

Personal freedom:

HERS: highly restricted; confined by job and the need to be at home with N.S. otherwise

N.S.: highly restricted

Initiation:

HERS: functional at work; restricted otherwise due to feelings of guilt that she should spend more time with N.S.

TABLE 8.3   *(continued)*

N.S.: minimal.
Use of time:
    HERS: too busy; excessive obligations to job or family; too little time for personal
        time, space or relaxation
    N.S.: too much unstructured and nonproductive time; watches TV
Public image:
    HERS: unchanged
    N.S.: conscious of his image in public
Self-image:
    HERS: unchanged in general; concerned that she's not doing enough or not doing
        things properly
    N.S.: diminished
Image of others:
    HERS: unchanged; somewhat surprised how others, e.g., N.S.'s former friends, have
        not been more present yet understanding why they wouldn't or couldn't be
    N.S.: unchanged
Comfort alone:
    HERS: unchanged; relishes such time when available
    N.S.: satisfactory to good
Comfort with family:
    HERS: unchanged
    N.S.: satisfactory, slightly reduced
Comfort with strangers:
    HERS: unchanged
    N.S.: minimal

mational content flowing back and forth. They were told that the use of drawing might seem awkward and unnatural at first but that with time and practice, this tool was generally comfortable and functional. More important, once comfort and ease were established, we could start to expand upon its use with other people and eventually move to exchanges outside the clinic and home. For several weeks, then, N.S. and his wife came to the clinic to observe how information might be exchanged through drawing.

Prioritization

At this point, N.S.'s prioritized list of preferences for remediation was (1) to talk better, (2) to communicate better, and (3) to be more involved in life. His wife's preferences were (1) to communicate better with N.S., (2) for N.S. to talk better, (3) for N.S. to be more involved in life, and (4) for her to have more personal freedom. The speech-language pathologist's list was (1) to have N.S. and his wife communicate better, (2) to get N.S. more involved in activities outside the home, and (3) to see if the latter might alleviate some of Mrs. S.'s current responsibilities for her husband. The absence of "talking better" from the clinician's list was because of two factors: (1) these skills were treated extensively during the first year post-onset with minimal return; and (2) N.S. was unable to hold onto an auditory-verbal trace internally for more than a couple of seconds.

The first order of business was to find common ground among the various priorities. N.S.'s prime concern, improving his speech, took precedence. Accordingly, the speech-language pathologist structured a home-based speech repetition drill from printed materials and supplemented it with a set of audio cassettes. All recommended verbal tasks were within N.S.'s capabilities and could be accomplished in the comfort of his home. He remained highly motivated to undertake this task. With that priority satisfied, the focus shifted to the next common objectives—facilitation of communication and re-establishment of activities outside the home.

Facilitation

The first several months of treatment were spent perfecting the use of drawing for communicative purposes. Initially, N.S. drew a variety of mock situations that were visually and semantically striking (e.g., spilling a glass of milk at the table this morning, finding a spider crawling on his arm this morning as he watched TV). When N.S. completed his drawings, Mrs. S. returned to the room and attempted to decipher her husband's depictions. Specific strategies were reviewed with Mrs. S. to aid her in deciphering N.S.'s drawings. Once comfortable and reasonably successful with this process, N.S. began drawing happenings from his daily life. Again, Mrs. S., naive to the content of these drawings, was aided in her efforts to extract the meaning from these messages.

In time, Mr. and Mrs. S. became proficient in this type of an exchange. As proficiency increased, N.S. independently began sketching more complex situations designed somewhat to stump the interpreter, a characteristic that continues today. At the moment, N.S.'s drawings are sophisticated visually and contextually. He readily draws from a couple of perspectives (above or from the side) upon request. Very seldom does it take more than a minute or two to derive meaning from his artistry.

With drawing secure as a viable communication tool at home, treatment moved to finding others, preferably strangers, who could acquire these same communicative skills. Efforts were made to secure communication partners for N.S. After considering various friends and volunteers from N.S.'s community, two such individuals were located. The two volunteers were enrolled in a training regimen comparable to Mrs. S.'s. Over several months, the communication partners perfected their skills in deciphering drawn messages from N.S. When all parties were comfortable with this process, the focus moved to activities of interest in the community.

Initially N.S. was familiarized with existing city bus routes. Over several months, his two communication partners escorted him to different parts of the city. They ensured that N.S. was able to transfer from one bus line to the next. Before too long, N.S. successfully traversed the entire community (of 50,000) unaided. His communication partners also observed that he was able to walk independently for short distances once at a destination. With these skills, N.S. could travel from home to the bus stops of his choice and then participate in planned activities.

Activities of choice were isolated next. By happenstance, the first activity was participating in a ceramics class that met within walking distance of his home. Shortly thereafter, he elected to begin making short visits to a local shopping mall, primarily to walk and look at items of interest, and interact with others.When the ceramics shop went out of business, N.S. and his communication partners set out to discover other activities. Swimming at the YWCA and an art course were targeted, both of which involved travel to a central downtown section of the city. Bus routes were reviewed and he was personally escorted to these locations by his communication partners. After a single chaperoned trip, each of these activities became a mainstay on N.S.'s weekly agenda and were managed independently. His swimming is now a biweekly event, and he reports increased strength and range of motion on his involved right side. His art classes are a permanent weekly event as well. Currently, his art work is on display in certain locations throughout the state. He reports occasional sales of these works.

Over a year ago, N.S. assumed still another activity. With the aid of his communication partners, he began volunteering at the Veterans Administration Hospital in Madison, Wisconsin. Initially, he wanted to escort patients to appointments in the hospital, but, given questions of gait stability and strength on his involved right side, he settled into assisting with certain housekeeping chores in the Rehabilitative Medicine Service. Not content with the degree of social isolation, he subsequently began playing checkers or chess with inpatients on medical wards. Although still highly restricted in his verbal output, N.S. carried a 5" × 8" index card with a brief explanation of his purpose in visiting patients on wards and the reason for his limited abilities to talk. He is now well-known, appreciated, and respected by staff and patients. His refined skills and reputation as a shark on the checkerboard may initially dissuade some patients from entering into this arena. But N.S.'s air of kindness and frivolity usually puts these fears to rest. Several months ago, N.S. and his wife attended an annual banquet at which he received a certificate for having surpassed 100 hours of volunteerism. He is currently arranging to spend a day volunteering at another nursing home in his own community, traveling the floors with his checker/chess set—if time will only permit!

Revision

N.S. and his wife's treatment plans were checked and revised periodically. As for N.S.'s speech, his printed materials and audio tapes were enlarged and changed several times. Once he began volunteering at the VA Hospital, which is located 50 miles from his home, his communication partners used the transit time to drill common functional phrases. For drawing, N.S. began to carry two 3" × 5" pocket notebooks; one is for drawing to communicate, and the other explains to naive, normal adults how to interpret these drawings. Although not yet a common communicative tool, he uses this technique occasionally with total strangers on daily visitations to the local shopping mall. In addition, he continues to draw three to five situational happenings weekly for his communication partners and the speech-language pathologist to review. As outlined earlier, numerous revisions were made to his outside activities. Changes were apparent in Mrs. S.'s lifestyle and well-being, too. She no longer acts on her earlier perception that she was responsible for N.S.'s daily routine.

Termination

N.S. has assumed a direction, a purpose, a control, an independence, and a responsibility for his life (Table 8.4). He and his wife do all of the work. Only on rare occasions do the communication partners and speech-language pathologist need to give a gentle nudge. N.S. maintains the momentum and force. Clearly, a direction and motion exist. Table 8.4 contains a current profile of the processing domains initially evaluated.

SUMMARY

At the beginning of this chapter, the question was posed: Why is it so difficult to establish trained communicative skills in natural settings? Physiologic limitations resulting from reduced higher cortical and cerebral functions may account for some of the lack of transference in adults with aphasia. However, it may well be that the omission of a comprehensive treatment plan that simultaneously addresses linguistic/communicative and psychosocial well-being, contributes equally, if not more so, to this shortcoming. If so, a key to transference may rest with a need to devise concurrent, integrated treatment plans for communication and well-being. As viewed here, this means striking a balance between what adults with aphasia and their prime caregivers see as being possible and what they are willing do. It is contingent on speech-language pathologists possessing and executing the best means possible for allowing these adults and their caregivers to reach their full potential. Most important, it is contingent on giving aphasic adults and their prime caregivers equal voice in the selection of treatment and how it should proceed. We, as practitioners, must be content to support and accept the form and content of a mutually enacted process.

TABLE 8.4   Post-Treatment Assessment of Disrupted Processes for N.S. and His Wife

1. Communication and Language

N.S. receptively

Speech: functional comprehension of everyday conversation; readily comprehends and responds to conversational exchanges; some difficulty if length or complexity is increased

Print: 90% accuracy with single-word (noun/verb) and short functional phrase comprehension; able to understand basic content from headlines of paper

Gestures: excellent recognition

Sketches: excellent recognition

N.S. expressively

Speech: more usage of common words and short phrases in spontaneous speech; still primarily uses a variety of short automatic, stereotypical utterances; no volitional confrontation naming but occasional names of people or places in free conversation; constant use of verbal repetition for short and longer words in free conversation

Writing: largely unchanged; recently started a home-writing program

Gestures: in free conversation, uses a host of gestures that are better differentiated and more appropriate to the context; periods where gestures can't be initiated or are too vague to be helpful

Drawing: draws communicatively all the time; keeps a daily log of "happenings" that are shared weekly with his communication partners and speech-language pathologist; uses drawing with his wife when unable to otherwise get his point across; carries a notebook with him that tells strangers how to interpret his drawings. Although limited, has drawn wants and needs to strangers

N.S.'s wife receptively

Speech: highly restricted but occasional verbal conveyance of content

Writing: nonfunctional

Gestures: improved usage and reliance on this; frequently is asked to show what he wants or needs

Drawing: backbone of exchanges when intent can't be discerned from speech or gesture; still small number of situations that can't be figured out even with drawing

N.S.'s wife expressively

Speech: improved ease of comprehension; still prime modality for imparting content to N.S.

Print: no need to use

Gestures: no need to use

Sketches: no need to use

2. Social Use of Communication

N.S.

Comfort: comfortable with wife, family, and other friends; reasonably comfortable with strangers (e.g., independently arranges all checkers and chess games with inpatients in medical center where he volunteers weekly)

Confidence: better than 95% confident of all content with wife and friends; 60% confident of content with strangers

Interactant Competence: excellent abilities for wife, communication partners and friends; strangers significantly less able but N.S. can now aid them in how to communicate with him

TABLE 8.4   *(continued)*

Conveyance: excellent with basic needs and wants, and basic content from his daily routine; more complex issues are still difficult but usually attainable through repeated trials; less able but improving with strangers

Initiation: initiates conversation constantly with familiar interactants; not hesitant, if the need exists, to do so with strangers

Maintenance: Does more (gestures, drawings) to maintain his part of an exchange with both family and strangers

N.S.'s wife

(HERS refers to wife's assessment of her abilities when conversing with N.S.; N.S. refers to wife's assessment of N.S.'s abilities to converse with her and others.)

Comfort:

HERS: much easier; greater chance for success and knowledge of what to do when "stuck" in an exchange; less frustration on N.S.'s part when communicating

N.S.: comfort with family and friends; reasonably so with strangers

Confidence:

HERS: fairly confident all crucial content can be conveyed

N.S.: same as her assessment; equally able with communication partners and friends; less so with strangers

Interactant Competence:

HERS: good to excellent in knowing how to extract content from exchange

N.S.: Views wife, communication partners and family as capable; others are still restricted in how to communicate with him although he can help them now

Conveyance:

HERS: gets almost everything across to her with time

N.S.: same as her assessment; communication partners and friends; less so with strangers

Initiation:

HERS: readily initiates conversations with her

N.S.: same as her assessment; equally quick to start exchange with communication partners and friends; less so with strangers but increasing in frequency

Maintenance:

HERS: still relies heavily on her to maintain direction and content but is better able to find ways of letting her know unknown parts

N.S.: same as her assessment; realizes that others can only do so much in an exchange; is accepting of what they can't do

3. Psychosocial Well-Being

N.S.

Purpose: good to excellent; now has a number of activities which he eagerly plans and looks forward to (e.g., swims twice weekly, volunteers at medical center weekly, attends art classes weekly)

Contentment: good to excellent; is happy with his daily routine but remains committed to future improvement

Personal freedom: excellent; is fully familiar with the bus system in his community; is able and does come and go as he pleases

Initiation: good to excellent; constantly expanding activities which he starts unaided

Use of time: excellent; remains occupied with designated activities or projects throughout the week

TABLE 8.4   *(continued)*

Public image: excellent; is out in public constantly without the aid of wife or communication partners

Self-image: good; has begun to recapture some of how he viewed himself before the stroke; some of his art work has been singled out for personal recognition

Image of others: excellent; constantly interacting with others

Comfort alone: excellent; is alone or with others he doesn't know throughout much of the day; enjoys that contact

Comfort with family: excellent; more interactive with family members

Comfort with strangers: good; not aggressive in seeking out strangers but not inhibited to interact with them

N.S.'s wife

(HERS refers to wife's assessment of herself; N.S. refers to wife's assessment of N.S.)

Purpose:

HERS: job continues to add new direction and purpose; previous "struggle" to find an equilibrium within relationship has lessened

N.S.: greatly changed and enhanced

Contentment:

HERS: satisfactory; able to devote more time to demands of job without feeling guilty; less concerned that N.S. will not be able to set a course of his own without her help

N.S.: greatly changed and enhanced; likes life

Personal freedom:

HERS: far less restricted due to concerns relating to N.S.; job and demands of daily living continue to restrict time and freedom

N.S.: greatly changed and enhanced; never at home

Initiation:

HERS: satisfactory; able to begin course work that would help at work

N.S.: constant

Use of time:

HERS: still very busy but greater comfort with that load; still value and need time for personal relaxation

N.S.: much of week is completely occupied with "chosen" activities

Public image:

HERS: unchanged

N.S.: greatly improved; is out in public all the time

Self-image:

HERS: slightly improved; less concerned that she can't do it all

N.S.: good; on the mend

Image of others:

HERS: unchanged; still favorable and thankful for those who have helped them along this path

N.S.: improved; more open with others

Comfort alone:

HERS: unchanged

N.S.: remains excellent

Comfort with family:

HERS: unchanged

TABLE 8.4 *(continued)*

N.S.: improved; more interactive
Comfort with strangers:
HERS: unchanged
N.S.: greatly changed and enhanced; spends much of day with strangers; not fearful at all

REFERENCES

Buck, M. (1968). *Dysphasia: Professional guidance for family and patient.* Englewood Cliffs, NJ: Prentice-Hall.

Byng, S., Kay, J., Edmundson, A., & Scotts, C. (1990). Aphasia tests reconsidered. *Aphasiology, 4,* 67–91.

Caramazza, A. (1989). Cognitive neuropsychology and rehabilitation: An unfulfilled promise? In X. Seron and G. Deloche (Eds.), *Cognitive approaches in neuropsychological rehabilitation.* Hillsdale, NJ: Lawrence Erlbaum Associates.

Darley, F.L. (1982). *Aphasia.* Philadelphia: W.B. Saunders.

Darley, F.L. (1991). I think it begins with an A. In T. Prescott (Ed.), *Clinical aphasiology* (Vol 20). Austin, TX: PRO-ED.

Davis, A., & Wilcox, M.J. (1985). *Adult aphasia rehabilitation.* San Diego: College-Hill Press.

Davis, G.A. (1986). Questions of efficacy in clinical aphasiology. In R.H. Brookshire (Ed.), *Clinical aphasiology conference proceedings* (pp. 154–162). Minneapolis: BRK.

Eisenson, J. (1984). *Adult aphasia.* Englewood Cliffs, NJ: Prentice Hall.

Goldstein, K. (1942). *After-effects of brain injuries in war.* New York: Grune & Stratton.

Herrmann, M., & Wallesch, C.W. (1989). Psychosocial changes and psychosocial adjustment with chronic and severe nonfluent aphasia. *Aphasiology, 3,* 513–526.

Herrmann, M., & Wallesch, C.W. (1990). Expectations of psychosocial adjustment in aphasia: A MAUT study with the Code-Muller scale of psychosocial adjustment. *Aphasiology, 4,* 527–538.

Holland, A. (1987). Functional/pragmatic communication in acquired adult neurogenic disorders: Clinical and contemporary issues. *Workshop at Speech and Stroke Centre,* North York/Toronto, Canada.

Kagan, A., & Gailey, G. (1993). *Functional is not enough: Training conversational partners for adults with aphasia.* In A. Holland and M. Forbes (Eds.), *World perspectives of aphasia.* San Diego: Singular Press.

Kearns, K. (1989). Methodologies for studying generalization. In: J. Spradlin & L.V. McReynolds (Eds.), *Generalization strategies in communication disorders.* Toronto: B.C. Decker.

Kimbarow, M.L. (1989, June). *The pragmatic paradox.* Presentation at Clinical Aphasiology Conference, Incline Village, NV.

Lesser, R. (1987). Cognitive neuropsychological influences on aphasia therapy. *Aphasiology, 1,* 189–200.

Lyon, J.G. (1989). Communicative partners: Their value in reestablishing communication with aphasic adults. In T. Prescott (Ed.), *Clinical aphasiology* (Vol 18). Boston: College-Hill Press.

Lyon, J.G. (1992). Communication use and participation in life for adults with aphasia in natural settings: The scope of the problem. *American Journal of Speech-Language Pathology, 1,* 7–14.

McNeil M. (1991). Toward the integration of resource allocation into a general theory of aphasia. In T. Prescott (Ed.), *Clinical aphasiology.* (Vol. 20). Austin, TX: PRO-ED.

Muller, D.J., & Code, C. (1983). Interpersonal perceptions of psychosocial adjustment to aphasia. In C. Code & D.J. Muller (Eds.), *Aphasia therapy.* London: Edward Arnold.

Roblin, W.J. (1984). Family therapy and the aphasic adult. In J. Eisenson (Ed.), *Adult aphasia.* Englewood Cliffs, NJ: Prentice-Hall.

Rosenbek, J.C., LaPointe, L.L., & Wertz, R.T. (1989). *Aphasia: A clinical approach.* Boston: College-Hill Press.

Sarno, M.T., & Hook, O. (1980). *Aphasia: Assessment and treatment.* New York: Masson Publishing USA.

Schuell, H., Jenkins, J.J., & Jimenez-Pabon, E. (1964). *Aphasia in adults: Diagnosis, prognosis and treatment.* New York: Hoeber Medical Division, Harper & Row.

Thompson, C.K. (1989). Generalization research in aphasia: A review of the literature. In T. Prescott (Ed.), *Clinical aphasiology* (Vol. 18). Boston: College-Hill Press.

Wohrborg, P. (1989). Aphasia and family therapy. *Aphasiology, 3,* 479-482.

Chapter 9

Pragmatic Assessment and Treatment for Aphasia

Audrey L. Holland

Language pragmatics concerns the use of language in context, as well as the role of language in communication. Because speech-language pathologists generally and clinical aphasiologists specifically are concerned with people who have deficits in language, these clinicians' interest in applying pragmatics to intervention comes as little surprise. In fact, concern with functional and communicative aspects of language disorders predated the explosion of interest in other branches of speech-language pathology. For example, Martha Taylor Sarno developed the Functional Communication Profile (1969) quite near the time at which the work of Searle (1969) galvanized pragmatic concerns. The Functional Communication Profile also antedated by at least 7 years the publication of Bates' *Language in Context* (1976), which crystallized the study of pragmatic aspects of children's language.

Thus, language pragmatics has been growing in importance for almost 20 years. During this time, pragmatic issues have come to be recognized as equally important to the study of language as are grammar, phonology, and lexical semantics. Much of this work has had direct clinical application to aphasia. The term *aphasia* is used here to denote the language disorder that accompanies focal brain lesions, affecting the language areas of the language-dominant hemisphere. Language disorders certainly occur following closed head injury, with its diffuse sites of damage. They also occur in dementing conditions, here again as the result of more diffuse damage. However, there is controversy regarding the appropriateness of describing these disorders with the term *aphasia*. One reason is that focal and diffuse damage appear to affect pragmatic aspects of language very differently. As we will see, the evidence suggests that pragmatic aspects of language are less vulnerable than other aspects to interference in focally engendered aphasia. However, pragmatic aspects are probably more vulnerable in the wake of generalized brain damage (Bayles & Kaszniak, 1987; Blanken,

Dittman, Haas, & Wallesch, 1987; Holland, 1982; Murdoch, 1990). Thus, treatments for the language disorders resulting from head injury or dementia that purport to capitalize on pragmatic strengths are not considered here.

This chapter describes the rationale and the research base for pragmatic approaches to assessment and therapy for aphasia. It explores standardized and observational approaches to assessing aphasia from a pragmatic perspective. Next, it briefly describes a few treatment approaches that have a pragmatic foundation. It concludes with notions about how work on pragmatic aspects of language can accompany treatment of syntactical, phonological, and lexical deficits in aphasia.

THE BASIS FOR PRAGMATIC APPROACHES

The rationale for pragmatic approaches to treatment comes from a number of sources. The most important is the relatively commonplace observation that aphasic people are maximally effective communicators when they can use their understanding of the way communication is conducted in everyday interactions. That is, aphasic people do better when they can capitalize on a message's verbal as well as its nonverbal context. They do better when they can be sure of their roles in a communicative situation, and when they can apply their unspoken knowledge of the way discourse is conducted and their knowledge of which scripts apply where and when.

This understanding is called *communicative competence.* It refers to a person's appropriate use of language and his or her understanding of the way the language works in social interactions within the speaker's culture (Hymes, 1972). Communicative competence appears to develop simultaneously with other language components. However, it seems less vulnerable than more formal components (e.g., lexicon, syntax, phonology) to damage by focal lesions in aphasia. Pragmatic skills certainly can be affected by focal brain damage; language structure and its use are clearly not doubly dissociated. Nevertheless, a substantial body of information supports the notion that pragmatic skills are relatively better preserved in aphasia than are lexical and syntactic components.

For example, aphasic individuals are sensitive to violations of politeness rules, as expressed in response to indirect requests (Wilcox, Davis, & Leonard, 1978). Despite linguistic limitations, aphasic patients can use compensatory strategies to convey intent (Glosser, Weiner, & Kaplan, 1986; Prinz, 1980). Even though they may confuse pronouns, aphasic patients use appropriate rules in their attempts at pronominalization (Kimbarow & Brookshire, 1982). Although breakdowns can (and do) occur frequently in conversations between aphasic and nonaphasic persons, and aphasic patients probably have a more limited repertoire of repair strategies, they use their repertories appropriately (Apel, Newhoff, & Browning-Hall, 1982). Further, in referential communication tasks, aphasics are as successful as nonaphasic individuals in identifying what information is crucial to communicate, although they are not as efficient or as accurate in communicating it (Busch, Brookshire, & Nicholas, 1989).

Word-retrieval deficits are a common impairment in aphasia. Yet most paraphasic errors are far from random and often show a surprising sensitivity to the linguistic demands of the situation. These errors support the notion that pragmatic skills are retained in aphasia. For example, the most conventional word-retrieval errors in confrontation naming are semantic paraphasia, regardless of the type of aphasia (LeDorze & Nespoulous, 1989), with in-class errors predominating (Marshall, 1976). Thus, the likelihood is that aphasic individuals will misname a "table" as a "bed" or a "chair," or that verbs will be replaced by other verbs in spontaneous speech, usually with appropriate inflectional morphology, except with agrammatical speakers. Similarly, patients with jargon aphasia generally speak within the phonological constraints of their native language (Buckingham & Kertesz, 1974). Agrammatical patients are also agrammatical within the constraints of the grammars of their languages (Bates & Wulfeck, 1989). Agrammatical aphasic patients manage to communicate salient and important aspects of their message (Doyle, Goldstein, & Bourgeois, 1987). In fact, some features of agrammatical output may represent a strategy for trading-off message saliency against ease of talking (Kolk & Van Grunsven, 1985). Further, even though gesture is symbolic communication, most patients who are free of limb apraxia can use gestures more effectively than they use speech or writing to communicate their messages (Duffy & Duffy, 1981).

Aphasic speakers seldom break cultural conventions in interpersonal interactions that define who may speak to whom, when to speak, and so forth. Patients with Wernicke's aphasia have been noted to follow conventional turn-taking rules when they talk to each other, although mutual difficulty in understanding renders their conversations somewhat disjointed (Schienberg & Holland, 1980).

Even patients with severe global aphasia can recognize their own language from foreign languages almost as well as normals can (Boller & Green, 1972; Green & Boller, 1974). Further, their nonverbal behavior is often used appropriately as compensation for verbal inadequacy (Herrman, Reichle, Lucius-Heone, Wallesch, & Johannsen-Horbach, 1988). Finally, it should be noted that clinicians and researchers implicitly rely on aphasic persons' knowledge of turn-taking rules almost automatically when they assess or provide therapy, and only infrequently have to mention these rules, even to patients who exhibit press-of-speech or have extensive global aphasia.

These studies confirm the notion that pragmatic components of aphasic language remain relatively intact. Another way to say this is that communicative competence in aphasia is probably more intact than is linguistic competence. Given the time-honored idea that a significant portion of aphasia therapy should be devoted to activities that maximize success, pragmatically based approaches are worthy of attention.

Another part of the rationale for pragmatic treatment for aphasia must be stated very carefully. Most carefully designed group and single-subject studies agree that aphasia therapy "works" (Wertz et al., 1986). Provided that clinical intervention with aphasic patients is systematic, relevant, frequent, applied to likely candidates, and performed by knowledgeable and empathic people, therapy should improve the aphasic condition. This does not mean that aphasia therapy overcomes aphasia in all cases. Therefore, the responsible aphasia clinician must also teach skills, strategies, and compensations that will be useful in circumventing some aspects of residual aphasia. Because pragmatically based approaches focus on communicative strengths, they have great compensatory potential. Many are designed to help aphasic patients when they experience communicative difficulty in their everyday activities. One aim of pragmatically oriented therapy is to help aphasic individuals accept the notion that language breakdowns, while unfortunate, are almost inevitable. The patient must also be taught to recognize these breakdowns when they occur, and then to use compensatory strategies.

FUNCTIONAL ASSESSMENT

Assessment of aphasic patients' pragmatic abilities requires a somewhat different slant on evaluation procedures, as well as different tools. A few standard measures are briefly described below. But less structured approaches, including observations of aphasic patients in communicative interactions, are also necessary.

Traditional aphasia tests focus on detailed description of the nonpragmatic components of the language deficits. Such measures are necessary prerequisites to pragmatic assessment. They form the background for defining the extent of need for pragmatic treatment and for describing the extent to which an aphasic patient is already compensating for deficits. If a given patient is making skillful adaptations to his or her deficits, pragmatic intervention techniques might be inappropriate. Conversely, the problem solving–oriented give-and-take of pragmatic intervention may well exceed the capabilities of the extensively globally impaired. The outcome of pragmatic assessment must be a careful weighing and balancing of aphasic strengths (usually pragmatic) and weaknesses (usually lexical, syntactic, phonologic) if one is to provide adequate intervention.

Standard Measures

Useful and interesting rating scales and evaluative approaches to measuring functional communication exist. These include Sarno's (1969) previously mentioned Functional Communication Profile (FCP), developed some years ago as an observational tool. The FCP requires clinicians to observe and then to rate functional adequacy of communicative behavior in a number of contexts. More recently, two new measures have been developed. The Amsterdam-Nijmegan Everyday Language Test (ANELT) by Blomert (1990) was designed to "measure verbal communicative behavior of aphasic patients as a function of the comprehensibility of the message and the intelligibility of the utterances for the listener." It uses a series of 10 scenarios of everyday activities, in which the aphasic patient is to provide an appropriate response. For example: "You see your neighbor walking by. You want to ask him/her to come visit sometime. What do you say?" Aphasic responses are scored according to criteria relating to the propositions employed by nonaphasic subjects in response to the ANELT items. The measure appears to be relatively easy to use. Unfortunately, it is limited to assessment of language production. The second recent measure is the Communicative Effectiveness Index (CETI) (Lomas et al., 1989). The CETI is a psychometrically well-designed 16-item rating scale, built on the aphasic person's family's perceptions of important communicative events, that was explicitly evaluated for its utility in measuring change in communication skills over time.

The test of Communicative Abilities of Daily Living (CADL) (Holland, 1980) provides direct measure of communication. This test uses simulated situations built into a scored interview procedure for measuring a number of aspects of functional communication. The test has been validated against observation of aphasic patients in actual everyday communications, and by correlation with formal language measures. Scoring is by the relative adequacy of communication performance, rather than accuracy of responses.

Observation

Direct observation is an important component of a pragmatic assessment. Such observations serve as the first step in helping the patient develop useful compensatory strategies for communicating. The aim is to create an inventory of the strategies that are used, as well as their relative effectiveness. Penn (1988) provides a comprehensive method for profiling communicative interaction in an interview. It is particularly beneficial to observe patients with their most typical communication partners (for example, spouses). This permits one to observe the relative sensitivity of the normal partner, as well as the strategies, both successful and unsuccessful, that these individuals use in communicating with the aphasic partner.

One is likely to find that some patients (and normal partners) use compensatory strategies naturally, spontaneously, and effectively. Others do not do so at all, seeming almost baffled by the communication barriers imposed by aphasia. Most patients and normal partners lie somewhere between these two extremes, using both effective and ineffective strategies, with mixed results. Later in this chapter, ways to apply these findings to treatment are discussed.

PRAGMATIC APPROACHES TO TREATMENT

A number of approaches can serve as examples of pragmatic treatment. Five approaches are described here, beginning with the most well-known: the procedure developed by Davis and Wilcox (1985) called "promoting aphasic communicative effectiveness" (PACE).

Promoting Aphasic Communicative Effectiveness

PACE is a format for clinical interaction designed to serve as a microcosm of a natural communication interchange. Implementation of PACE procedures is guided by principles of normal communicative interaction in which (1) new information is exchanged, (2) the patient can choose any communicative modality to convey a message, (3) clinician and patient participate equally as senders and receivers of information, and (4) the natural feedback of communicative interactions in everyday life provides the sender with feedback on whether or not a message is successfully communicated.

In a typical PACE interaction, the patient and therapist might communicate what objects are depicted on each of a stack of cards, placed face down, between the two participants. What is on the cards is not known to either participant. Let us say that the patient picks up a picture of a bull. He communicates the content by saying "It's a bell." The clinician's natural response would be to say something like "Oh, you have a picture of a bell." The patient can here correct the therapist by indicating no, for example, by gesturing a pair of horns, and the therapist can modify the statement as a function of this new input. Then the roles are reversed and the therapist chooses a card, communicates its contents, and so forth.

PACE activities are intended to provide communicative practice using a variety of modes of communication, illustrating to the aphasic patient alternative methods of effective communication. A feature of the paradigm is that therapist-as-sender behavior serves to influence patient-as-sender behavior. This provides a dramatic way for the therapist to teach effective communication.

Teaching Compensatory Strategies

A second pragmatic approach involves teaching compensatory strategies. This approach stems from the work of Whitney (1975). As suggested earlier, communicative strategies are devices that are useful for getting messages across, despite grammatical or lexical errors that occur in talking. Penn (1988) provides a comprehensive list of compensatory strategies that have been noted to occur in the verbal and nonverbal communication attempts of aphasic patients. A limited sampling of talking strategies includes simplifying messages, elaborating on them or repeating them, circumlocuting, and using placeholders and fillers to signal ongoing lexical searching.

Comprehension strategies involve techniques that aphasic patients might use for encouraging their nonaphasic conversation partners to modify their own messages to maximize their comprehensibility. Included here are devices such as teaching aphasic patients to ask nonaphasic speakers to speak more slowly, or to simplify or elaborate on their messages. Still other compensatory strategies include augmenting verbal messages by nonverbal means, or using writing to augment messages transmitted verbally. Such strategies are the focus of the observations described earlier.

Although all of the strategies listed above can potentially increase the aphasic patient's ability to communicate more effectively, there are also some strategies that are ineffective. Some simply do not work, others are inefficient, and others might be overused and their effectiveness decreased as a result. An example is an aphasic patient who does not switch topics with facility and tends to monopolize the conversation to avoid this problem.

For patients who have shown themselves to be minimally artful, didactic instruction might be necessary. An effective approach is to set up and then to require from the patient specific use of some strategies in very contextually constrained drills. For patients who have only limited understanding of compensations, the extent of effectiveness should be very directly and carefully explained, and then tasks devised to require the patient to use the strategies. Later, tasks that use the strategies in less controlled and guided contexts are imposed. All must be extended to conversation eventually. The method described next is an attempt to provide such training.

Conversational Coaching

The third example of a pragmatic approach is conversational coaching. This includes preparation of a short (i.e., six-to-eight-utterance) monologic script that is written to be slightly too difficult for the patient to produce. The script is designed to force the patient to use the strategies worked on previously (usually in the ways described earlier in this chapter). It is intended to be a bridging framework to initiate transfer of strategy use to patient-generated conversation. Once the script is prepared, the clinician and patient practice the script. The therapist suggests how strategies might be used to convey the script's content, and he or she guides the patient in performing it. Then a family member, who does not know the script, is called into the room, and the patent communicates the content while being coached by the clinician.

The clinician also coaches the family members to practice those strategies to maximize the patient's ability to communicate. Family members are also coached to ask questions, to guess, and so forth. Frequent checks on comprehension are made by having the family member repeat what the patient says. All of this is videotaped, and when the patient finishes the script, the clinician, family member, and patient view the tape and discuss it. The purpose of this discussion is to heighten awareness of both the aphasic patient and the family member as to which strategies were most effective, and why. The viewing and discussion also provide the therapist with further insight into ways that he or she might more effectively train the patient.

Next, the entire procedure is repeated with an unfamiliar person as the audience, and patient, therapist, and spouse again review the videotape, with the same goal. It should be noted that there are several contextual ways in which the difficulty of the task can be modified. First, the level of sophistication and familiarity of the listener can be varied. Second, scripts themselves can vary in informativeness, and therefore ease of decipherability. The easiest ones consist of old, known information; harder ones consist of new information; the most difficult ones comprise improbable events or gossip.

Conversational coaching is a formal approximation to communication in the environment outside the clinic. The messages themselves comprise controlled discourse, and family members and aphasic patients are the targets of treatment. Finally, the use of unfamiliar listeners extends the generalizability of the approach. The method is quite new, and only limited data concerning its effectiveness have been generated. Nevertheless, the use of videotape makes it possible to compare pre- and post-coaching sessions for the frequency and ease with which strategies are used, and pre- and post-coaching changes have been demonstrated. One patient has even been noted to use his scripts, when they are interesting and meaningful to him, as conversational devices with his family and friends, although this was never an intent of the method.

Using a Behavior Modification Method to Train Requesting

Behavior modification can also be used to achieve changes in pragmatic skills. Doyle, Goldstein, Bourgeois, and Nakles (1989) developed a rigorous behavioral approach for teaching aphasic individuals to make requests, and to ask questions of listeners. This work was first tested using a multiple baseline design across behaviors and subjects. Because one purpose was to demonstrate generalization beyond the treatment setting, multiple trainers were involved for each of the four subjects with which the approach was validated. Weekly sessions of 5-minute conversational interaction with trainers and with unfamiliar persons were used as probes in this study. Maintenance and follow-up work indicated increases in requesting that brought aphasics' requesting attempts within the range of those of normal speakers observed under the same probe conditions. These data attest to the efficacy of the approach.

Behavior modification generates requests through the following sequence. First, three conversational topics—personal information, leisure activities, and health—were chosen, and a list of prompts for use by the trainer were chosen. (For example, "You could ask where I work.") These prompts introduced topics and subtopics about which the subjects could request information and keep the conversation on topic. When necessary, the prompts were used in a random order by trainers after a particular topic was introduced. "Requests for information" were defined as "the conversational or elocutionary act of soliciting information or acknowledgment." Requests were also required to be intelligible, to be on the topic specified, to contain a question morpheme and a content word, or to end with a rising inflection. Note that grammatical accuracy was not required, nor even differentially reinforced. Each training session consisted of 20 trials per day, three times a day over 36–40 weeks, with probe sessions occurring weekly.

Even more impressive than the behavioral data were Doyle and colleagues' ecological validity data, showing statistically significant changes in talkativeness, inquisitiveness, and conversational success. Doyle notes that the method is more successful for aphasic pragmatic awareness. That is, sharing already-known information is essentially pragmatically inappropriate, and this is apparently recognized by aphasic patients using the technique, since the topics of Doyle's training contained information that was of communicative value to strangers, not to individuals who already knew the patient.

Working with Internal Language

A final pragmatic approach is more of an idea than a fulfilled treatment procedure. All of the approaches described above are to some extent therapist-driven in the sense that the language to be worked with, even the PACE cards chosen for sending "unknown information," are largely selected in advance by the clinician. Is this pragmatically defensible? It is not likely that therapists are clairvoyant. Chances are they do not know the words nor the intentions that their patients wish to convey. Rather, ideas and notions internal to the patient are the subjects of his or her aphasic struggle. Techniques that enhance and provide for patient-motivated language, such as one might find in incorporating natural conversation into therapy, or specifying the semantic field, but not the actual words from that semantic field for retrieval by the aphasic patient, are substantially within the pragmatic purview. So is the use of patient-generated diaries or personal oral histories. One pertinent feature of pragmatic approaches is that they specifically devote time to the content that the patient feels is important to convey.

Combining Pragmatic Approaches with More Direct
Language Treatment

The following comments represent a personal view of the most satisfactory way to conduct pragmatically appropriate speech and language therapy for aphasic patients. It should be clear that treatment requires not only pragmatic tactics, but other methods geared to other components of the problems faced by the aphasic individual. Even the most traditional methods can probably be refreshed by ensuring that the core content of training materials include useful, everyday materials. Most pragmatically astute therapists would not hesitate to use melodic intonation therapy (Helm-Estabrooks & Albert, 1991), as well as direct work on reading and writing (using functional language, where possible, of course), to name just a few. Also useful in conjunction with pragmatic approaches are visualization and relaxation techniques designed to reduce the stress that magnifies linguistic problems.

Exciting new therapy approaches are emerging from cognitive neuropsychology, exemplified by the work of Byng (1988), Behrman (1987), dePartz (1986), and their colleagues. Working from models designed to be very specific about the exact locus of linguistic breakdowns, these methods have solid rationales, display problem-specific creative inventiveness, and are quite principled in substantiating therapeutic gains by presenting relevant efficacy data. To date, much of this work centers on sentence processing and reading, but it has important implications for the development of techniques for working with other aspects of the aphasia spectrum, such as word-retrieval deficits, as well. Howard and colleagues (Howard & Orchard-Lisle, 1985; Howard, Patterson, Franklin, Orchard-Lisle, & Morton, 1985) and Lesser (1989) provide important and promising insights in this latter regard.

These approaches from cognitive neuropsychology can be quite comfortably combined with pragmatic approaches. One reason is that they are so specifically deficit-centered. This is just the opposite of the strength-centered pragmatic approach, but together, the approaches can result in a fairly comfortable balance between the molar and the more molecular components of language. A second reason for their compatibility is that most of the approaches depend on the patient's ability to engage in quite active problem-solving. That is, patients seem to be required to use the rest of their brains to overcome deficits in very specific but stimulating and innovative ways. If such is the case, then it can be argued that, like the pragmatic approaches, the successful use of approaches based in cognitive neuropsychology relies partly on residual skills, an aphasic patient's ability to understand the nature of their language deficits, and their communicative competence.

Second, it is necessary to view aphasia as a family problem, not a problem faced by a single individual. Therefore, a significant amount of treatment time must be devoted to counseling patients and families, whenever possible.

Finally, it is not clear how one determines the apportioning of clinical time among the pragmatic, the more direct linguistic, and the counseling aspects of aphasia treatment. Such apportioning probably depends on the nature of the aphasia, the characteristics of the aphasic individual, and even the characteristics of the therapist. However, maintaining a delicate balance among these elements, as described by Lyon in Chapter 8, is likely to be an important aspect of successful therapy. This is an important topic that needs further exploration.

In essence, reliance on pragmatic methods should be limited by common sense. A monolithic approach to aphasia treatment is probably never profitable to the patient. However, pragmatic considerations should almost always be a feature of treatment. This is because talking about what one wishes to talk about—not processing sentences, or retrieving words, or articulating correctly—is the primary goal of clinical intervention in aphasia.

CONCLUSIONS

Pragmatic approaches have a place in treating the aphasic patient. Neither the extent of their utility nor the forms that pragmatic treatment might take are as yet fully explicated. However, it is likely that some of these principles and some treatments stemming from them might not only be elaborated for aphasic individuals in the next decade, but find a place in the treatment regimens of adults who suffer from other types of speech and language disorders as well.

REFERENCES

Apel, K., Newhoff, M., & Browning-Hall, J. (1982, November). Contingent queries in Broca's aphasia. Paper presented at the annual meeting of the American Speech-Language-Hearing Association, Toronto.

Bates, E. (1976). *Language in context: The acquisition of pragmatics.* New York: Academic Press.

Bates, E., & Wulfeck, B. (1989). Comparative aphasiology: A cross-linguistic approach to language breakdown. *Aphasiology, 3,* 111–145.

Bayles, K., & Kaszniak, A. (1987). *Communication and cognition in normal aging and dementia.* Boston: Little, Brown.

Behrman, M. (1987). The rites of righting writing: Homophone remediation in acquired dysgraphia. *Cognitive Neuropsychogy, 4,* 365–384.

Blanken, G., Dittman, J., Haas, J., & Wallesch, C.W. (1987). Spontaneous speech in senile dementia and aphasia: Implication for a neurolinguistic model of language production. *Cognition, 27,* 247–274.

Blomert, L. (1990). What functional assessment can contribute to setting goals for aphasia therapy. *Aphasiology, 4,* 307–320.

Boller, F., & Green, E. (1972). Comprehension in severe aphasia. *Cortex, 8,* 382–394.

Buckingham, H., & Kertesz, A. (1974). A linguistic analysis of fluent aphasia. *Brain and Language, 1,* 143–161.

Busch, C., Brookshire, R., & Nicholas, L. (1989). Referential communication by aphasic and nonaphasic adults. *Journal of Speech and Hearing Disorders 53,* 475–482.

Byng, S. (1988). Sentence processing deficits: Theory and therapy. *Cognitive Neuropsychology, 5,* 629–676.

Davis, G., & Wilcox, M.J. (1985). *Adult aphasia rehabilitation: Applied pragmatics.* San Diego: College-Hill.

dePartz, M. (1986). Re-education of a deep dyslexic patient: Rationale of the methods and results. *Cognitive Neuropsychology, 3,* 149-177.

Doyle, P., Goldstein, H., & Bourgeois, M. (1987). Experimental analysis of syntax training of Broca's aphasia: A generalization and social validation study. *Journal of Speech and Hearing Disorders, 52,* 143–155.

Doyle, P., Goldstein, H., Bourgeois, M., & Nakles, K. (1989). Facilitating generalized requesting behavior in Broca's aphasia: An experimental analysis of a generalization training procedure. *Journal of Applied Behavior Analysis, 22,* 157–170.

Duffy, R., & Duffy, J. (1981). Three studies of deficits in pantomimic expression and pantomimic recognition in aphasia. *Journal of Speech and Hearing Research, 24,* 70–84.

Glosser, G., Weiner, M., & Kaplan, E. (1986). Communicative gestures in aphasia. *Journal of Speech and Hearing Disorders, 27,* 345–359.

Green, E., & Boller, F. (1974). Features of auditory comprehension in severely impaired aphasics. *Cortex, 10,* 133–145.

Helm-Estabrooks, N., & Albert, M. (1991). *Manual of aphasia therapy.* Austin, TX: PRO-ED.

Herrman, M., Reichle, T., Lucius-Heone G., Wallesch, C.W., & Johannsen-Horbach, H. (1988). Nonverbal communication as a compensatory strategy for severely nonfluent aphasics—A quantitative approach. *Brain and Language, 33,* 41–54.

Holland, A. (1980). Communicative abilities in daily living: A test of functional communication for aphasic adults. Baltimore: University Park.

Holland, A. (1982). When is aphasia aphasia? The problem of closed head injury. In R. Brookshire (Ed.), *Clinical aphasiology conference proceedings.* Minneapolis: BRK Publishers.

Howard, D., & Orchard-Lisle, V. (1985). On the origin of semantic errors in naming: Evidence from the case of a global aphasic. *Cognitive Neuropsychology, 1,* 163–190.

Howard, D., Patterson, D., Franklin, S., Orchard-Lisle, V., & Morton, J. (1985). The facilitation for picture naming in aphasia. *Cognitive Neuropsychology, 2,* 49–80.

Hymes, D. (1972). Toward ethnographies of communication: The analysis of communicative events. In P.P. Giglioli (Ed.), *Language and social context.* Middlesex, CT: Penguin.

Kimbarow, M., & Brookshire, R. (1982). The influence of communication context on aphasic speakers' use of pronouns. In R. Brookshire (Ed.), *Clinical aphasiology conference proceedings.* Minneapolis: BRK Publishers.

Kolk, H., & Van Grunsven, M. (1985). Agrammatism is a variable phenomenon. *Cognitive Neuropsychology, 2,* 347–384.

LeDorze, G., & Nespoulous, J.L. (1989). Anomia in moderate aphasia: Problems in accessing the lexical representation. *Brain and Language, 37,* 381–400.

Lesser, R. (1989). Some issues in the neuropsychological rehabilitation of anomia. In X. Seron & G. Deloche (Eds.), *Cognitive approaches in neuropsychological rehabilitation.* Hillside, NJ: Lawrence Erlbaum.

Lomas, J., Pichard, L., Bester, S., Elbard, H., Finlayson, A., & Zoghaib, C. (1989). The communicative effectiveness index: Development and psychometric evaluation of a functional communication measure for adult aphasia. *Journal of Speech and Hearing Disorders, 54,* 113–24.

Marshall, R. (1976). Word retrieval of aphasic adults. *Journal of Speech and Hearing Disorders, 41,* 444–451.

Murdoch, B. (1990). *Acquired speech and language disorders.* London: Chapman and Hall.

Penn, C. (1988). The profiling of syntax and pragmatics in aphasia. *Clinical Linguistics and Phonetics, 2,* 179–207.

Prinz, P. (1980). A note on requesting strategies in adult aphasics. *Journal of Communication Disorders, 13,* 65–73.

Sarno, M.T. (1969). *Functional communication profile.* New York: Institute for Rehabilitation Medicine.

Schienberg, S., & Holland, A. (1980). Conversational turn taking in Wernicke's aphasia. In R. Brookshire (Ed.), *Clinical aphasiology conference proceedings.* Minneapolis: BRK Publishers.

Searle, J.R. (1969). *Speech acts.* London: Cambridge University Press.

Wertz, R.T., Weiss, D., Aten, J., Brookshire, R., Garcia-Bunuel, L., Holland, A., Kurtzke, J., LaPointe, L., Milianti, F., Brannegan, R., Greenbaum, H., Marshall, R., Vogel, D., Carter, J., Barnes, J., & Goodman, R. (1986). Comparison of clinic, home and deferred language treatment for aphasia: Veterans Administration cooperative study. *Archives of Neurology 43,* 653–658.

Whitney, J. (1975). *Developing aphasics' use of compensatory strategies.* Paper presented at the annual meeting of the American Speech-Language-Hearing Association, Washington, DC.

Wilcox, M.J., Davis, G.A., & Leonard, L.B. (1978). Aphasics' comprehension of contextually conveyed requests. *Brain and Language, 6,* 362–377.

Chapter 10

Treatment of Auditory Comprehension Impairment

Robert S. Pierce and Janet P. Patterson

Auditory comprehension impairments are common in aphasia. Almost all aphasic adults have difficulty understanding some aspects of a speaker's message. This chapter discusses variables that affect how well aphasic adults comprehend messages. Typically, an auditory comprehension treatment task requires a patient to demonstrate understanding of a specific component of an auditory stimulus, such as a single word, a sentence, or a narrative. Accordingly, this chapter is organized around the domains of single words, sentences, and narratives. This is not to say that these domains represent an invariant hierarchy of difficulty, because they do not. Nor does it suggest that variables that affect comprehension accuracy are active in only one of these domains, because they are not.

SINGLE-WORD LEVEL

Semantic Dimensions

Words can be ranked along many semantic dimensions. For example, Toglia and Battig (1978) obtained ratings from college students for 2,854 words on several semantic dimensions including familiarity, meaningfulness, concreteness, imagery, and categorization (the ability to identify a superordinate category for a word). Two main higher-order semantic dimensions emerged. One consisted of concreteness, imagery, and categorization. The other consisted of familiarity and meaningfulness. In addition, Toglia and Battig reported that frequency of occurrence could be added to this second dimension because it correlates strongly with familiarity.

The finding that these two semantic dimensions somewhat independently influence word ranking in normal persons suggests that they could exert related but potentially distinct effects on comprehension accuracy in patients with aphasia. Researchers have long recognized that word frequency influences single-word comprehension; higher-frequency words are comprehended more accurately than are lower-frequency words (Schuell, Jenkins, & Landis, 1961). Shewan and Bandur (1986) recommended this continuum as a basis for selecting words to emphasize in treatment. In addition, the dimension of concreteness also influences comprehension accuracy (Goldstein, 1948). What is not known is the extent to which these two dimensions influence comprehension independently of each other.

The application of these dimensions to individual patients is not without problems. One difficulty relates to the nature of the norms themselves. Toglia and Battig (1978) stress that "any reliability or validity of these mean ratings is not indicative of high consistency between individual subjects on the ratings given to any particular word" (p. 14). Accordingly, a word that is high in familiarity for one person may be lower on this dimension for another person. Clearly, each person's experiences in life will determine the vocabulary to which she or he is most familiar. This is particularly important since recent research suggests that familiarity may be more important than frequency of occurrence for successful comprehension, at least for patients with severe aphasia (Wallace & Canter, 1985; Van Lancker & Klein, 1990). Another problem is that frequency counts typically do not account for the homographic nature of words. Many words have a number of distinct meanings of which some are more typical than others. Pierce (1984) demonstrated that aphasic patients comprehend typical meanings more accurately than nontypical meanings. For example, while the word *bank* has a high frequency of occurrence, aphasic subjects' success at comprehending it depends on whether it refers to a place to store valuables or the side of a river. Francis and Kucera (1982) corrected for this problem to some extent by providing frequency counts based on a word's grammatical role.

Even if clinicians use these continua as rough guidelines for selecting treatment items, the question remains as to how far along them to go. Clinicians commonly emphasize comprehension of high-frequency words with more severely impaired patients. However, as comprehension skills improve, treatment emphasis often changes to tasks involving sentences and other aspects of the comprehension process, while work on individual words becomes de-emphasized. It is not clear whether this is appropriate. It may be beneficial to continue emphasizing the comprehension of specific words by the systematic introduction of less frequently occurring or less familiar vocabulary. This may be particularly important because aphasic patients' comprehension of sentential and discourse material relies greatly on the application of semantic and contextual knowledge, of which word meanings are a major component. This issue is discussed in the following sections of this chapter.

Semantic Knowledge

When treating comprehension by asking patients to select from among an array of pictures based on the spoken word, performance accuracy is influenced by the nature of the pictures in the array. Using arrays of five pictures, Butterworth, Howard, and McLoughlin (1984) found that aphasic patients performed similarly to normals when the pictures were unrelated to each other. However, when the arrays contained pictures that were semantically related (e.g., different members of the same category), the aphasic patients' performance was significantly impaired. These authors suggest that aphasic patients are capable of only superficial semantic analysis. That is, they appreciate some semantic features of words but not others. For example, appreciation of the superordinate feature of *fruit* would be sufficient to distinguish the word *apple* from *horse, comb,* and *ball* but not from *orange, grape,* and *banana.* This type of confusion among semantically related words is reported frequently in the literature (Gainotti, Miceli, Caltagirone, Silveri, & Musullo, 1981; Gardner, Albert, & Weintraub, 1975; Lesser, 1974; Pierce, Jarecki, & Cannito, 1990; Pizzamiglio & Appicciafuoco, 1971).

Whether semantically related arrays cause particular problems also depends on the size of the arrays. Pierce et al. (1990) found that patients with aphasia did significantly worse with related arrays compared to unrelated arrays when the array size was six and eight pictures but not when the array size was either two or four pictures. The smaller array sizes may reduce the demands on stimulus retention and visual scanning so that more processing attention can be devoted to semantic analysis. Accordingly, patients can conduct a finer semantic analysis, which allows them to successfully distinguish among the pictures. Alternatively, a superficial semantic analysis may be sufficient to distinguish from among a small array of pictures while a more detailed analysis is required for choosing from among a larger set of pictures.

These studies raise the issue of what aphasic patients know about the words that they appear to comprehend. Many years ago, Goodglass and Baker (1976) reported that there are holes in the semantic fields of some aphasic patients. That is, patients know some semantic associations but not others. If a patient demonstrates comprehension of the word *chair* by pointing to the correct picture on the word discrimination subtest of the Boston Diagnostic Aphasia Examination (BPAE) (Goodglass & Kaplan, 1983), what does that patient know about chairs? Does the patient with poorer comprehension skills know only enough about chairs to pick the correct picture? Does the patient with better comprehension skills know much more about chairs than the patient with poorer comprehension, although both can choose the correct picture on the BDAE? Does having a richer knowledge of concepts represented by specific words contribute in any meaningful way to the notion of better comprehension skills? The answers to these questions could have significant impact on how we assess and treat single-word comprehension skills in aphasic patients (see Germani and Pierce, 1995).

Contextual Influences

The traditional assessment of single-word comprehension in contextually barren environments may not provide a complete indication of aphasic patients' comprehension skills. Words are usually encountered within some context that supports their meaning. That context can make it easier for aphasic patients to comprehend the words. Clark and Flowers (1983) found that a supportive linguistic context (e.g., "Which one is the book that you read?") generated significantly better comprehension accuracy for aphasic patients than did the same target word without the context ("Which one is the book?"). Pierce and Beekman (1985) found that a target noun in a sentence was comprehended more accurately when a preceding supportive sentence was provided than when it was not. Similar benefits accrued when the supportive information occurred after the target utterance, but not when the target utterance was simply repeated once (Pierce, 1988).

Brookshire (1987) suggests that context improves the comprehension of target information because it allows the listener to ignore the target and respond based on the context alone. Work by Clark and Flowers (1983) argues against that notion. They found that the items containing the target plus the contextual support (e.g., "Which one is the book that you read?") were comprehended significantly more accurately than those items with just the contextual information ("Which is the one you read?"). Improved comprehension derives from an interaction between the target and the contextual information, rather than either one on its own. Interestingly, the use of redundant vocabulary is a common modification made by nonaphasic speakers when talking to aphasic patients (Gravel & LaPointe, 1983; Linebaugh, Pryor, & Margulies, 1983).

To date, the positive benefit of contextual influences has been strongest in aphasic patients with relatively poor comprehension skills. As discussed previously, it is possible that these patients have impoverished semantic representations. Perhaps the context emphasizes semantic features that are not activated independently. This enriched semantic representation might lead to better comprehension. In the psycholinguistic literature, Barsalou (1982) and Greenspan (1991) have argued that concepts are composed of context-independent and context-dependent attributes. Context-independent attributes are activated regardless of the context and serve as the core meaning of a word. Context-dependent attributes compose the sense of a word (Anderson, 1990), becoming activated only if the context emphasizes them. Pierce and Townsend (1990) demonstrated that in patients with dementia of the Alzheimer's type, context-independent attributes lose their independence; that is, their activation becomes sensitive to the context. A similar process may occur in patients with aphasia. Germani (1994) report-

TABLE 10.1   A Hierarchy of Difficulty From Easiest to Most Difficult of Different Syntactic Constructions

Negatives
Gender
Reflexives
Prepositions
Tense
Word order
Relative clauses

ed that more semantic features were available to aphasia patients when supportive context was present.

Finally, it should be noted that context does not always improve comprehension. It can make comprehension worse. Pierce and DeStefano (1987) found that aphasic patients could accurately select responses from an array of seemingly unrelated words because the surrounding narrative contexts were weak. However, the patients did significantly worse when the word choices became more related by virtue of logically fitting with stronger, more predictive contexts. These findings also highlight the interactions that can occur among the factors that influence comprehension of single words in patients with aphasia.

SENTENTIAL LEVEL

When aphasic patients are asked to comprehend sentences, a number of factors emerge that are not pertinent at the single-word level. These include syntax, sentence length, memory, speaking rate, and quantity of information.

Syntax

Aphasic patients have difficulty deriving meaning from the syntax of a sentence. This is not an all-or-none phenomenon, and some syntactic constructs are more difficult than others. Table 10.1 contains a general hierarchy of difficulty as suggested by a number of studies (Butler-Hinz, Waters, & Caplan, 1990; Lesser, 1974; Naeser, Mazurski, Goodglass, Peraino, Laughlin, & Leaper, 1987; Parisi & Pizzamiglio, 1970; Pierce, 1983; Sherman & Schweickert, 1989). The exact order of difficulty varies across studies and across patients. However, in general, negatives, gender, and some prepositions are easier to comprehend, while relative clauses, tense, and word order are more difficult. Difficulty comprehending syntax is not confined to aphasic patients with poor comprehension skills, or those with agrammatism. It occurs in patients with all types of aphasia, including those with better overall comprehension skills (Ansell & Flowers, 1982; Peach, Canter, & Gallaher, 1988; Pierce, 1983).

The traditional way of assessing syntactic comprehension in isolated sentences may overestimate the severity of the deficit. One reason relates to the allocation of processing resources. When sentences containing a complex syntactic structure (e.g., John was hit by Mary) are presented in isolation, aphasic patients must attend to the meaning of the lexical items (John, hit, Mary) as well as to the relationship among them (Mary was the agent and John was the object). These demands often exceed aphasic patients' capabilities, and their processing of the syntactic relationship suffers (Peach et al., 1988). However, when these sentences are preceded by narratives that identify the characters and predict the forthcoming action (but do not predict the syntactic relationship of who will be the agent and who will be the recipient of the action), aphasic patients comprehend the syntax of the sentences more accurately (Cannito, Jarecki, & Pierce, 1986; Hough, Pierce, & Cannito, 1989). Presumably, since the patients already know the key lexical items and the probable action based on the narrative, they can devote less processing attention to them in the target sentences and more to identifying the syntactic relationship. In normal daily communication, it is unusual for sentences to contain all "new" information. Typically, sentences contain mostly "old" information with a bit of "new" information added. In the previous sentence, the listener would probably have already known that John and Mary were involved in the act of hitting. Only in the traditional treatment paradigm would aphasic listeners have to process an entire sentence as if it were "new" information.

In contrast, single-sentence nonpredictive contexts do not significantly enhance the comprehension of reversible sentences (Pierce & Wagner, 1985). It is possible that single-sentence contexts do not provide sufficient exposure to key lexical items to alleviate forthcoming processing demands.

Aphasic patients also comprehend difficult syntactic relationships more accurately if the surface structure of the sentences identifies those relationships clearly. For example, the sentences below generated three significantly different levels of comprehension accuracy ("a" was the most difficult and "c" was the easiest) (Pierce, 1981; Pierce, 1982):

a. The man washed the car.
b. The man has washed the car.
c. The man has already washed the car.

Difficulty both in comprehending past tense and in recognizing that the sentence is in the past tense contributed to the impairment in understanding sentence "a." The additional surface structure markers in "b" and "c" made it easier for aphasic patients to recognize that the sentence is in the past tense. Similar results were found for future tense and reversible passive constructions.

Aphasic patients can use semantic and pragmatic strategies to work around their problems in comprehending syntax. As might be expected, the more difficulty patients have with syntax, the more they rely on semantic/pragmatic strategies (Sherman & Schweickert, 1989). Aphasic patients comprehend reversible sentences, where world knowledge predicts that one agent/object relationship is more plausible than the other (e.g., The cat lies in wait for the mouse.), more accurately than they do sentences where both agent/object relationships are equally plausible (e.g., The soldier charms the girl.) (Deloche & Seron, 1981). Sentences that are nonreversible based on semantic constraints (e.g., The flower was picked by the girl) are significantly easier to comprehend than are reversible sentences (e.g., The man was kissed by the woman) (Caramazza & Zurif, 1976; Heilman, Scholes, & Watson, 1976; Sherman & Schweickert, 1989).

The surrounding context can also generate plausibility. Reversible sentences that are difficult for aphasic patients to comprehend in isolation are significantly easier when preceded or followed by single sentences or narration that predict a particular agent/object relationship (Hough et al., 1989; Pierce, 1988; Pierce & Beekman, 1985; Pierce & Wagner, 1985). For example, the sentence "John was hit by Mary" would be comprehended more accurately if the listener knew that John had a black eye. Again, researchers have questioned whether this type of predictive context facilitates comprehension because it allows listeners to simply ignore the target information and respond based solely on the context (Brookshire, 1987; Huber, 1990). Using a reading comprehension task, Germani and Pierce (1990) found that aphasic patients performed as well when predictive narrative contexts were presented by themselves as they did when the reversible target sentences were presented by themselves. However, they did significantly better when the two were presented together. This supports the notion, mentioned above, that contextual facilitation relies on an interaction between target and context.

Caplan and Evans (1990) highlighted the power of semantic/pragmatic strategies. They tested aphasic patients who performed poorly on context-free sentence-level tests of syntactic comprehension. These patients did equally well at comprehending stories that were composed of either syntactically simple sentences or syntactically complex sentences that were semantically or pragmatically constrained. If one accepts the notion that daily communication environments typically contain semantic and pragmatic constraints, then one could argue that comprehension deficits for the type of syntactic structures discussed in this section do not play a prominent role in aphasic patients' functional comprehension skills.

Length, Amount of Information, Speaking Rate, and Memory

The relationship between sentence length, amount of information, and memory is cloudy at best. Kearns and Hubbard (1983) provided a hierarchy

Table 10.2   A Hierarchy of Auditory Comprehension Tasks From Easiest to More Difficult

Point to one common object by name.
*Point to one common object by function.
Point in sequence to two common objects by function.
*Point in sequence to two common objects by name.
Point to one object spelled by examiner.
Point to one object described by the examiner with three descriptors ("Which one is white, plastic, and has bristles?").
Follow one-verb instruction ("Pick up the pen").
Point in sequence to three common objects by name.
Point in sequence to three common objects by function.
Carry out two-object location instructions ("Put the pen in front of the knife").
*Carry out, in sequence, two-verb instruction ("Point to the knife. Turn over the fork").
Carry out, in sequence, two-verb instructions, with time constraint ("Before you pick up the knife, hand me the fork").
*Carry out three-verb instructions ("Point to the knife. Turn over the fork. Touch the pencil").

*Represents four levels of significantly different performance accuracy.
Source: Modified from K.F. Kearns, D. Hubbard. (1983). A Comparison of Auditory Comprehension Tasks in Aphasia. In R.K. Brookshire (Ed.), *Clinical Aphasiology*. Minneapolis: BRK Publishers.

of stimuli difficulty based on commands (Table 10.2). This overall hierarchy reflects increased length, amount of information, the fact that verbs are often more difficult to comprehend than nouns, and grammatical complexity.

Increasing length does not necessarily impair comprehension. If sentence length is increased to reduce grammatical complexity without adding any new information, the longer sentences may be easier to understand. For example, longer, less complex sentences such as, "The man was greeted by his wife and he was smoking a pipe" are significantly easier for aphasic subjects to comprehend than their shorter but more complex counterparts, "The man greeted by his wife was smoking a pipe" (Goodglass et al., 1979). However, if sentence length increases because of the addition of nonredundant information, then comprehension for some aphasic patients can suffer. Curtis, Jackson, Kempler, Hanson, and Metter (1983) systematically varied the influence of length and syntactic complexity using stimuli exemplified in Table 10.3. Of their 10 aphasic patients, four demonstrated a length effect, four demonstrated a syntax effect, and the other two showed a mixed pattern. None of these groups were homogeneous with relationship to aphasia type.

Sensitivity to increased length based on the inclusion of nonredundant information may relate to memory. It is well established that aphasic patients have deficits in verbal short-term memory (Albert, 1976; Martin & Feher, 1990; Tandridag, Kirshner, & Casey, 1987). Martin and Fehr (1990) demonstrated that aphasic patients' sequential short-term memory skills related to their comprehension accuracy of commands of increasing length based on nonredundant information (similar to those in Table 10.3). This is

TABLE 10.3   Examples of Stimuli

4-word sentences
Touch the red circle.
Touch the yellow square.
Touch each yellow one.
Touch the square quickly.

5-word sentences
Touch the large green circle.
Touch the small blue circle.
Touch only two big ones.
Touch one that isn't white.

8-word sentences
Touch the yellow circle and the red square.
Touch the green square and the blue circle.
Touch the blue circle with the red square.
Except for the green one, touch the circles.

10-word sentences
Touch the small yellow circle and the large green square.
Touch the small blue square and the small yellow circle.
Pick up all the circles except the yellow one.
If there is a yellow square, touch the green circle.

Source: Modified from S. Curtis, C.A. Jackson, D. Kempler, W.R. Hanson, & E.H. Metter. (1983). Length vs. Structural Complexity in Sentence Comprehension in Aphasia. In R.K. Brookshire (Ed.), *Clinical Aphasiology*. Minneapolis: BRK Publishers.

not too surprising, given the similarity between the two types of stimuli. However, sequential short-term memory was not related to the patients' ability to comprehend sentences containing more complex syntax (see also McCarthy & Warrington, 1987). Grogan and Pierce (1991) used a test of working memory during reading with aphasic patients. This test, modeled after Daneman and Green (1986), tapped the retention of information along with the processing of new sentential information. Daneman and Carpenter (1980) found that working memory in normal subjects strongly related to their reading comprehension level. However, Grogan and Pierce did not find a significant relationship between aphasic patients' performance on their working memory test and the comprehension of newspaper articles.

Memory may play a role in the comprehension of strings of nonredundant information, such as Token Test-type commands (Martin and Fehr, 1990). However, these types of stimuli have questionable ecological validity. Memory appears to play a more limited role in comprehending the type of linguistic information typically encountered in daily life. McCarthy and Warrington (1990) suggest that memory's primary role in language comprehension occurs when patients must backtrack over a spoken message in order to rethink or reorganize the information. This can occur when expectations generated by a sentence are violated or when additional cognitive operations, such as comparative judgments, must be applied to the information in the sentence. Memory limitations may also explain why aphasic patients sometimes benefit from others speaking slower. If their rate of processing cannot keep up with the rate of presentation, they have difficulty retaining the information in order to process it retrospectively.

NARRATIVE LEVEL

While there are several models of narrative text processing in normal individuals (Frederickson, 1975; Frederickson, Bracewell, Breuleux, & Renaud, 1990; Thorndyke, 1977; van Dijk & Kintsch, 1983), they all have a common tenet: a text consists of information that is greater than the sum of its lexical and grammatical parts. Comprehension of narrative text requires integration of information derived both from the text and from other sources. Accordingly, many factors, such as characteristics of the text, contextual and extralinguistic variables, and individual processing strategies can influence comprehension. In designing treatment programs, clinicians can maximize opportunities for success in text comprehension by carefully considering these factors (Ulatowska & Chapman, 1989).

Characteristics of the Text

Cohesion is one feature that can be manipulated within a text. Cohesive passages contain word-level ties across sentence boundaries (Halliday & Hasan, 1976), which connect sentences in the passage and allow a listener to integrate new information and predict upcoming events. Matthews (1981), using a story retelling task, reported that cohesive texts were comprehended more accurately by adults with aphasia than were noncohesive texts. Huber and Gleber (1982), however, reported that linguistic cohesion did not affect performance on a scrambled story task. Their aphasic subjects did equally well at recognizing the information about the gist of a text in both high- and low-cohesion conditions.

　　Coherence in a passage links idea units. Texts can be locally coherent over a span of several adjacent sentences, and globally coherent across an entire text (Davis & Wilcox, 1985). Wegner, Brookshire, and Nicholas (1984) examined recognition of main ideas and details in coherent and noncoherent passages and found that, for subjects with aphasia, coherence did not affect the comprehension of main ideas, but did affect the comprehension of details. Contrary to expectations, comprehension of details was more accurate in the noncoherent passages than in the coherent passages. The authors suggested that the details in the noncoherent passages were more like lists of unrelated words, having little semantic overlap, which may be easier to retain than lists of related words.

　　An alternative explanation relates to aphasic adults' retained ability to recall more first- and second-level propositions (more important constructions located higher in the hierarchical representation of a passage) than third-level propositions (less important propositions located lower in the hierarchy) (Patterson, 1990). Because noncoherent passages contain several different topics, the amount of information about each topic is reduced and typically placed higher in the hierarchy. By virtue of this placement, the information is better retained.

Adults with aphasia demonstrate preserved knowledge of the hierarchical structure of narratives. Information higher in the hierarchical representation (that is, main ideas) (Wegner et al., 1984), first- or second-level propositions (Patterson, 1990), or highly salient information units (Ernest-Baron, Brookshire, & Nicholas, 1987), is recalled better than information lower in the hierarchy such as details (Wegner et al., 1984), third-level propositions (Patterson, 1990), or information units with low salience (Ernest-Baron et al., 1987). Comprehension of narrative passages can be aided by using an initial teaching strategy that accentuates the division between higher- and lower-order information within passages. Later treatment goals and materials might increase the amount or complexity of information within passages, thus reducing or clouding the division between levels of information.

Narratives frequently include information that is both directly and indirectly stated. Comprehension of indirectly stated information typically requires inference by the listener. Brookshire and Nicholas (1984, 1986) investigated comprehension of both types of statements in persons with aphasia. Comprehension of the main ideas of a passage was unaffected by whether the information was directly or indirectly stated. Contradictory results were noted for the details of a passage; in one study, details were unaffected by statement type (Brookshire & Nicholas, 1984), but in another (Nicholas & Brookshire, 1986) details were comprehended more accurately when directly stated than when indirectly stated. The authors related the distinction to the degree of inferencing required. Indirectly stated details that required more inferencing by listeners were more difficult to comprehend than were the directly stated details. Details that required less inferencing were not. Accordingly, the degree of difficulty of questions used to assess narrative comprehension may be varied by whether they refer to main ideas or details, and the amount of inferencing required to obtain the details from the narrative.

Contextual and Extralinguistic Variables

The well-documented influence of contextual variables in comprehension (van Dijk & Kintsch, 1983) is considered relevant to developing treatment programs for adults with aphasia (Brookshire, 1987; Nicholas & Brookshire, 1986). Using van Dijk and Kintsch's model as a guide, three sources contributing to comprehension can be identified: the textbase, situational knowledge, and world knowledge. Each of these sources can be manipulated in treatment, allowing clients to take advantage of all available information during comprehension.

The textbase consists of information obtained directly from the narrative. Information in the textbase is converted from surface structure to propositional form, and stored in memory for later retrieval. Aspects of the textbase from which information can be derived were presented in previous sections.

Situational knowledge affects comprehension at two points. At the early stages of input, it provides a framework to assist in the organization of incoming information. Following text presentation, situational knowledge contributes to the creation of a mental representation of the text (van Dijk & Kintsch, 1983). Adults with aphasia have shown intact situational knowledge for several text formats, including procedural discourse (Ulatowska, Allard, & Chapman, 1990; Ulatowska, Doyel, Stern, Haynes, & North, 1983; Ulatowska, North, & Macaluso-Haynes, 1981), narrative discourse (Ulatowska, North, & Macaluso-Haynes, 1981; Chapman & Ulatowska, 1989) and scripts (Armus, Brookshire, & Nicholas, 1989). The clinician might capitalize on this ability to use situational knowledge by identifying the overall structure of narratives to be presented so that the adult with aphasia may know what to expect.

World knowledge is defined as one's storehouse of information and includes generally accepted information and individual memories. World knowledge can facilitate comprehension of a text. Within world knowledge are subsets of specialized information referred to as domain knowledge (Yekovich, Walker, Ogle, & Thompson, 1990). Domain knowledge, too, can be manipulated in aphasia to build comprehension skills. Stimulus passages can be designed to take advantage of a client's knowledge by using familiar topics to develop strategies for comprehending less familiar text material.

Processing at the sentential and narrative levels can influence each other. For example, processing requirements at the microlinguistic level (sentence level) can be reduced by using syntactically simple sentence structure (few clauses or embedded phrases), thereby allowing more processing to be devoted to the macrolinguistic level. Those processing strategies used at the macrolinguistic level to create a narrative macrostructure or gist can also be applied to more syntactically complex passages, thus reducing the need to comprehend the syntax of each sentence. Huber (1990) and Caplan and Evans (1990) suggest that the macrostructure of a passage is often strong enough to override sentential features, making comprehension of a narrative possible without full comprehension of each sentence.

The rate of text input can influence comprehension. Nicholas and Brookshire (1986) reported that comprehension was facilitated by slowing the rate of presentation and pausing between sentences. However, the effect was inconsistent across subjects and trials.

Strategies to Aid Comprehension

One strategy most helpful in comprehending a text is identifying the theme or gist of the text. Aphasic listeners benefit from thematic information equally well whether it occurs at the beginning or at the end of a narrative (Hough, 1990). In addition, delayed recall of narrative information is greatly improved by the presentation of thematic information as a cue (Patterson, 1990). Treatment goals that incorporate identification of the theme of a passage may be valuable in helping aphasic adults more efficiently create and retain a text macrostructure.

Adults with aphasia remain sensitive to the distinction between main ideas and details of a text (Ernest-Baron et al., 1987; Glosser & Deser, 1990; Huber, 1990; Ulatowska et al., 1990; Wegner et al., 1984). Because they arrange propositions into a hierarchy and retain information better from higher in the hierarchy than lower in the hierarchy (Ernest-Baron et al., 1987; Glosser & Deser, 1990; Patterson, 1990), treatment might emphasize the more central propositions (main ideas and important details) that should be arranged at the higher levels, and then progress to the less central (and presumably less important) details.

Narratives contain both directly and indirectly stated information. Indirectly stated information requires inference before comprehension (Siefert, 1990). Van den Broek (1990) stated that backward inferences connect given and new information, while forward inferences allow the prediction of upcoming text. Treatment techniques to develop the use of inferences might include direct instruction, providing examples, presenting questions that elicit inference, and cuing. Treatment could progress from the provision of strong and direct information in the early stages to minimal assistance at later stages in treatment. The degree of required inferencing can also be varied from minimal to more extensive.

SUMMARY

Many factors influence comprehension in aphasic adults. The specific factors that are relevant to a particular task depend on whether the patient is asked to demonstrate comprehension of a single word, a sentence, or a narrative. To complicate matters, factors may be relevant for a particular target utterance presented in one condition but not another. For example, syntactic complexity has a significant impact on comprehension accuracy at the level of single sentences but frequently has little impact on the comprehension of sentences contained within narratives. An awareness by the clinician of these factors and how they influence performance will improve the quality of treatment for auditory comprehension deficits in adults with aphasia.

REFERENCES

Albert, M. (1976). Short-term memory and aphasia. *Brain and Language, 3,* 26–33.

Anderson, R.C. (1990). Inferences about word meanings. In A.C. Graesse & G.H. Bower (Eds.), *Inferences and text comprehension.* New York: Academic Press.

Ansell, B.J., & Flowers, C.R. (1982). Aphasic adults' use of heuristic and structural linguistic cues for sentence analysis. *Brain and Language, 16,* 61–72.

Armus, S.R., Brookshire, R.H., & Nicholas, L.E. (1989). Aphasic and nonbrain-damaged adults' knowledge of scripts for common situations. *Brain and Language, 36,* 518–528.

Barsalou, L. (1982). Context-independent and context-dependent information in concepts. *Memory and Cognition, 10,* 82–93.

Brookshire, R.H. (1987). Auditory language comprehension disorders in aphasia. *Topics in Language Disorders, 8*(1), 11–23.

Brookshire, R.H., & Nicholas, L.E. (1984). Comprehension of directly and indirectly stated main ideas and details in discourse by brain-damaged and nonbrain-damaged listeners. *Brain and Language, 21,* 1–36.

Butler-Hinz, S., Waters, G., & Caplan, D. (1990). Characteristics of syntactic comprehension deficits following closed head injury versus left cerebrovascular accident. *Journal of Speech and Hearing Research, 33,* 269–280.

Butterworth, B., Howard, D., & McLoughlin, P. (1984). The semantic deficit in aphasia: The relationship between semantic errors in auditory comprehension and picture naming. *Neuropsychologia, 22,* 409–429.

Cannito, M., Jarecki, J., & Pierce, R. (1986). Effects of thematic structure on syntactic processing in aphasia. *Brain and Language, 27,* 38–49.

Caplan, D., & Evans, K.L. (1990). The effects of syntactic structure on discourse comprehension in patients with parsing impairments. *Brain and Language, 39,* 206–234.

Caramazza, A., & Zurif, E.B. (1976). Dissociation of algorithmic and heuristic processes in language comprehension: Evidence from aphasia. *Brain and Language, 3,* 572–582.

Chapman, S.B., & Ulatowska, H.K. (1989). Discourse in aphasia: Integration deficits in processing reference. *Brain and Language, 36,* 651–668.

Clark, A.E., & Flowers, C.R. (1983). The effect of semantic redundancy on auditory comprehension in aphasia. In R.K. Brookshire (Ed.), *Clinical aphasiology.* Minneapolis: BRK Publishers.

Curtis, S., Jackson, C.A., Kempler, D., Hanson, W.R., & Metter, E.H. (1983). Length vs. structural complexity in sentence comprehension in aphasia. In R.K. Brookshire (Ed.), *Clinical aphasiology.* Minneapolis: BRK Publishers.

Daneman, M., & Green, I. (1986). Individual differences in comprehending and producing words in context. *Journal of Memory and Language, 25,* 1–18.

Daneman, M., & Carpenter, P.A. (1980). Individual differences in working memory and reading. *Journal of Verbal Learning and Verbal Behavior, 19,* 450–460.

Davis, G.A., & Wilcox, M.J. (1985). *Adult aphasia rehabilitation: Applied pragmatics.* San Diego: College-Hill Press.

Deloche, G., & Seron, X. (1981). Sentence understanding and knowledge of the world: Evidence from a sentence-picture matching task performed by aphasic patients. *Brain and Language, 14,* 57–69.

Ernest-Baron, C.R., Brookshire, R.H., & Nicholas, L.E. (1987). Story structure and retelling of narratives by aphasic and nonbrain-damaged adults. *Journal of Speech and Hearing Research, 30*, 44–49.

Francis, W.N., & Kucera, H. (1982). *Frequency analysis of English usage: Lexicon and grammar.* Boston: Houghton-Mifflin.

Frederickson, C.H. (1975). Acquisition of information from discourse: Effects of repeated exposure. *Journal of Verbal Learning and Verbal Behavior, 14*, 158–169.

Frederickson, C.H., Bracewell, R.J., Breuleux, A., & Renaud, A. (1990). The cognitive representation and processing of discourse: Function and dysfunction. In Y. Joanette & H. Brownell (Eds.), *Discourse ability and brain damage: Theoretical and empirical perspectives.* New York: Springer-Verlag.

Gainotti, G., Miceli, G., Caltagirone, C., Silveri, M.C., Masullo, C. (1981). The relationship between the type of naming error and semantic-lexical discrimination in aphasic patients. *Cortex, 17*, 401–409.

Gardner, H., Albert, M.L., Weintraub, S. (1975). Comprehending a word: The influence of speed and redundancy on auditory comprehension in aphasia. *Cortex, 11*, 155–162.

Germani, M. (1994). Semantic attribute knowledge in aphasia: the effects of context. Paper presented to the American Speech-Language-Hearing Association, New Orleans.

Germani, M., & Pierce, R. (1990). *Contextual influence in reading comprehension of adults with aphasia.* Paper presented to the American Speech-Language-Hearing Association, Seattle.

Germani, M., & Pierce, R. (1995). Semantic attribute knowledge in adults with right and left hemisphere damage. *Aphasiology, 9,* 1–21.

Glosser, G., & Deser, T. (1990). Patterns of discourse production among neurological patients with fluent language disorders. *Brain and Language, 40*, 67–89.

Goldstein, K. (1948). *Language and language disturbances.* New York: Grune & Stratton.

Goodglass, H., & Baker, E. (1976). Semantic field, naming, and auditory comprehension in aphasia. *Brain and Language, 3*, 359–374.

Goodglass, H., & Kaplan, E. (1983). *The assessment of aphasia and related disorders* (2nd ed.). Philadelphia: Lea & Febiger.

Goodglass, J., Blumstein, S.E., Gleason, J.B., Hyde, M.R., Green, E., & Statlender, S. (1979). The effect of syntactic encoding on sentence comprehension in aphasia. *Brain and Language, 7*, 201–209.

Gravel, J., & LaPointe, L.L. (1983). Length and redundancy in health care providers' speech during interactions with aphasic and nonaphasic individuals. In R.K. Brookshire (Ed.), *Clinical aphasiology.* Minneapolis: BRK Publishers.

Greenspan, S. (1991). Semantic flexibility and referential specificity of concrete nouns. *Journal of Memory and Language, 25*, 539–557.

Grogan, S., & Pierce, R. (1991). *Influence of working memory on newspaper text comprehension in aphasia.* Paper presented to the Ohio Speech and Hearing Association. Akron, OH.

Halliday, M.A.K., & Hasan, R. (1976). *Cohesion in English.* London: Longman.

Heilman, K.M., Scholes, R.J., & Watson, R.T. (1976). Defects of immediate memory in Broca's and conduction aphasia. *Brain and Language, 3*, 201–208.

Hough, M.S. (1990). Narrative comprehension in adults with right and left hemisphere brain-damage: Theme organization. *Brain and Language, 38*, 253–277.

Hough, M., Pierce, R., & Cannito, M. (1989). Contextual influences in aphasia: Effects of predictive versus nonpredictive narratives. *Brain and Language, 36*, 325–334.

Huber, W. (1990). Text comprehension and production in aphasia: Analysis in terms of micro- and macrostructure. In Y. Joanette & H. Brownell (Eds.), *Discourse ability and brain damage: Theoretical and empirical perspectives*. New York: Springer-Verlag.

Huber, W., & Gleber, J. (1982). Linguistic and nonlinguistic processing of narratives in aphasia. *Brain and Language, 29*, 1–18.

Kearns, K.P., & Hubbard, D. (1983). A comparison of auditory comprehension tasks in aphasia. In R.K. Brookshire (Ed.), *Clinical aphasiology*. Minneapolis: BRK Publishers.

Lesser, R. (1974). Verbal comprehension in aphasia: An English version of three Italian tests. *Cortex, 10*, 247–263.

Linebaugh, C., Pryor, A., & Margulies, C. (1983). Picture descriptions by family members of aphasic patients to aphasic and nonaphasic listeners. In R.K. Brookshire (Ed.), *Clinical aphasiology*. Minneapolis: BRK Publishers.

Martin, R.C., & Feher, E. (1990). The consequences of reduced memory span for the comprehension of semantic versus syntactic information. *Brain and Language, 38*, 1–20.

Matthews, C. (1981). *Factors influencing the recall of stories by aphasics*. Paper presented to the American Speech-Language-Hearing Association, Los Angeles.

McCarthy, R.A., & Warrington, E.K. (1987). The double dissociation of short term memory for lists and sentences: Evidence from aphasia. *Brain, 110*, 1545–1563.

McCarthy, R.A., & Warrington, E.K. (1990). *Cognitive neuropsychology: A clinical introduction* (pp. 292–295). New York: Academic Press.

Naeser, M.A., Mazurski, P., Goodglass, H., Peraino, M., Laughlin, S., & Leaper, W.C. (1987). Auditory syntactic comprehension in nine aphasia groups (with CT scans) and children: Differences in degree but not order of difficulty observed. *Cortex, 23*, 359–380.

Nicholas L.E., & Brookshire R.H. (1986). Consistency of the effects of rate of speech on brain-damaged adults' comprehension of narrative discourse. *Journal of Speech and Hearing Research*, 29, 462–470.

Parisi, D., & Pizzamiglio, L. (1970). Syntactic comprehension in aphasia. *Cortex, 6*, 204–215.

Patterson, J.P. (1990). *Memory for narrative discourse in adults with mild linguistic impairment following left or right cerebrovascular accident*. Unpublished doctoral dissertation, Kent State University, Ohio.

Peach, R.K., Canter, G.J., & Gallaher, A.J, (1988). Comprehension of sentence structure in anomic and conduction aphasia. *Brain and Language, 35*, 119–137.

Pierce, R. (1981). Facilitating the comprehension of tense related sentences in aphasia. *Journal of Speech and Hearing Disorders, 46*, 364–368.

Pierce, R. (1982). Facilitating the comprehension of syntax in aphasia. *Journal of Speech and Hearing Research, 24*, 408–412.

Pierce, R. (1983). A study of sentence comprehension of aphasic subjects. In R.K. Brookshire (Ed.), *Clinical aphasiology*. Minneapolis: BRK Publishers.

Pierce, R. (1984). Comprehending homographs in aphasia. *Brain and Language, 22*, 339–349.

Pierce, R. (1988). Influence of prior and subsequent context on comprehension in aphasia. *Aphasiology, 2*, 577–582.

Pierce, R., & Beekman, L. (1985). Effects of linguistic and extralinguistic context on semantic and syntactic processing in aphasia. *Journal of Speech and Hearing Research, 28,* 250–254.

Pierce, R., & DeStefano, C. (1987). The interactive nature of auditory comprehension in aphasia. *Journal of Communication Disorders, 20,* 15–24.

Pierce, R., Jarecki, J., & Cannito, M. (1990). Single word comprehension in aphasia: Influence of array size, picture relatedness and situational context. *Aphasiology, 4,* 155–165.

Pierce, R., & Townsend, M. (1990). *Context independent and dependent semantic representation in dementia.* Paper presented to the American Speech-Language-Hearing Association, Seattle.

Pierce, R., & Wagner, C. (1985). The role of context in facilitating syntactic decoding in aphasia. *Journal of Communication Disorders, 18,* 203–214.

Pizzamiglio, L., & Appicciafuoco, A. (1971). Semantic comprehension in aphasia. *Journal of Communication Disorders, 3,* 280–288.

Schuell, H.M., Jenkins, J.J., & Landis, L. (1961). Relationships between auditory comprehension and word frequency in aphasia. *Journal of Speech and Hearing Research, 4,* 30–36.

Sherman, J.C., & Schweickert, J. (1989). Syntactic and semantic contributions to sentence comprehension in agrammatism. *Brain and Language, 37,* 419–439.

Shewan, C., & Bandur, D. (1986). *Treatment of aphasia: A language-oriented approach.* Austin, TX: PRO-ED.

Siefert, C.M. (1990). Content-based inferences in text. In A.C. Graesser & G.H. Bower (Eds.), *Inferences and text comprehension.* San Diego: Academic Press.

Tandridag, O., Kirshner, H.S., & Casey, P.F. (1987). Memory function in aphasic and nonaphasic stroke patients. *Aphasiology, 1,* 201–214.

Thorndyke, P.W. (1977). Cognitive structures in comprehension and memory of narrative discourse. *Cognitive Psychology, 9,* 77–110.

Toglia, M.P., & Battig, W.F. (1978). *Handbook of semantic word norms.* New York: John Wiley & Sons.

Ulatowska, H.K., Allard, L., & Chapman, S.B. (1990). Narrative and procedural discourse in aphasia. In Y. Joanette & H. Brownell (Eds.), *Discourse ability and brain damage: Theoretical and empirical perspectives.* New York: Springer-Verlag.

Ulatowska, H.K., & Chapman, S.B. (1989). Discourse considerations for aphasia management. *Seminars in Speech and Language, 10,* 298–314.

Ulatowska, H.K., Doyel, A.W., Stern, R.F., Haynes, S.M., & North, A.J. (1983). Production of procedural discourse in aphasia. *Brain and Language, 18,* 315–341.

Ulatowska, H.K., North, A.J., & Macaluso-Haynes, S.M. (1981). Production of narrative and procedural discourse in aphasia. *Brain and Language, 13,* 345–371.

van den Broek, P. (1990). Casual inferences and the comprehension of narrative texts. In A.C. Graesser & G.H. Bower (Eds.), *Inferences and text comprehension.* San Diego: Academic Press.

van Dijk, T.A., & Kintsch, W. (1983). *Strategies of discourse comprehension.* New York: Academic Press.

Van Lancker, D., & Klein, K. (1990). Preserved recognition of familiar personal names in global aphasia. *Brain and Language, 39,* 511–529.

Wallace, G., & Canter, G. (1985). Effects of personally relevant language materials on the performance of severely aphasic individuals. *Journal of Speech and Hearing Disorders, 50,* 385–390.

Wegner, M.L., Brookshire, R.H., & Nicholas, L.E. (1984). Comprehension of main ideas and details in coherent and noncoherent discourse by aphasic and non-aphasic listeners. *Brain and Language, 21*, 37–51.

Yekovich, F.R., Walker, C.H., Ogle, L.T., & Thompson, M.A. (1990). The influence of domain knowledge on inferencing in low-aptitude individuals. In A.C. Graesser & G.H. Bower (Eds.), *Inferences and text comprehension*. San Diego: Academic Press.

Chapter 11

Model-Based Approach to Rehabilitation of Acquired Reading Disorders

Sharon E. Moss

Treatment of acquired reading disorders in adults has rarely been based on an understanding of the underlying mechanisms of the deficit. In recent years, however, studies in cognitive neuropsychology have led to an increased understanding of language processing (Morton & Patterson, 1980; Newcombe & Marshall, 1980). Consequently, some clinicians now consider cognitive neuropsychological models as an integral part of the assessment and treatment of patients. The purpose of this chapter is to describe a model-based approach to treating reading disorders in brain-injured adults. This discussion is confined to linguistic disorders in processing single words in order to more effectively describe the theoretical foundation of the model.

COGNITIVE NEUROPSYCHOLOGICAL MODELS AS A BASIS FOR TREATMENT

Research in cognitive neuropsychology has provided models of complex reading tasks and a means of hypothesizing specific impairments that can more fully explain patterns of performance observed following brain injury (Funnell, 1983; Schwartz, Saffran, & Marin, 1980). These models have many similarities. One similarity is the underlying assumption of modularity; that is, that separable components are responsible for different aspects of processing. Researchers believe that a functional model for single-word reading is organized such that disruption of an individual component of the model does not lead to a complete dissolution of processing (Howard & Patterson, 1989).

There are many reasons for basing treatment on a well-articulated model. First, researchers believe that deficits tend to be highly selective, and that the effectiveness of treatment of these deficits is maximized when treatment objectives are based on precise knowledge of the integrity of a patient's processing system. Therefore, the model allows for a clear understanding of the disruption underlying each patient's errors, and thus leads to the identification of specific processes that must be improved or circumvented for the patient to respond correctly in a given task (Hillis, 1990). Before implementing an intervention program, the impaired components of the patient's processing system, along with those that are operating with at least partial efficiency, must be identified (Howard & Patterson, 1989). The model can guide clinicians' selection of a strategy from among those in their repertoire or can aid in designing original interventions (Hillis, 1990).

A second reason for using processing models to design treatment is that in addition to offering hypotheses about the individual components of the reading system, models can provide important information about how these components intercommunicate.

In summary, to maximize the benefits of treatment, the assessment of each patient's specific pattern of performance should be based on a detailed processing model. Treatment should be directed at the underlying deficit(s) identified, and designed such that treatment efficacy can be subsequently evaluated.

NEUROPSYCHOLOGICAL MODEL OF READING: MULTIPLE-ROUTE APPROACH

Acquired reading disorders were one of the first areas to be subjected to intense investigation from a cognitive neuropsychological perspective. Consequently, many types of syndromes have been identified, each presenting with different symptoms, interpretations, and implications for theories of normal reading (Ellis & Young, 1988).

There are a number of theories that have been proposed to account for reading in normal adults. One view is that reading involves multiple processing pathways. That is, there are several strategies thought to be responsible for oral reading of single words. Recently, cognitive neuropsychological models have been proposed that incorporate multiple levels of reading processes to account for normal reading (Margolin, 1984; Morton, 1980). A simplified sketch of the processes thought to be involved in word recognition is presented in Figure 11.1. The implication is that (1) each of the components and communicating pathways is necessary to account for the pronunciation or comprehension of normal adult readers, and (2) each process or pathway is interdependent in normal activity and functions with the other parts of the system but is separately susceptible to malfunction from brain damage (Ellis & Young, 1988).

The functions of each component of the model are summarized below. The *visual perceptual analysis system* is believed to have three functions:

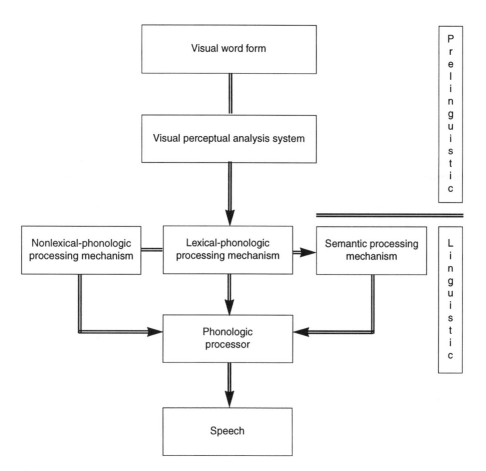

Figure 11.1   *Functional model for recognizing and comprehending written words.*

(1) to identify the component letters of an item (words, nonwords, letter strings), (2) to encode each letter for its position within the word, and (3) to perceptually group those letters that belong together as part of the same word. Word length generally has little effect on the recognition of familiar words, as evidenced by the parallel and simultaneous identification of several letters at a time by the visual perceptual analysis system (Ellis & Young, 1988). Processing within this system is thought to be prelinguistic (perceptual) in nature. That is, the processing of information takes place at primary and secondary cortical levels. There is no linguistic analysis of written words. Rather, printed material is transformed into a representation that is acceptable to the linguistic processing mechanism.

For word production to occur, the visual perceptual analysis system must first identify the component letters. The letters ("graphemes") must then be converted into sounds ("phonemes"). The function of the *nonlexical-phono-*

logic recoding mechanism is to translate unfamiliar grapheme strings into phoneme strings (Ellis & Young, 1988). The nonlexical-phonologic recoding mechanism allows letter-to-sound conversions, enabling an individual to read aloud nonwords, regularly spelled words, and function words (Table 11.1).

A reader's previously stored information about word pronunciation (i.e., lexical knowledge) is housed in the *lexical-phonologic processing mechanism*. As written words become familiar to a reader, this mechanism establishes pronunciational representations of those words. Thus, skilled readers who have learned to recognize many thousands of words "by sight" have a representation for each word in their visual input lexicon, each representation being activated specifically by its own written word (Ellis & Young, 1988). Individuals can read aloud regularly spelled and rule-governed words better than they can irregularly spelled words.

Representations of word meanings are contained within the *semantic processing mechanism*, thereby allowing the reader to comprehend the meanings of printed words in the absence of identifying information about pronunciation. This mechanism is thought to correspond to the "semantic memory" component of many cognitive theories of memory (Ellis & Young, 1988). In essence, words are "remembered" or recognized as familiar so that their meanings can be accessed. Processing within the nonlexical-phonologic, lexical-phonologic, and semantic processing mechanisms is thought to be linguistic in nature. That is, the processing takes place at cortical levels involved in the analysis of single words, including phonologic, semantic, and lexical.

The *phonologic processor* stores representations of spoken words. These representations are activated when a word is to be spoken, thus making the spoken form of a word available to a speaker (Ellis & Young, 1988).

SYNDROMES IDENTIFIED: ACQUIRED READING DISORDERS

Cognitive neuropsychological studies of reading suggest at least four major patterns of acquired reading disorder. These linguistic (as opposed to prelinguistic) disorders are differentiated on the basis of the sensitivity of the patient's reading performance to various dimensions of the word to be read (i.e., word length, regularity of grapheme-to-phoneme correspondence, word concreteness/imageability) (Patterson, 1981).

Individuals presenting with *deep dyslexia*, for example, have an intact semantic processing mechanism but impaired nonlexical-phonologic recoding and lexical-phonologic processing mechanisms. The most salient feature of this syndrome is the presence of semantic paralexias (i.e., production of a word semantically related to target) (Table 11.2). This feature may reflect an underlying disorder of concept arousal and word retrieval. Neither of these components, however, are considered specific to visual processing (Coltheart, Patterson, & Marshall, 1980). The assumption is that deep dyslexia represents

TABLE 11.1   Examples of Word Types

Nonwords	trad pable manver tralf intret
Regularly spelled words	transfer neglect forget vent mask
Irregularly spelled words	mischief tomb deny heir answer
Rule-governed words	ritual debt sign limb foreign
Function words	both whom thus always shall
Content words	general club church trial history
Homophonic words	mail/male hoes/hose cord/chord pain/pane sea/see
Pseudohomophonic words	coam/comb yott/yacht bild/build rapt/wrapped bomm/bomb
Homographic-nonhomophonic words	refuse: I refuse to continue the game. lead: Lead is a heavy metal. conduct: He will conduct the band. minute: Wait a minute. object: I object to that.

TABLE 11.2   Characteristics of Dyslexia

Processing mechanism	Deep	Surface	Phonologic	Semantic
Nonlexical-phonologic processing mechanism	Impaired	Spared	Impaired	Spared
Lexical-phonologic processing mechanism	Impaired	Impaired	Spared	Spared
Semantic processing mechanism	Spared	Impaired	Spared	Impaired

an inability to gain access to, or to create, phonologic (speech-based) representations. The individual can no longer use grapheme-to-phoneme rules of conversion. Other symptoms include: (1) inability to read nonwords and pseudohomophones, (2) sensitivity to word meaning, (3) insensitivity to spelling regularity and word length, and (4) better performance on irregularly spelled words, content words, nouns, and imageable words than on homophonic, pseudohomophonic, and other words (Marshall & Newcombe, 1973; Patterson & Marcel, 1977; Richardson, 1975; Shallice & Warrington, 1975).

The second of the four syndromes identified in the literature is *surface dyslexia*, in which the nonlexical-phonologic recoding mechanism is spared but the lexical-phonologic and semantic processing mechanisms are impaired. The most salient feature of this syndrome is the presence of a "regularity" effect; that is, regular words are read more accurately than are irregularly spelled or rule-governed words. This syndrome may represent limited visual access to the lexicon, resulting in a forced reliance on phonologic decoding; hence, the regularity effect. (Marshall & Newcombe, 1973). Other symptoms include (1) sensitivity to word length and part of speech; (2) insensitivity to word meaning; (3) better performance on nonwords, concrete words, and function words; and (4) phonetically accurate misspellings (Deloche, Andreewsky, & Desi, 1982; Kremin, 1980).

Individuals presenting with *phonologic dyslexia* have intact lexical-phonologic and semantic processing mechanisms but an impaired nonlexical-phonologic recoding mechanism. The most salient feature of this syndrome is a severe impairment of the ability to read nonwords, with a concomitant sparing of the ability to read real words aloud. Phonologic alexia may represent an inability to use grapheme-to-phoneme conversion rules (Beauvois & Derouesne, 1979). Other symptoms of this syndrome include (1) inability to read pseudohomophones, (2) sensitivity to word meaning, (3) insensitivity to spelling regularity, and (4) better performance on high-frequency words and content words.

Individuals diagnosed with *semantic dyslexia* present with a sparing of the nonlexical-phonologic recoding and lexical-phonologic processing mechanisms but impairment of the semantic processing mechanism. The most salient feature of this syndrome is apparent normal reading accompanied by an inability to comprehend irregularly spelled words. This syndrome may represent an inability to gain access to a word's phonologic and semantic representations (Schwartz, Marin, & Saffran, 1979). Other symptoms include (1) inability to dissociate synonyms (same meaning) or homophones (same sound) and (2) inability to categorize words based on meaning.

MODEL-SPECIFIC APPROACH TO TREATMENT

Features That Make Mechanisms Unique

Specific features make each mechanism unique. Clinicians should be aware of these features as they select how stimuli are presented and the form of the desired response. Stimuli may be presented manually via flash cards, tachistoscope, or computer; clinician creativity is responsible for any manipulations within task design.

When treating the impaired *nonlexical-phonologic processing mechanism*, the clinician should select items (nonwords or words) that have a direct grapheme-to-phoneme correspondence. The objective of these tasks is for the individual to make a phonologic comparison or decision about the stimuli independent of meaning. Stimuli should (1) rely strictly on phonologic analyses without meaning required and (2) require visual analysis (analytical) at the level of the single grapheme. These tasks require an unlimited exposure rate. That is, the duration (length of time) for stimulus presentation is unlimited. Thus, nonwords (e.g., *vatter, blime*) may be selected as stimuli for this task; real words having a direct grapheme-to-phoneme correspondence (e.g., *stand, open*) are also useful.

When treating the impaired *lexical-phonologic processing mechanism*, the clinician should select stimuli that require a lexically based phonological analysis and do not require a semantic analysis. Stimuli should (1) have a direct visual-to-lexical correspondence and (2) require visual analysis at a syllabic-to-whole-word level. The length of time stimulus item should be presented is from 500 to 600 msec. Therefore, any real word (e.g., *veteran, limb*) can be used as a stimulus for this type of task, as long as the purpose of the task is simply to read the word aloud and not derive meaning.

When treating the impaired *semantic processing mechanism*, the clinician should select stimuli that only require semantic analysis and not phonologic or lexical analysis. In this case, access of semantic information occurs prior to lexical or phonologic processing. Stimuli should (1) have a direct visual-to-meaning correspondence and (2) require a visual analysis (gestalt). Stimuli for these tasks should be presented at a rate of 350 msec. Therefore, real words (e.g., *match, reign, aisle*) are used as stimuli for this type of task as long as the analysis is semantic and not phonologic.

In summary, treatment objectives may be changed depending on the mechanism being addressed. When treating the impaired nonlexical-phonologic recoding mechanism, exposure rate (the amount of time stimulus item is presented) is unlimited. The latency of response (the amount of time taken by patient to respond) is not a critical measure. When treating the impaired lexical-phonologic and semantic processing mechanism, objectives focus on gradually decreasing latency of response. Exposure rate is decreased as success (acceptable level of performance) is achieved. In each case, the primary goal is to increase accuracy level. Criteria for success vary depending on each patient's need. However, when treating higher-level patients, the clinician may choose to refocus treatment objectives such that accuracy level is maintained rather than increased.

Illustration of Tasks

Examples of tasks designed to treat each of the three aforementioned mechanisms, as well as a combination of impaired mechanisms, are provided below. For each task, task administration procedures, method of scoring, and sample stimuli are explained.

Nonlexical-Phonologic Processing Mechanism

The objective of both of the following tasks is to increase accuracy while forcing a phonologic analysis of the stimulus word. The scoring criterion is percentage of correct responses.

   1.   *Phoneme production*: The individual is presented with a grapheme and asked to produce the corresponding phoneme. Sample stimuli include B, P, K, L, T.
   2.   *Read aloud nonwords*: The individual reads aloud a set of nonwords. Sample stimuli include: BLIB, GORT, SLIG, DREK, RILK.

Lexical-Phonologic Processing Mechanism

The objective of both of the following tasks is to increase accuracy while decreasing response latency and exposure rate. The scoring criteria are exposure rate, latency of response, and percentage of correct responses.

   1.   *Rhyme recognition*: The individual is presented with four pairs of words. In each pair, the stimulus word is followed by a visually dissimilar rhyme, a visually similar nonrhyme, a visually similar rhyme, and a visually dissimilar nonrhyme. Each pair is presented visually for a predetermined amount of time. The individual responds "yes" or "no" if the stimulus rhymes with its mate. Sample stimuli include pore/boar; pour/hour; pore/more; pore/hour; dime/thyme; dime/dame; dime/time; dime/door.
   2.   *Homophone match*: The individual is presented a stimulus word for a predetermined amount of time, then two other words, one a homophone,

the other a word visually similar to the homophonic pair. The individual determines which of the two words following the stimulus sounds the same as the stimulus. Sample sequences (stimuli italicized) include: *pain*, pine, pane; *all*, awl, ale; *rye*, rue, wry.

Semantic Processing Mechanism

The objective of both of the following tasks is to maintain or increase accuracy while decreasing response latency and exposure rate. Scoring criteria are exposure rate, latency of response, and percentage of correct responses.

    1. *Homophone definition*: The individual is visually presented one of a pair of homophones as a stimulus followed by three multiple-choice words: a semantic associate (e.g., "a word whose meaning is associated with the stimulus"), a semantic/phonologic foil (e.g., "a word whose meaning is associated with the homophone of the stimulus"), and an unrelated foil (e.g., "a decoy whose meaning is unrelated to either homophome"). Stimuli are presented for a predetermined exposure rate. The individual identifies the response word that is the semantic associate of the stimulus word. Sample sequences (stimuli italicized) include *reign*, queen, cloud, baseball; *ate*, food, number, raise; *suite*, room, sugary, glue.

    2. *Semantic decision*: The individual is presented a stimulus word for a predetermined exposure rate and identifies which of two categories the stimuli belongs to. Sample stimuli include: (food/nonfood) beans, apple, chairs, nurses; (animal/vegetable) bird, monkey, potato, celery; (female name/male name) Vicky, Victor, Iris, Ike.

Combination

On some occasions, distinguishing impairment of an isolated system is not possible. Therefore, tasks can be designed to treat two mechanisms concurrently.

Nonlexical-Phonologic/Lexical-Phonologic Processing Mechanisms. The objective of both of the following tasks is to increase accuracy while making phonological analyses of the stimuli. The scoring criterion is percentage of correct responses.

    1. *Read aloud functors*: The individual is presented a set of functors to be read aloud. Sample stimuli include of, is, the, upon, after.

    2. *Synonym identification*: The individual is graphically presented two words (both of them real), one of which is read aloud by the examiner. The individual identifies the word presented orally. Sample stimuli include: sad/grim; enemy/rival; chum/pal; short/small; look/see.

Lexical-Phonologic/Semantic Processing Mechanisms.   The objective of both of the following tasks is to increase accuracy while decreasing the time allotted to complete the task. The scoring criteria are: time allotted to complete task, time used to complete task, and percentage of correct responses.

    1.   *Read aloud irregular words*: The individual is provided a predetermined amount of time in which to read a set of irregularly spelled words. The allotted time is systematically decreased contingent upon accuracy. Sample stimuli include: ocean, cuisine, rhyme, dinosaur, simile. This task may also be used with rule-governed words.
    2.   *Lexical decision*: The individual is presented a stimulus at a predetermined exposure rate. The individual determines whether the stimulus is a "word" or "nonword," a choice that should involve lexical decision-making strategy. Sample stimuli include: ugly, flad, jury, itch, tord.

    In summary, reading tasks that incorporate specific word types as stimuli in specific tasks can be used to treat impairment of a particular mechanism. The above list of word types is not meant to be exhaustive but rather an initial point of reference. The tasks demonstrate how specific word types may be effective stimuli through their ability to address the inherent features of the mechanism described. Finally, the importance of stimuli lies not only in the selection of words, but in how they are used.

Case Presentation

This section describes an intervention study designed to improve the reading ability of a patient with surface dyslexia. The underlying cause of the deficit was identified and a plan for intervention was developed. The extent to which the intervention was of benefit with regard to the previously described model of normal word recognition was also addressed.
    A 25-year-old right-handed woman was seen for language evaluation 18 months postinjury. She had completed 3 years of college as an English literature major. Results of our reading assessment performed at that time were consistent with surface dyslexia. The patient could read nonwords aloud surprisingly well. The regularity of grapheme-to-phoneme correspondence significantly affected her performance on reading real words aloud; her accuracy decreased significantly as spelling regularity decreased. The type of errors made on reading aloud irregularly spelled words (for example, reading *colonel* as *colonial*) reflected an attempt to project a direct grapheme-to-phoneme correspondence that was not present. On all tasks, the patient read slowly and wrote with her finger while reading, which she said helped her to "sound out" words.
    The treatment program was implemented at 24 months postinsult. As noted previously, the distinctive features of the impaired semantic processing mechanism include (1) semantic analysis before phonologic access, (2) rapid response and presentation time, and (3) relative indifference to ortho-

graphic irregularities. Our primary purpose was to determine the efficacy of treating the deficient semantic mechanism in a patient possibly relying on the nonlexical-phonologic mechanism for reading.

Therefore, tasks were designed to reflect the distinctive features of the semantic processing mechanism. These included a forced semantic analysis of words presented at set presentation speeds (i.e., semantic categorization tasks); reading of irregular words during a minimum presentation interval (i.e., reading of irregular words task); and correct selection of homophones within the context of written paragraphs (i.e., homophone selection task).

This patient's performance on post-test measures indicated a decrease in reading time without a compromise of accuracy of performance. The percentage of accuracy scores either remained stable or increased. We concluded that for this patient, the treatment was effective in forcing more rapid processing speeds while maintaining an appropriate level of accuracy (90%). The treatment may have forced more reliance on the deficient semantic processing mechanism and allowed less reliance on the nonlexical-phonologic processing mechanism.

SUMMARY

Recently, attempts have been made to combine cognitive neuropsychological theory and therapeutic intervention. Recommendations regarding treatment are based primarily on the nature of the underlying mechanism of a deficit. The attempts have been largely successful in demonstrating significant improvement in the treated behavior. These successes suggest several conclusions. Areas of dysfunction can be defined based on a model describing normal cognitive functioning. Second, treatment programs designed to address a specific function can be developed and implemented. Finally, the extent to which an intervention plan is successful can be evaluated with respect to a given model (Lesser, 1989). Ideally, information presented in this chapter should be adapted to address the patient's specific day-to-day needs and alexia severity level.

REFERENCES

Beauvois, M.F., & Derouesne, J. (1979). Phonological alexia: Three dissociations. *Journal of Neurology, Neurosurgery, and Psychiatry 42*, 1115–1124.

Coltheart, M., Patterson, K., & Marshall, J.C. (Eds.). (1980). *Deep dyslexia*. London: Routledge & Kegan Paul.

Deloche, G., Andreewsky, E., & Desi, M. (1982). Surface dyslexia: A case report and some theoretical implications to reading models. *Brain and Language, 15*, 11–32.

Ellis, A.W., & Young, A.W. (1988). *Human cognitive neuropsychology*. London: Erlbaum.

Funnell, E. (1983). Phonological processes in reading: New evidence from acquired dyslexia. *British Journal of Psychology, 74,* 159–180.

Hillis, A.E. (1990, October). *Relationship between a model of the naming process and treatment of naming deficits.* Paper presented at the Academy of Aphasia, Baltimore, MD.

Howard, D., & Patterson, K. (1989). Models for therapy. In X. Seron & G. Deloche (Eds.), *Cognitive approaches in neuropsychological rehabilitation.* Hillsdale, NJ: Lawrence Erlbaum.

Kremin, H. (1980). *Case study of a patient with surface dyslexia.* Paper presented at the Meeting of the International Neuropsychological Society, Chianciano-Terme, Italy.

Lesser, R. (1989). Some issues in the neuropsychological rehabilitation of anomia. In X. Seron. & G. Deloche (Eds.), *Cognitive approaches in neuropsychological rehabilitation.* Hillsdale, NJ: Lawrence Erlbaum.

Margolin, D.I. (1984). The neuropsychology of writing and spelling: Semantic, phonological, motor, and perceptual processes. *Quarterly Journal of Experimental Psychology, 36A,* 459–489.

Marshall, J.C., & Newcombe, F. (1973). Patterns of paralexia: A psycholinguistic approach. *Journal of Psycholinguistic Research, 2,* 175–199.

Morton, J. (1980). The logogen model and orthographic structure. In U. Frith (Ed.), *Cognitive processes in spelling.* London: Academic Press.

Morton, J., & Patterson, K.E. (1980). A new attempt at an interpretation or an attempt at a new interpretation. In M. Coltheart, K. Patterson, & J. C. Marshall (Eds.), *Deep dyslexia.* London: Routledge & Kegan Paul.

Newcombe, F., & Marshall, J.C. (1980). Transcoding and lexical stabilization in deep dyslexia. In M. Coltheart, K. Patterson, & J. C. Marshall (Eds.), *Deep dyslexia.* London: Routledge & Kegan Paul.

Patterson, K. (1981). Neuropsychological approaches to the study of reading. *British Journal of Psychology, 72,* 151–174.

Patterson, K.E., & Marcel, A.J. (1977). Aphasia, dyslexia and the phonological coding of written words. *Quarterly Journal of Experimental Psychology, 29,* 307–318.

Richardson, J.T.E. (1975). The effect of word imageability in acquired dyslexia. *Neuropsychologia, 13,* 281–288.

Schwartz, M.F., Marin, O.S.M., & Saffran, E. (1979). Dissociations of language function in dementia. *Brain and Language, 7,* 277–306.

Schwartz, M.F., Saffran, E.M., & Marin, O.S. (1980). Fractionating the reading process in dementia: Evidence for word-specific print-to-sound associations. In M. Coltheart, K. Patterson, & J. C. Marshall (Eds.), *Deep dyslexia.* London: Routledge & Kegan Paul.

Shallice, T. & Warrington, E.K. (1975). Word recognition in a phonemic dyslexic patient. *Quarterly Journal of Experimental Psychology, 27,* 187–199.

Chapter 12

Treatment of Verbal Apraxia in Broca's Aphasia

Thomas P. Marquardt and Michael P. Cannito

Apraxia of speech—impairment due to left hemisphere brain damage in the ability to carry out programmed articulatory movements in the absence of neuromuscular deficits—is a controversial disorder. Several investigators (e.g., Johns & Darley, 1970; Wertz, LaPointe, & Rosenbek, 1984) view apraxia as a distinctive speech disorder that may occur independently from aphasia. In contrast, Marquardt (1982) argued that the dense connectivity of neural circuitry subserving communication precludes the development of a speech disorder separate from other language deficits associated with focal lesions of the dominant hemisphere. We will assume a middle ground in this controversy. In most cases, in our view, apraxia of speech is a primary characteristic of a syndrome of deficits associated with anterior left hemisphere brain damage most frequently described as *Broca's aphasia*. From a treatment standpoint, focusing treatment for these patients then requires that we deal with deficits in speech motor programming typical of apraxia and with deficits in language expression characteristic of nonfluent aphasia.

Our basic philosophy of treatment is that the clinician's first task is to ensure that the patient has a reliable means of communication, regardless of the output modality used. Compensatory communication strategies, augmentative communication systems, and focused speech-based treatment techniques all have a place. The subsequent goals of treatment are to make the patient's communication system more efficient and to reduce the communicative demands by requiring the audience to assume a greater portion of the information-exchange burden. Implicit in this stage of treatment is that the type of treatment is determined by the severity of the disorder and the communication needs of the patient. Before we take up a more detailed consideration of assessment and treatment of verbal apraxia and expressive language disorders, we first describe the salient characteristics of these disorders.

LESION SITE

Verbal apraxia and nonfluent aphasia result from damage to the anterior left hemisphere. The lesion typically includes Broca's area (posterior portion of the third frontal convolution) but is not limited to that site. Mohr (1976), in a review of lesions associated with Broca's aphasia, concluded that the damage includes a wide range of contiguous tissue surrounding Broca's area. Marquardt and Sussman (1984) found that nine patients with verbal apraxia (in a study of 15) had a concentration of lesions extending from the posterior frontal lobe to the anterior parietal lobe and superior temporal lobe including the insula and opercula. Six of the subjects did not have lesions that extended to the cortical surface. Similarly, Kertesz (1979) reported variations in lesion sites for patients with Broca's aphasia that focused on the posterior frontal lobe and later described (Kertesz, 1984) 10 patients with apraxia secondary to subcortical lesions. What might be concluded from these studies is that nonfluent aphasia results from lesions to the anterior dominant hemisphere for speech and language, but that the lesion is not limited to Broca's area or cortical structures alone.

DISORDERS OF ORAL EXPRESSION: RELATIONSHIP OF APRAXIA AND APHASIA

One generally held view, as noted earlier, is that apraxia of speech may occur as a disorder independent of expressive language disorders (Johns & Darley, 1970; Kent & Rosenbek, 1983). Few would argue, however, that finding a patient with deficits limited to speech output processing alone is unusual at best. In most cases, the patient with an anterior left hemisphere lesion will demonstrate a constellation of disorders typical of Broca's aphasia. Included are agrammatical speech, word-finding deficits, prosodic abnormalities, and marked deficits in the production of speech sounds. While we recognize that language deficits of the syndrome have a potent impact on rehabilitation of the patient with Broca's aphasia, our discussion will focus on speech deficits, including articulatory characteristics and prosodic abnormalities.

CHARACTERISTICS OF APRAXIA OF SPEECH

Articulation

Apraxia of speech includes deficits in speech sound production and in prosody. Typically, the speech of the apractic patient is effortful and variable with groping for articulatory positions and sequences of movements for speech sound production. Speech rate is slowed and there are changes in prosody related to intonation and stress. The patient is aware that efforts to produce sounds and sequences of speech sounds are in error, but may not be able to correct them with repeated trials.

Darley (1984) noted that the preponderance of errors in apraxia are consonant substitutions, additions, and repetitions. Specific characteristics include an increase in errors with increases in the motoric complexity required for the production of the sound. Therefore, there is a higher frequency of errors on singleton consonants than vowels, more errors on affricates and fricatives, and most difficulty on consonant clusters. Although not a consistent finding (e.g., Dunlop & Marquardt, 1977), errors occur more often in word initial position. Phonemes with a high frequency of occurrence in the language are less often misarticulated and sequencing errors (anticipatory, reiterative, metathesis) are observable but have a low incidence. Among other attributes, Darley noted that apractic patients demonstrate a marked discrepancy between automatic-reactive speech and more volitional production, they make more articulation errors on imitation than spontaneous production, and their speech production accuracy is affected by word abstractness and length.

The characteristics of apraxia of speech recently have come under more careful scrutiny because the data in support of salient descriptors of the disorder have a direct bearing on the issue of whether or not apraxia of speech can occur independently of brain-damage–based language disorders (Lesser, 1978). If speech production is conceptualized as a multilevel process with premotor and motor stages, it might be argued that phonemic substitutions would dominate the error patterns of patients with damage to brain areas responsible for language-based selection and sequencing of phonemes, but distortion errors would have a higher incidence in patients with damage to neural structures responsible for the programming and execution of speech sound production.

There is substantial support for this revised view of the phonetic errors of apractic speakers from both transcription and physiological/acoustic studies. Square, Darley, and Sommers (1982) found that the dominant type of errors for three apractic speakers based on a large corpus of data derived from imitation, oral reading, and confrontation naming was distortions. Odell, McNeil, Rosenbek, and Hunter (1990) investigated consonant articulation in four apractic speakers using narrow transcription. Distortions constituted the largest percentage of errors (25%), followed by omissions (9%), substitutions (6%), distorted substitutions (6%), and additions (5%). Fifty-four percent of the consonants were produced correctly. Other findings of importance "were that errors did not preferentially appear in word-initial position, that affricate and fricative sounds were not markedly more vulnerable to disruption than other sounds, and that the frequency of errors did not increase with increasing length of the speech unit" (p. 356).

Physiological and acoustic studies of articulation in apraxia and aphasia are not without methodological problems (Sussman, Marquardt,

MacNeilage, & Hutchinson, 1988) but have added a highly useful window for better understanding articulatory dynamics in apraxia of speech. Fromm, Abbs, McNeil, and Rosenbek (1982), in a physiological study of speech muscle function and movement, found that 95% of the substitution and addition errors were produced with one or more neuromuscular abnormalities and hypothesized that segmental errors in apraxia were due to neuromotor execution and programming deficits rather than problems with phonological selection. Other studies have shown that apractic patients demonstrate delayed onset of coarticulatory gestures (Ziegler & von Cramon, 1985, 1986), reduced accuracy of articulatory movements (Harmes et al., 1984; Kent & Rosenbek, 1983), changes in the timing relationship of laryngeal and upper airway movements reflected in voice onset time (Baum, Blumstein, Naeser, & Palumbo, 1990; Blumstein, Cooper, Zurif, & Caramazza, 1977), and reduced ability to compensate for novel constraints on the articulatory mechanism (Sussman, Marquardt, Hutchinson, & MacNeilage, 1986).

The foregoing studies suggest that the most prominent features of apraxia of speech in nonfluent aphasia stem from disrupted programming and execution of speech movements, although problems in the selection and sequencing of speech segments also may be observable (Kent & Rosenbek, 1983). The expected patterns of error will depend on the degree to which premotor and motor aspects of speech production are affected by the site and extent of brain damage. For a more detailed discussion of these issues, see Rosenbek, Kent, and LaPointe (1984), and Pierce (1991).

Prosody and Fluency

Prosody is that aspect of the phonology of a language that accounts for the rhythms and melodies of speech. It encompasses such suprasegmental variables as stress, intonation, juncture, and rate of speaking. While it is less well understood than the segmental aspects (i.e., phonemes and allophones) of language, prosody is known to convey a variety of structural, functional, and affective information in linguistic communication. A consideration of prosody is clinically important because nonfluent aphasics with apraxia exhibit a diverse assortment of expressive prosodic abnormalities that interfere with communication. In addition, several specific treatment approaches to be presented have been motivated by prosodic notions. It is not clear at present which dysprosodic elements are attributable to the aphasia or to the apraxia, and no attempt will be made to differentiate them in the following discussion.

Broca's aphasia is a nonfluent aphasia. Deal & Cannito (1991) have pointed out that it is diagnostically important to differentiate between *nonfluency* and *dysfluency* in aphasic patients. While they often co-occur, the two phenomena can also be demonstrated differentially in individual patients. Nonfluent speech is slow, labored, dysprosodic, reduced in quantity (both overall and in terms of phrase length), and agrammatical (Benson, 1979). Dysfluency, in contrast, implies stuttering-like behaviors such as sound and syllable repetitions, blocks, prolongations and dysrhythmic phonations. Nonfluency is an expressive language disorder; dysfluency a motor control problem. In nonfluent aphasia with apraxia of speech, both components are commonplace. Various investigators have noted the marked prevalence of stuttering-like dysfluencies in association with articulatory programming problems of apraxia of speech (Johns & Darley, 1970; Trost, 1971; Yairi, Gintautas, & Avent, 1981) often accompanied by Broca's aphasia. This was so much the case that Johns and Darley (1970) observed that apractic subjects "as a group, do a creditable job of miming secondary stutterers, both acoustically and behaviorally" (p. 580). Yairi et al. (1981) reported that the overall mean frequency per 100 words of dysfluency in Broca's aphasia was 16.03, in comparison to a normal control group mean of 5.13 and a nonaphasic brain damaged group mean of 5.59. Individual frequencies for the Broca's aphasic subjects ranged from 5.40, which was quite normal, to 38.50, which was more than three standard deviations above the normal mean. A breakdown by dysfluency type for the aphasic subjects was 8.40 for interjections, 3.18 for revisions, 1.53 for disrhythmic phonation, 1.13 for word repetitions, 0.89 for part word repetitions, 0.52 for phrase repetitions, and 0.34 for tense pauses. These values were all significantly higher than those of normal controls and nonaphasic brain-damaged subjects. Canter (1971) suggested that "apraxic stuttering" should be regarded as a differentiated subtype of acquired neurogenic dysfluency (in contrast to aphasic and dysarthric subtypes); however, emerging evidence has not supported such classifications. See Deal and Cannito (1991) for additional discussion.

Abnormalities of speaking rate are characteristic of both Broca's aphasic and verbal apractic patients. Nonfluent aphasics have been reported to generally exhibit a speaking rate of less than 50 words per minute, which was significantly slower than that of both Wernicke's aphasics and normal subjects (Benson, 1979). Broca's aphasics are also known to speak telegraphically, using one- to three-word utterances, with hesitant speech initiation and prolonged pauses between words. Kent and Rosenbek (1983) reported acoustical findings for a group of mildly aphasic patients with significant apraxia of speech. These investigations recognized that some clinicians might regard the patients as "mildly Broca's aphasics"; however, they were not agrammatical and their most salient clinical finding was the articulation disorder. Sentence durations produced by these patients, without exception, exceeded those of control subjects by more than two standard deviations. In many cases, differences greater than 10 standard deviations were reported. To account for these durational differences, both articulatory prolongation and syllable segregation were demonstrated. *Articulatory prolongation* was defined as "a lengthening of steady-state segments and the intervening transitions," whereas *syllable segregation* was defined as "a pattern of temporally separated or isolated syllables" (Kent & Rosenbek, 1983, p. 233).

Increased word durations with dramatically prolonged interword pauses have also been reported of more classic, agrammatical Broca's aphasics (Danly & Shapiro, 1982). Some investigators have attributed the rate abnormalities of apraxia to compensation for articulatory difficulty, while others have posited them to be primary symptoms (Kent & Rosenbek, 1982). Increased hesitation behavior in the spontaneous speech of nonfluent aphasics as a function of more active lexical searching (relative to fluent aphasics) has also been hypothesized (Hoffmann, 1980).

Stress and Intonation

The integrity of the stress system has not been well studied in verbal apraxia/Broca's aphasia, but some relevant data have emerged. In addition to overall lengthening of vocalic nuclei, there is, in verbal apraxia, a greater prolongation of unstressed syllables (Kent & Rosenbek, 1983). It must be remembered, however, that the percept of word level stress arises from a complex interaction of fundamental frequency, duration, and intensity (Beckman, 1986). Kent and Rosenbek (1983) reported "a flattening of intensity envelope" across sequences of syllables, such that syllables that are normally reduced (e.g., function words), were, in verbal apraxia, abnormally intense. This might also have a neutralizing effect on stress. Odell, McNeil, Rosenbek, and Hunter (1991) reported a high incidence of perceived stress placement errors in imitative word productions of four apraxic patients. The interactive roles of fundamental frequency, duration, and intensity were investigated in three apraxic and three normal subjects of Colson, Luschei, and Jordan (1986). They found no difference in the perceived accuracy of stress placement for imitative nonsense disyllables (e.g., /pəkʌ/) between groups. Whereas the apraxics tended to neutralize duration differences between stress and unstressed syllables, they compensated by exaggerating fundamental frequency differences. Given the discrepancy between the Odell et al. and Colson et al. studies, further investigation of stress marking in apraxia appears to be needed.

While there is some evidence suggesting that Broca's aphasics exhibit impaired syllabic stress, there is also evidence to support a facilitative influence of stress on speech production. Goodglass, Fodor, and Schulhoff (1967) demonstrated in 10 Broca's aphasics that when function words occur in a stressed position within a sentence (e.g., "Aren't they hungry"), they are far less likely to be deleted than when they occur in an unstressed position. A similar effect has been reported with respect to segmental articulatory accuracy. In a group of 11 Broca's aphasics with verbal apraxia, Nichols (1979) found that accuracy was greater in stressed than unstressed syllables, and the effect was most powerful in phrase initial position.

Intonation refers to the pattern of pitch changes across an utterance, and impairments in this domain have traditionally been considered a defining feature of Broca's aphasia (Benson, 1979). Acoustical studies of Broca's intonation as represented by voice fundamental frequency (fo) have been some-what equivocal. Ryalls (1987) found that the fo range was abnormally restricted in Broca's aphasia. Similarly, Cooper, Soares, Nicol, Michelow, and Goloskie (1984) reported a compression of fo peaks relative to normal. Paradoxically, Danley and Shapiro (1982) observed exaggerated fo variation in Broca's aphasics. Danly and Shapiro (1982) demonstrated relatively nor-mal intonation features of terminal fall and declination of fo for shorter utterances. However, they found that for longer utterances, Broca's aphasics were only able to produce declination over short phrases, having to reset their declination repeatedly across the utterance. These investigators also observed that Broca's aphasics used "continuation rises," which in normals signal that a sentence is not finished, suggesting that this may be a compen-sation for their hesitant speech. Intonation findings in apraxia of speech have also been somewhat equivocal. Kent & Rosenbek (1983) report relative-ly normal terminal falls in their mildly aphasic, apractic sample. In contrast, Keatley (1979) found that mild to moderate Broca's aphasics with apraxia of speech exhibited abnormal terminal fo contours.

In summary, patients with apraxia and nonfluent aphasia demonstrate impaired ability to program movements reflected in a high incidence of phonetic (subphonemic) errors and disrupted prosody. Specific treatment approaches for these deficits are discussed following a review of assess-ment procedures.

ASSESSMENT AND DIAGNOSIS

Evaluation of verbal apraxia and nonfluent aphasia will include assessment of both the speech and language components of the disorder. We have found it useful to use an aphasia battery in order to provide a broad-based descrip-tion of the disorder plus additional measures that focus on specific aspects of speech motor programming deficits. It is assumed that this assessment will be included in a broader program of evaluation that includes acquisi-tion of case history information relative to educational history, medical information, and results from neurological assessment and neurodiagnostic tests to provide a full complement of clinical data to provide a context for differential diagnosis. The aphasia test battery chosen is a matter of clinical preference. Certainly, long-used tests such as the Minnesota Test for the Differential Diagnosis of Aphasia (Schuell, 1965), the Boston Diagnostic Aphasia Examination (Goodglass & Kaplan, 1983), the Porch Index of Communicative Ability (PICA) (Porch, 1971), or the Western Aphasia Battery (Kertesz, 1982) will provide a broad description of the communica-tion disorders.

We have found it useful to administer the Communicative Abilities in Daily Living test (Holland, 1980) or the Functional Communication Profile (Sarno, 1969) in addition to a battery that details the speech and language deficits in order to provide a more complete picture of the relative degree of communication impairment. It is expected that performance on standardized aphasia batteries provides information on the degree of difficulty in the performance of specific tasks, but it does not provide data on how well the patient is able to communicate in everyday situations. The use of these functional measures yields at least some preliminary data on how well the patient is able to meet his or her daily communication needs. Several assessment batteries have been developed to assess the relative degree of verbal, oral, and limb apraxia. DeRenzi, Pieczuro, and Vignolo (1966), for example, developed procedures to assess oral and limb apraxia, and Rosenbek and Wertz (1976) developed a modified assessment instrument for limb, oral, and verbal apraxia. Dabul (1979) compiled a group of tasks including diadochokinetic rate, increasing word length, limb apraxia and oral apraxia, latency and utterance time for polysyllabic words, repeated trials test, and an inventory of articulation characteristics of apraxia to determine the presence and severity of apraxia. Finally, DiSimoni (1989) developed a test instrument, the Comprehensive Apraxia Test (CAT), that focuses on oral and verbal apractic deficits. Included are six subtests that assess oral postures and movements, vowels in isolation, alternate motion rates, production of syllables and production of utterances of increasing length, and a nonsense disyllable contextual interference subtest used to assess the effects of context on errors.

Administration of the aphasia test batteries plus careful exploration of possible oral and verbal apractic deficits using one of the above protocols should yield a large corpus of clinical data for differential diagnosis and specification of the aphasic/apractic involvement. The diagnosis is based on history, documented site of lesion, and speech and language characteristics.

TREATMENT

The first goal of treatment, as we noted earlier, is to provide a reliable means of communication. Quite obviously, the type of communication used will depend on the patient's residual ability and the communicative setting. Based on the assessment and additional observation, a communication system can be explored. For the patient with severe apraxia, this may take the form of a yes/no gesture system or a simplified communication board with pictures and alphabet. For the less impaired patient, verbal expression with some compromises on accuracy, speed, and length may be more appropriate. There also should be a careful exploration of communication contexts. We have found it helpful to provide a daily log of communicative situations, the type of communication used, and the success of the patient in meeting communication needs. Checklists (e.g., Chapey, 1986) that explore speech and language behaviors in detail also may be of value.

A second focus of treatment is to make the patient's communication system more efficient. If the patient is using a communication board with some residual verbal expression, then improved word retrieval and/or articulatory programming will have the effect of increasing the speed and flexibility of the patient's communication system. Similarly, teaching of an increased number of gestures for a patient with a manual communication system will increase the communicative facility of this patient.

The third goal of treatment is to increase communicative interaction. A frequent problem with many patients with aphasia is that they are reactive but infrequently initiate communication. An important function of the treatment program is to develop communication strategies to enhance the exchange of information with the aphasic patient.

Developing a Functional Communication System

Counseling

Brain damage results in a large number of emotional and psychological responses in the patient and family (e.g., Biorn-Hansen, 1957; Kinsella & Duffy, 1980; Turnblom & Myers, 1952; Zraick & Boone, 1991). Included are role changes, guilt feelings, altered social life, and oversolicitousness of the family. These feelings and reactions may have dramatic effects on the patient's motivation and self-esteem and cannot be underestimated as important factors in rehabilitation. However, our discussion here is limited to the counseling of the patient, family, and rehabilitation personnel as it relates to communication.

The patient should be counseled about what has happened. Frequently the patient is informed about the fact that he or she has had a stroke at a time when that information cannot be fully comprehended. The type and extent of communication problem should be reviewed carefully and over a period of time in terms most likely to be understood by the patient. A treatment action plan should be proposed and agreed on so that the clinician and patient are partners in the process. The family should be provided with comparable information about the communication problem but will also need guidance about the most effective means to communicate with the patient. The intent of this counseling is to provide information about the communication disorder, the best ways to communicate with the patient, and methods to reduce the communicative burden for the patient by assuming a larger portion of the communication load. Rehabilitation staff should be counseled about communication limits of the patient and optimal means of conveying information in multistep occupational therapy, physical therapy, and nursing-related tasks.

Functional Responses

Holland (1978) indicated that functional responses are based on three considerations: (1) the strategies used by the patient to communicate, (2) compromises on accuracy acceptable to the patient and family, and (3) the use of alternative forms of communication. In verbal apraxia, functional responses are strategies the patient uses to convey information regardless of the modality used. In treatment terms, this means that compensatory strategies used by the patient should be evaluated to determine which should be reinforced and capitalized on. At the initial stage of treatment, any and all responses that are effective in meeting this goal are reinforced as long as they allow reliable communication to take place. Acceptable responses may include gestures, letter boards, single-word responses, and written words. For the recovering patient these strategies may be a prelude to completely verbal responses. For the severely impaired patient, this may be the end-product of the rehabilitation effort.

Compensatory strategies can be taught. The patient may be instructed to nod his or her head to indicate a positive or negative response if verbal responses are not differentiated. Other examples are to teach the patient to carry identifying information like a driver's license to answer questions about his date of birth, address, and age; using symbolic gestures in lieu of verbal responses that are not understood; and writing the first letter of words that he is attempting to produce.

Augmentative communication may have a major role at this stage of rehabilitation. Picture and letter boards offer the patient the opportunity to convey information in other than verbal terms. Simple communication devices of this type are the instruments of choice for patients at early stages of recovery; more sophisticated devices are perhaps most appropriate for patients who do not develop functional oral communication but who have good auditory comprehension.

Approaches Based on Articulatory Accuracy

Several treatment paradigms for verbal apraxia are predicated on direct behavioral modification of impaired ability to produce articulatory movements. To a large extent, these are modifications of treatment programs for children with delayed articulatory development. Their use for patients with verbal apraxia is reviewed in detail by Wertz et al. (1984) and Square-Storer (1989). In general, there is a hierarchical ordering of the tasks, working from productions that are articulatorily least complex and most visible to those that are more complex and less visible.

Phonetic Placement

The phonetic placement approach, initially described by Van Riper and Irwin (1958), is familiar to most clinicians. It involves describing to the patient what placement is required for the production of a sound accompanied by pictures of the articulator positions and movements. For example, in the development of the bilabial voiceless stop /p/, the position of the lips at closure, the development of intraoral pressure, and the rapid opening for the production of a transient noise burst would be described with the aid of pictures and drawings. If the patient was unable to produce the stop after several trials, manual manipulation of the lips would be undertaken to provide tactile and kinesthetic cues associated with the movements. We have found this approach to be helpful in establishing highly visible anterior stops and fricatives, but it is less successful with speech sounds heavily context-dependent in their production, such as semivowels. Similarly, in patients with severe apraxia and stereotyped output, a large investment of time may be required to produce a limited repertoire of words.

Phonetic Derivation

Phonetic derivation (Van Riper & Irwin, 1958), is the production of a speech sound that the patient cannot correctly articulate from another that he or she can produce correctly. It frequently is used in combination with phonetic placement since the derived sound will have important features in common with its counterpart. For example, if the patient has difficulty producing the voiced bilabial stop /b/ but can correctly produce its cognate /p/, then using tactile feedback by placement of the patient's hand on his or her larynx, beginning voicing, and then continuing through the articulatory movements for production of /p/ would result in the production of /b/, albeit with an abnormally long prevoicing time.

Integral Stimulation

Another treatment for verbal apraxia based on imitative articulation training for children (Milisen, 1954) is integral stimulation (Rosenbek, Lemme, Ahern, Harris, & Wertz, 1973). Its primary features are the maximizing of sensory information (visual, auditory, tactile) with gradual reduction in the "aid" provided by the clinician. Integral stimulation provides the cornerstone of the well known "eight-step continuum" for the treatment of apraxia of speech, beginning with "Watch me and listen to me," as the clinician and patient simultaneously produce words followed by presentation of the stimulus with a delayed response by the patient as the clinician mimes the production. Steps three through five involve integral stimulation followed by delayed production by the patient without visual and auditory cues, repeated production of the word or phrase by the patient without auditory or visual cues by the clinician, and presentation of a visual stimulus and simultaneous production of the utterance by the clinician and patient, respectively. Steps six through eight remove the integral stimulation cues. The final steps are production of the utterance by the patient after a visual stimulus has been presented and removed, production of the stimulus in response to a question, and appropriate use of the word or phrase in situational context.

Sequencing of Speech Sounds

Dabul and Bollier (1976) argued that a primary problem for the patient with apraxia was the inability to produce sequences of syllables. They developed a multistep approach based on nonsense syllables to deal specifically with this deficit. Patients are first taught to produce individual speech sounds that are under voluntary control through phonetic placement or derivation at a 90% criterion level. The patient then learns to produce each sound in rapid succession before attempting to master a second sound. The sounds are then integrated into nonsense disyllables beginning with CVCV shapes but progressing to more complex syllable forms such as CVC and nonsense syllables with different consonants and vowels in the syllable series. At this point, the patient has sound production under voluntary control and can progress to a word level.

PROMPT System of Therapy

*P*rompts for *R*estructuring *O*ral *M*uscular *P*honetic *T*argets (PROMPTS) "is a dynamic tactile and kinesthetic-based articulatory-prosodic treatment strategy for the enhancement of motor speech production" (Square, Chumpelik, Morningstar, & Adams, 1986, p. 221). The system of treatment uses multiple tactile cues applied to the face and under the chin to prompt place of production, nasality, manner of production, phoneme duration, degree of jaw opening, and tense-lax distinctions. A different prompt is used to cue each of the English phonemes. The prompts may be strung together to cue a syllable, word, or phrase that is produced with an articulatory pattern similar to the model produced by the clinician. Square et al. (1986) reported that the PROMPT system was highly effective for training minimal pairs, multisyllabic words and functional phrases for patients with apraxia of speech.

Traditional Apraxia Therapy

An amalgam of the preceding approaches to treatment is included in what might best be termed traditional therapy for verbal apraxia (Darley, Aronson, & Brown, 1975). Included are a series of tasks, hierarchically arranged by difficulty, that encompasses integral stimulation, phonetic placement, combination of phonemes into nonsense syllables of increasing complexity for repeated production, and carry-over to phrases and sentences. Throughout the program there is a focus on repetitive drill, feedback, working on visible sounds first, self-correction, and progression to increasingly longer utterances.

Prosodically Oriented Treatment Approaches

Treatment approaches related to prosodic variables can be subdivided into two broad categories: (1) direct intervention for dysprosodic aspects of production, in which abnormalities of stress, rate, intonation, and timing become the *targets* of treatment; and (2) remediation strategies for apraxic articulation, wherein prosodic or suprasegmental variables are used as *facilitators* of more accurate production. This distinction appears to be an outgrowth, to some extent, of whether one views the dysprosody of Broca's aphasia/verbal apraxia as a primary symptom (Kent & Rosenbek, 1983) or a compensatory strategy (Johns & Darley, 1970). It is also possible that both mechanisms may contribute to dysprosody in an individual patient and may therefore be differentially addressed in treatment.

Direct intervention for prosodic abnormalities has not been well-studied and relatively little information is available on the topic. Robin, Klouda, and Hug (1991) take the position that remediation of neurogenic dysprosody in general should be regarded as a legitimate treatment goal because of the importance of prosody in interpersonal communication. These authors provide a comprehensive program for the assessment, treatment, and counseling of patients afflicted with neurogenic dysprosody, emphasizing the importance of acoustical instrumentation for diagnostic quantification and for biofeedback in therapy. They also present specific case data. The reader is referred to Robin et al. (1991) for more in-depth discussion.

Abnormalities of speaking rate and rhythm are frequently related to dysfluency, which is common in Broca's aphasia with apractic speech. Deal and Cannito (1991) outlined treatment approaches that have been used in association with acquired neurogenic dysfluency. These can generally be categorized as focusing either on *management of the underlying pathology* or *direct symptom modification* of dysfluent speech. Managing the underlying pathology includes enhancement of the physiological substrate, by means of drugs, surgery, or protheses, as well as the traditional speech-language therapies for aphasia, dysarthria, or apraxia of speech. Direct symptom modification approaches borrow directly from the rich literature available on the treatment of stuttering, and include either stuttering modification (e.g., breathing, relaxation) or fluency shaping (e.g., prolonged speech) techniques. With regard to selection of a particular treatment strategy, Deal & Cannito (1991) suggest that traditional aphasia and motor speech evaluations, used in conjunction with the neurodiagnostic data, will determine the presence of classical aphasias, dysarthrias, or apraxia of speech. Faced with dysfluency in the presence of these primary communicative deficits, addressing the primary deficit first may be the preferred procedure.

Early in treatment, a primary deficit such as Broca's aphasia/verbal apraxia is probably more disruptive to interpersonal communication than is dysfluency alone, and the dysfluency will often (but not always) resolve as the primary deficit resolves. Further, direct symptom modification of dysfluency by methods derived from developmental stuttering literature tend to be cognitively or linguistically demanding and therefore may be more appropriate to a later stage of recovery. Helm-Estabrooks (1986) noted that "successful management of neurogenic stuttering requires differential treatment as well as differential diagnosis" (p. 211). In a survey of practicing clinicians who provide direct therapy for acquired neurogenic stuttering, Market, Montague, Buffalo, and Drummond (1990) reported that approximately 78% favor slow rate, 58% favor easy onset/air flow, 28% favor attitude/relaxation, and 17% favor Van Riperian methods as preferred treatment strategies. As the clinical database increases, clinicians may anticipate increasing guidance for remediation of dysprosodic/dysfluent patients. In the meantime, the current state of the art largely remains trial-and-error experimentation with individual cases.

In contrast to the foregoing, there is substantial literature related to the use of prosodic variables as facilitators of apraxic speech output. This treatment orientation includes such widely used strategies as melodic intonation and singing therapies, auditory rhythmic stimulation therapies, altered rate, increased loudness, and the use of contrastive stress (Darley, 1984). All of these approaches are rooted in the assumption that prosodic abilities, with the exception of articulatory timing, are relatively spared in Broca's aphasia/verbal apraxia and can therefore be exploited as an organizational scaffolding for impaired articulation.

Melodic intonation therapy (MIT) and other singing therapies are rooted in the notion that the right hemisphere is preferentially involved in the processing of melodies and intonation contours, as well as the common clinical finding that the ability to sing, chant, or hum is relatively well preserved in many left-hemisphere–damaged aphasic patients (Sparks, Helm, & Albert, 1974). Historically, aphasiologists have emphasized the importance of singing as a component of aphasia rehabilitation. Unfortunately, however, improved word production in the context of singing popular tunes or jingles does not typically transfer to propositional connected speech. MIT was developed to capitalize on the relatively intact melodic abilities of aphasic patients as a facilitator of improved verbal expression for severe nonfluent aphasics who are not "global" in the extent of their impairment. In its most current version, MIT has been described as a "hierarchically structured program that is divided into three levels" (Helm-Estabrooks & Albert, 1991, p. 208). Each level has highly elaborated substeps, and a detailed scoring procedure is used to determine when specific criteria are met for advancement through the program. Initially, short high-probability sentences are musically intoned. A gradual progression through stages of increasing difficulty leads to more complex sentences that are first intoned, then spoken with prosodic exaggeration, then produced normally. When utterances are melodically intoned they are produced slowly using continuous phonation but normal stress with a combination of high and low notes. During melodic intonation the clinician taps the patient's left hand in unison with each syllable produced. The first level of the MIT progression is the most heavily clinician-assisted and has easier response requirements on the part of the patient. At this level, the patient moves from humming to unison singing, to immediate repetition, to response to a probe question. The second level increases task complexity by introducing response delays, after which the patient attempts to intone the words without verbal assistance (although tapping assistance continues to be provided). At this level, the patient moves from observation of the stimulus item introduced by the clinician, to unison production with fading, to delayed repetition, to response to a probe question. Level three is the most difficult stage, wherein sentence complexity is increased and a return to normal prosody is the ultimate goal. Rhythm and stress continue to be exaggerated but the songlike tonal quality of the previous stages is eliminated (i.e., "speech song"). At this level, the patient moves from delayed repetition with melodic intoning, to introduction of "speech song" with fading, to delayed spoken repetition, to response to a probe question. For a comprehensive description of this program, the reader is referred to Helm-Estabrooks and Albert (1991) and Sparks and Holland (1976).

The MIT program is especially recommended for Broca's aphasics with apraxia of speech who have mild to moderate auditory comprehension impairment, poor repetition, as well as good motivation and attention span. Treatment efficacy appears to be favorable with appropriate candidates and has been evaluated in Albert, Sparks, and Helm (1973), Sparks et al. (1974), and Naeser and Helm-Estabrooks (1985). The elaborately hierarchical structure of MIT appears to be important, inasmuch as simple imitation of melodically intoned sentences (without preliminary training steps) has been shown to be detrimental rather than beneficial to articulation in apraxia of speech subjects (Tonkovich & Marquardt, 1977). Specific suggestions for custom tailoring MIT plans for individual patients have been provided by Marshall and Holtzapple (1976).

An alternative form of singing therapy found to be effective with an individual apractic/aphasic patient was reported by Keith and Aronson (1975). The patient was able to imitate well-known song lyrics and sing completions to sentences sung by the clinician. The patient was also able to sing short functional phrases and was encouraged to do so in the hospital ward, and afterward at home. At follow-up approximately 1 year later, test performance on the PICA had improved substantially and the patient was able to speak spontaneously in most situations, albeit with aphasic errors of grammar and word choice.

Auditory rhythmic stimulation and other rate control therapies appear to address the articulatory initiation and timing deficits of verbal apraxia. Auditory rhythmic stimulation, using a device such as a metronome or a pulsed-tone generator, imposes an external temporal stimulus around which the patient may organize syllable articulation. Shane and Darley (1978) reported no significant effect on articulatory accuracy for either fast or slow rates of rhythmic stimulation in eight mildly aphasic subjects with apraxia of speech. Using a multiple-baseline, single-subject design with one apractic patient, Dworkin, Abkarian, and Johns (1988) reported dramatic improvement of articulatory accuracy with metronome stimulation in polysyllabic words and sentences. Therapeutic gains did not transfer, however, to sentence production in the absence of metronome stimulation. It is noteworthy that in this study the metronome did not immediately facilitate multisyllabic productions but came to do so over several training sessions. This may explain the disparity between Dworkin et al. (1988) and Shane & Darley (1978); the latter was a single-shot experiment without a long-term treatment component.

Other forms of rate control have also been suggested. Southwood (1987) used single subject multiple baseline designs to demonstrate a systematic decrease in articulation errors as a consequence of prolonged speech in two residual aphasics with mild-to-moderate apraxia of speech. Pacing is a form of rate control in which an external timing signal is imposed by the patient using a pacing board as a prosthetic aid (Helm-Estabrooks, 1986). Darley (1984) has suggested that "slowing down rate will . . . almost surely . . . permit a more accurate imitation of the stimulus" (p. 300). In contrast, Johns and Darley (1970) reported that their apractic subjects produced markedly fewer articulation errors and became more intelligible when instructed to speak as rapidly as possible. Because rate control is an easy and inexpensive clinical manipulation, continued experimentation with its use with individual patients seems warranted. Available data, however, do not support widespread, indiscriminate application.

The method of contrastive stress enjoys some popularity among experienced clinicians who treat apraxia. Tonkovich and Marquardt (1977) demonstrated a facilitative effect of stressed syllables on articulatory accuracy during sentence imitation with 10 apraxia of speech subjects. Darley (1984) suggested that the technique is useful in facilitating apractic articulation by manipulating "elements of pitch, loudness and time to highlight a syllable or word" (p. 300). Rosenbek (1985) suggests that contrastive stress is a valuable technique because "apraxia of speech is both an articulatory and a prosodic disturbance" (p. 296). Thus, contrastive stress drills are intended to ameliorate both difficulties simultaneously. In this technique, the clinician typically presents a stimulus sentence (e.g., "Jill kicked Jack"), uttering each word slowly with equivalent stress. The client then produces the sentence in response to question stimuli provided by the examiner (e.g., "Who kicked Jack?"), in which the client emphasizes the word that is highlighted by the information requested in the interrogative stimulus. The procedure lends itself to the development of phonological and syntactic hierarchies and has the added benefit of facilitating grammatical production (Goodglass et al., 1967). In addition, the approach enjoys face validity due to the fact that stressed syllables are normally pronounced with greater articulatory precision and less profound accommodation and reduction effects than are their unstressed counterparts.

A previously unpublished study by Nichols (1979) focused specifically on the hypothesis that stress facilitates production accuracy in 11 individuals with Broca's aphasia and apraxia of speech. Sixty-four phrases, each composed of three monosyllabic words conforming to four stress patterns, were presented via videotape for the aphasic subjects to imitate. Production errors due to phonetic inaccuracy or word substitution and omission were noted. Given equal numbers of stressed and unstressed syllables pooled across contours, the mean number of word production errors in stressed syllables was 26.55 (S.D. = 15.96) and 33.36 in unstressed syllables (S.D. = 33.36). This difference was statistically significant. Within all four stress contours, error means for unstressed syllables always exceeded error means for stressed syllables.

In their single case study, Dworkin et al. (1988) also demonstrated an initial facilitative stress effect and gradual sustained improvement across sessions on contrastive stress drills. Interestingly, their patient demonstrated equivalent degrees of generalization of therapeutic gains to conversational speech for both neutrally stressed sentences produced with metronome stimulation and sentences produced with contrastive stress.

Gestural Reorganization

The positive treatment gains resulting from use of a pacing board and melodic intonation therapy reflect the facilitatory effect of simultaneous limb and oral motor activity. In effect, more intact limb function is used to reorganize speech motor activity by pairing moment-to-moment gestural movements to speech production in order to generate intersystemic reorganization, "the rebuilding of speech by the introduction into the act of speaking a system or sets of responses in a unique form or with a unique regularity" (Rosenbek, Collins, & Wertz, 1976, p. 256). Motor activities vary in meaningfulness and range from tapping (MIT), to finger counting (Simmons, 1978), to the use of more meaningful gestures. Skelly, Schinsky, Smith, and Fust (1974) taught American Indian Sign (AMERIND) to a group of six patients with apraxia. They found that the patients made progress in using speech while they produced accompanying signs. Additionally, they found marked improvements in PICA verbal subtest scores when pre-training and post-training scores were compared. Performance improved 1.60–7.07 points on the verbal subtests while gestural subtest score changes during the 6-month period were minimal (0.03–1.62 points).

Volitional Sentence Production

It should be recognized that, in apraxia of speech patients with significant aphasic impairment, the inability to talk may be as much due to sentence formulation difficulty as to the articulation disorder. Approaches that stress volitional production of selected sentences for functional communication appear to address both of these issues simultaneously. Foremost of these is the well known eight-step continuum procedure originated by Rosenbek et al. (1973). This approach relies heavily on the technique of integral stimulation and the patient's ability to imitate words and phrases in a highly structured clinical situation. Unlike segmental approaches discussed previously, whole utterance approaches are communication centered and are accepting of "a variety of articulation errors and even telegraphic utterances if failure to do so inordinately delays the patients' use of meaningful, useful utterances" (Rosenbek et al., 1973. p. 471). The eight-step continuum consists of a series of activities of increasing difficulty noted earlier. In addition to the specific steps, a variety of other facilitative techniques, both segmental and prosodic, are employed liberally as needed. The technique proved to be useful for two of three moderately aphasic/apractic patients studied by Rosenbek et al. Subsequently, Deal and Florance (1978) developed a modified version of the eight-step continuum in which step utilization was tailored to the individual, and they demonstrated its utility with four severely nonfluent patients who had suffered left cerebrovascular accidents (the extent of aphasia was not documented). The ultimate goal of treatment in both of these studies was functional communication in the home environment. Although the program purports to address articulatory variables, the extent to which sentence formulation processes were also stimulated has not been determined. A similar but highly streamlined approach, using simple sentence repetition for highly individualized utterances that were motivating to the patient (e.g., "I want a cold Bud"), has also been reported (Marshall, 1986).

Other whole utterance approaches have more directly targeted sentence formulation processes. Florance and Deal (1979a) describe a "conversational program" developed for a severely nonfluent-patient with moderate aphasia and apraxia of speech. The program was designed to (1) teach sentences, (2) establish conversational units, and (3) stimulate purposeful conversational speech at home. The program was structured in four units. First, the patient read sentences with clinician cueing as needed until a criterion of 80% correct sentence production (i.e., one error or less) on two uncued trials was achieved. Second, the same procedure was used to train sentences corresponding to a script for ordering in a restaurant. Initially, the patient used trained utterances to respond to a clinician-initiated restaurant dialogue. Later, any appropriate response was encouraged. Third, a conversational unit was developed around a blackjack game. Finally, a conversational unit was developed around making inquiring telephone calls. Dramatic improvement across sessions was demonstrated for each unit. In addition, a home program was incorporated with the patient's spouse serving as interlocutor and monitor of progress. During the treatment period over 100 novel utterances were recorded outside of therapy.

Florance and Deal (1979b) elaborated and refined their conversational program, reporting pre- and post-treatment results for 15 "nonverbal stroke patients," with severely nonfluent output consisting of recurrent utterances or verbal stereotypes, relatively intact comprehension, and apraxia of speech. The treatment consisted of three steps. First, target utterances were trained, using a combination of auditory and graphic stimulation with visual cueing. Second, a "pseudo conversational procedure" was employed in which the patient initially responds to pre-established questions, followed later by interactions in which the patient was encouraged to provide any appropriate response. Third, a generalization step uses information regarding the patient's "immediate needs and communicative desires." From this a scripted conversational interaction was developed in which the patient responds to a logical series of coordinated questions. As a result of this program, significant gains were reported for PICA overall and verbal scores, as well as increases in utterance length and information conveyed in spontaneous speech.

A somewhat different approach to improving functional verbal expression in a Broca's aphasic patient with apraxia was reported by Kearns (1986a). The goal of treatment was to facilitate spontaneous verbal elaboration of information, defined as a number of intelligible, relevant content words per response. The program employs a six-step sequence of verbal elaboration of patient-initiated responses to action pictures. A single-subject multiple-baseline design was used to demonstrate significant gains in treatment that were subsequently maintained and which generalized to untreated items. Significant gains in PICA verbal subtests were also observed across pre- to post-testing. This study emphasized the importance of "loose training," wherein patient-initiated responding and creative language are encouraged. In general, the volitional sentence production or whole utterance approaches appear efficacious for many patients and are easily integrated with other facilitative techniques. The importance of ongoing training for transfer of these utterances into the home or other functional environment cannot be overemphasized.

Functional Approaches

The third goal of treatment is the development of interactive communication skills at the highest level of efficiency for the patient. Several treatment approaches may aid in evolving communication skills that are interactive and not simply reactive. We have found that the use of Promoting Aphasics' Communicative Effectiveness (PACE) (Wilcox & Davis, 1978) is helpful in the early stages of treatment for demonstrating a full range of communication options by modeling information transfer through multiple modalities. We have also found it effective in a broader context wherein the patient is asked to communicate information to conversational partners other than the clinician.

PACE is based on four principles: (1) new information is conveyed by the patient or clinician during each communication turn; (2) any modality or combination of modalities may be used to convey the information; (3) the patient and clinician are equal communication partners; and (4) feedback is provided by the clinician regarding the success of the information transfer.

We have found this approach helpful in initial treatment because it fosters compensatory strategies that focus on the success of communication rather than on verbal accuracy (Holland, 1978). A second beneficial feature of the approach is that it requires that the patient actively convey information rather than serving as a reactive partner.

A second functional approach that allows the patient to try new communicative behaviors in a controlled setting is group aphasia therapy (Kearns, 1986b; Marquardt, 1982). This setting is particularly effective for apractic patients because they are better receivers than senders of information. The content units of the sessions can be geared to the interests of the patients in the group in an attempt to foster communication content of maximal interest to the participants.

SUMMARY

There is a richness and diversity to the treatment of patients with verbal apraxia and Broca's aphasia that is perhaps unmatched in the rehabilitation of adults with neurogenic disorders. This chapter has focused on treatment for impaired speech production, but it is important to note that approaches as diverse as electromyographic feedback (McNeil, Prescott, & Lemme, 1976) and American Indian Hand Talk (Skelly, 1979) also may have an important role. Treatment paradigms are built on the type and severity of the disorder and the therapy approaches that prove to be most beneficial to the patient.

REFERENCES

Albert, M.L., Sparks, R., & Helm, N.A. (1973). Melodic intonation therapy. *Archives of Neurology, 29*, 130–131.

Baum, S., Blumstein, S., Naeser, M., & Palumbo, C. (1990). Temporal dimensions of consonant and vowel production: An acoustic and CT scan analysis of aphasic speech. *Brain and Language, 39*, 33–56.

Beckman, M.E. (1986). *Stress and nonstress accent.* Dordrecht, Holland: Foris Publications.

Benson, D.F. (1979). *Aphasia, alexia and agraphia.* New York: Churchill Livingstone.

Biorn-Hansen, V. (1957). Social and emotional aspects of aphasia. *Journal of Speech and Hearing Disorders. 22*, 53–59.

Blumstein, S., Cooper, W., Zurif, E., & Caramazza, A. (1977). The perception and production of voice-onset-time in aphasia. *Neuropsychologia, 15*, 371–383.

Canter, G.J. (1971). Observations on neurogenic stuttering: A contribution to differential diagnosis. *British Journal of Disorders of Communication, 6*, 139–143.

Chapey, R. (1986). The assessment of language disorders in adults. In R. Chapey (Ed.), *Language intervention strategies in adult aphasia* (pp. 81–104). Baltimore: Williams & Wilkins.

Colson, K., Luschei, E., & Jordan, L. (1986). Perceptual and acoustic analyses of stress patterning in apraxic and normal speech. In R.H. Brookshire (Ed.), *Clinical aphasiology conference proceedings* (pp. 281–290). Minneapolis: BRK Publishers.

Cooper, W., Soares, C., Nicol, J., Michelow, D., & Goloskie, S. (1984). Clausal intonation after unilateral brain damage. *Language and Speech, 27*, 17–24.

Dabul, B. (1979). *Apraxia battery for adults.* Austin, TX: PRO-ED.

Dabul, B., & Bollier, B. (1976). Therapeutic approaches to apraxia. *Journal of Speech and Hearing Disorders, 41*, 268–276.

Danly, M., & Shapiro, B (1982). Speech prosody in Broca's aphasia. *Brain and Language, 16*, 171–190.

Darley, F.L. (1984). Apraxia of speech: A neurogenic articulation disorders. In H. Winitz (Ed.), *Treating articulation disorders: For clinicians by clinicians* (pp. 289–305). Austin, TX: PRO-ED.

Darley, F., Aronson, A., & Brown, J. (1975). *Motor speech disorders.* Philadelphia: Lea & Febiger.

Deal, J., & Cannito, M. (1991). Acquired neurogenic dysfluency. In D. Vogel & M. Cannito (Eds.), *Treating disordered speech motor control: For clinicians by clinicians* (pp. 217–239). Austin, TX: PRO-ED.

Deal, J.L., & Florance, C. (1978). Modification of the eight-step continuum for treatment of apraxia of speech in adults. *Journal of Speech and Hearing Disorders, 43*, 89–95.

DeRenzi, E., Pieczuro, A., & Vignolo, L. (1966). Oral apraxia and aphasia. *Cortex, 2*, 50–73.

DiSimoni, F. (1989). *Apraxia of speech: Theoretical and practical considerations.* Dalton, PA: Praxis House Publishers.

Dunlop, J., & Marquardt, T. (1977). Linguistic and articulatory aspects of single word productions in apraxia of speech. *Cortex, 13*, 17–39.

Dworkin, J.P., Abkarian, G.G., & Johns, D.F. (1988). Apraxia of speech: The effectiveness of a treatment regimen. *Journal of Speech and Hearing Disorders, 53*, 280–292.

Florance, C., & Deal, J. (1979a). A treatment protocol for nonverbal stroke patients. In R. Brookshire (Ed.), *Clinical aphasiology: Conference proceedings* (pp. 59–67). Minneapolis: BRK Publishers.

Florance, C.L., & Deal, J.L. (1979b) Treatment for apraxia of speech: A conversational approach. *Ohio Journal of Speech and Hearing, 14*, 184–191.

Fromm, D., Abbs, J., McNeil, M., & Rosenbek, J. (1982). Simultaneous perceptual-physiological method for studying apraxia of speech. In R.H. Brookshire (Ed.), *Clinical aphasiology: Conference proceedings* (pp. 251–262). Minneapolis: BRK Publishers.

Goodglass, H., Fodor, I., & Schulhoff, C. (1967). Prosodic factors in grammar-evidence from aphasia. *Journal of Speech and Hearing Research, 10*, 5–20.

Goodglass, H., & Kaplan, E. (1983). *The assessment of aphasia and related disorders.* Philadelphia: Lea & Febiger.

Harmes, S., Daniloff, R.G., Hoffman, P.R., Lewis, J., Kramer, M.B., & Absher, R. (1984). Temporal and articulatory control of fricative articulation by speakers with Broca's aphasia. *Journal of Phonetics, 12*, 367–385.

Helm-Estabrooks, N. (1986). Diagnosis and management of neurogenic stuttering in adults. In K.O. St. Louis (Ed.), *The atypical stutterer: Principles and practices of rehabilitation* (pp. 193–217). Orlando, FL: Academic Press.

Helm-Estabrooks, N., & Albert, M. (1991). *Manual of aphasia therapy.* Austin, TX: PRO-ED.

Hoffmann, E. (1980). Speech control and paraphasia in fluent and nonfluent aphasics. In H.W. Dechert & M. Raupach (Eds.), *Temporal variables in speech: Studies in honor of Frieda Goldman-Eisler* (pp, 121–127). The Hague: Mouton.

Holland, A. (1978). Functional communication in the treatment of aphasia. In L. Bradford (Ed.), *Communicative disorders: An audio journal for continuing education.* New York: Grune & Stratton.

Holland, A. (1980). *Communicative abilities in daily life.* Baltimore: University Park Press.

Johns, D., & Darley, F. (1970). Phonemic variability in apraxia of speech. *Journal of Speech and Hearing Research, 13,* 556–583.

Kearns, K.P. (1986a) Systematic programming of verbal elaboration skills in chronic Broca's aphasia. In R.C. Marshall (Ed.), *Case studies in aphasia rehabilitation: For clinicians by clinicians* (pp. 225–243). Austin, TX: PRO-ED.

Kearns, K.P. (1986b). Group aphasia therapy: Theoretical and practical considerations. In R. Chapey (Ed.), *Language intervention strategies in adult aphasia* (pp. 304–318). Baltimore: Williams & Wilkins.

Keatley, M.A. (1979). A comparison of intonational contours in subjects with apraxia of speech and normals. *Aphasia-Apraxia-Agnosia, 1,* 30–42.

Keith, R.L., & Aronson, A.E. (1975). Singing as therapy for apraxia of speech and aphasia: Report of a case. *Brain and Language, 2,* 483–488.

Kent, R.D., & Rosenbek, J.C.(1982). Prosodic disturbance and neurologic lesion. *Brain and Language, 15,* 259–291.

Kent, R.D., & Rosenbek, J.C. (1983). Acoustic patterns of apraxia of speech. *Journal of Speech and Hearing Research, 26,* 231–249.

Kertesz, A. (1979). *Aphasia and associated disorders.* New York: Grune & Stratton.

Kertesz, A. (1982). *Western aphasia battery.* New York: Grune & Stratton.

Kertesz, A. (1984). Subcortical lesions and verbal apraxia. In J. Rosenbek, M. McNeil, & A. Aronson (Eds.), *Apraxia of speech: Physiology-Acoustics-Linguistics-Management* (pp. 73–90). San Diego: College-Hill Press.

Kinsella, G., & Duffy, R. (1980). Attitudes toward disability expressed by spouses of aphasic patient. *Scandinavian Journal of Rehabilitation Medicine, 12,* 129–132.

Lesser, R. (1978). *Linguistic investigations of aphasia.* London: Arnold.

Market, K.E., Montague, J.C., Buffalo, M.D., & Drummond, S.S. (1990). Acquired stuttering: Descriptive data and treatment outcome. *Journal of Fluency Disorders, 15,* 21–33.

Marquardt, T. (1982). Acquired neurogenic disorders. Englewood Cliffs, NJ: Prentice-Hall.

Marquardt, T., & Sussman, H. (1984). The elusive lesion-apraxia of speech link in Broca's aphasia. In J. Rosenbek, M. McNeil, & A. Aronson (Eds.), *Apraxia of speech: Physiology-Acoustics-Linguistics-Management* (pp. 91–112). San Diego: College-Hill Press.

Marshall, N., & Holtzapple, P. (1976). Melodic intonation therapy: Variations on a theme. In R. Brookshire (Ed.), *Clinical aphasiology: Conference proceedings* (pp. 115–139). Minneapolis: BRK Publishers.

Marshall, R.C. (1986). A case for flexibility. In R.C. Marshall (Ed.), *Case studies in aphasia rehabilitation: For clinicians by clinicians* (pp. 197–213). Austin, TX: PRO-ED.

McNeil, M., Prescott, T., & Lemme, M. (1976). An application of electromyographic biofeedback to aphasia/apraxia treatment. In R. Brookshire (Ed.), *Clinical aphasiology: Conference proceedings* (pp. 151–165). Minneapolis: BRK Publishers.

Milisen, R. (1954). A rationale for articulation disorders. *Journal of Speech and Hearing Disorders, 4,* 6–17.

Mohr, J. (1976). Broca's area and Broca's aphasia. In H. Whitaker & H.A. Whitaker (Eds.), *Studies in neurolinguistics (Vol 1,* pp. 201–235). New York: Academic Press.

Naeser, M., & Helm-Estabrooks, N. (1985). CT scan lesion localization and response to melodic intonation therapy with nonfluent aphasia cases. *Cortex, 21,* 203–223.

Nichols, D. (1979). *Verbal expression in aphasia: Effects of prosodic stresses.* Unpublished Masters Thesis. University of Texas at Austin.

Odell, K., McNeil, M., Rosenbek, J., & Hunter, L. (1990). Perceptual characteristics of consonant productions by apraxic speakers. *Journal of Speech and Hearing Disorders, 55,* 345–359.

Odell, K., McNeil, M., Rosenbek, J., & Hunter, L. (1991). Perceptual characteristics of vowel and prosody production in apraxic, aphasic, and dysarthric speakers. *Journal of Speech and Hearing Research, 34,* 67–80.

Pierce, R. (1991). Apraxia of speech versus phonemic paraphasia: Theoretical, diagnostic, and treatment considerations. In D. Vogel & M. Cannito (Eds.), *Treating disordered speech motor control: For clinicians by clinicians* (pp. 185–216). Austin, TX: PRO-ED.

Porch, B.E. (1971). *Porch index of communicative ability* (2nd Edition). Palo Alto, CA: Consulting Psychologists Press.

Robin, D.A., Klouda, G.V., & Hug, L.N. (1991). Neurogenic disorders of prosody. In D. Vogel & M.P. Cannito (Eds.), *Treating disordered speech motor control: For clinicians by clinicians* (pp. 241–271). Austin, TX: PRO-ED.

Rosenbek, J.C. (1985). Treating apraxia of speech. In D.F. Johns (Ed.), *Clinical management of neurogenic communicative disorders* (pp. 267–312). Austin, TX: PRO-ED.

Rosenbek, J., Collins, M., & Wertz, R. (1976). Intersystemic reorganization for apraxia of speech. In R. Brookshire (Ed.), *Clinical aphasiology: Conference proceedings* (pp. 255–260). Minneapolis: BRK Publishers.

Rosenbek, J., Kent, R., & LaPointe, L. (1984). Apraxia of speech: An overview and some perspectives. In J. Rosenbek, M. McNeil, & A. Aronson (Eds.), *Apraxia of Speech: Physiology-Acoustics-Linguistics-Management* (pp. 1–72). San Diego: College-Hill Press.

Rosenbek, J., Lemme, J., Ahern, M., Harris, E., & Wertz, R. (1973). A treatment for apraxia of speech in adults. *Journal of Speech and Hearing Disorders, 38,* 462–472.

Rosenbek, J., & Wertz, R. (1976). *Veterans Administration workshop on motor speech disorders,* Madison, Wisconsin.

Ryalls, J.H. (1987). Vowel production in aphasia: towards an account of the consonant-vowel dissociation. In J.H. Ryalls (Ed.), *Phonetic approaches to speech production in aphasia and related disorders* (pp. 23–43). Austin, TX: PRO-ED.

Sarno, M. (1969). The functional communication profile. *New York University Medical Center Rehabilitation Monograph, 42.*

Schuell, H. (1965). *Minnesota test for the differential diagnosis of aphasia.* Minneapolis: University of Minnesota Press.

Shane, H.C., & Darley, F.L. (1978). The effect of auditory rhythmic stimulation on articulatory accuracy in apraxia of speech. *Cortex, 14,* 444–450.

Simmons, N. (1978). Finger counting as an intersystemic reorganizer in apraxia of speech. In R. Brookshire (Ed.), *Clinical aphasiology: Conference proceedings* (pp. 174–179). Minneapolis: BRK Publishers.

Skelly, M. (1979). *Amer-Ind gestural code.* New York: Elsevier.

Skelly, M., Schinsky, L., Smith, R., & Fust, R. (1974). American Indian Sign (Amerind) as a facilitator of verbalization for the oral verbal apraxic. *Journal of Speech and Hearing Disorders, 39,* 445–456.

Southwood, H. (1987). The use of prolonged speech in the treatment of apraxia of speech. In R. Brookshire (Ed.), *Clinical aphasiology: Conference proceedings* (pp. 277–287). Minneapolis: BRK Publishers.

Sparks, R., Helm, N. & Albert, M. (1974). Aphasia rehabilitation resulting from melodic intonation therapy. *Cortex, 10,* 303–316.

Sparks, R.W., & Holland, A.L. (1976). Method: Melodic intonation therapy for aphasia. *Journal of Speech and Hearing Disorders, 41,* 287–292.

Square, P., Darley, F., & Sommers, R. (1982). An analysis of the productive errors made by pure apractic speakers with differing loci of lesions. In R. Brookshire (Ed.), *Clinical aphasiology: Conference proceedings* (pp. 245–250). Minneapolis: BRK Publishers.

Square, P., Chumpelik, D., Morningstar, D., & Adams, S. (1986). Efficacy of the PROMPT system of therapy for the treatment of acquired apraxia of speech: A follow-up investigation. In R. Brookshire (Ed.), *Clinical aphasiology: Conference proceedings* (pp. 221–226). Minneapolis: BRK Publishers.

Square-Storer, P. (Ed.). (1989). *Acquired apraxia of speech in aphasic adults.* New York: Taylor & Francis.

Sussman, H., Marquardt, T., Hutchinson, J., & MacNeilage, P. (1986). Compensatory articulation in Broca's aphasia. *Brain and Language, 27,* 56–74.

Sussman, H., Marquardt, T., MacNeilage, P., & Hutchinson, J. (1988). Anticipatory coarticulation in aphasia: Some methodological considerations. *Brain and Language, 35,* 369–379.

Tonkovich, J., & Marquardt, T. (1977). The effects of stress and melodic intonation on apraxia of speech. In R. Brookshire (Ed.), *Clinical aphasiology: Conference proceedings* (pp. 97–102). Minneapolis: BRK Publishers.

Trost, J.E. (1971, November). *Apraxic dysfluency in patients with Broca's aphasia.* Paper presented at the Annual Convention of the American Speech and Hearing Association, Chicago.

Turnblom, M., & Myers, J. (1952). A group discussion program with the families of aphasic patients. *Journal of Speech and Hearing Disorders, 17,* 393–396.

Van Riper, C., & Irwin, J. (1958). *Voice and articulation.* Englewood Cliffs, NJ: Prentice-Hall.

Wertz, R., LaPointe, L., & Rosenbek, J. (1984). *Apraxia of speech in adults: The disorder and its management.* New York: Grune & Stratton.

Wilcox, J., & Davis, G., (1978). *Promoting aphasics' communicative effectiveness (PACE).* Memphis, TN: Memphis State University.

Yairi, E., Gintautas, J., & Avent, J.R. (1981). Disfluent speech associated with brain damage. *Brain and Language, 14,* 49–56.

Ziegler, W., & von Cramon, D. (1985). Anticipatory coarticulation in a patient with apraxia of speech. *Brain and Language, 26,* 117–130.

Ziegler, W., & von Cramon, D. (1986). Disturbed coarticulation in apraxia of speech. *Brain and Language, 29,* 34–47.

Zraick, R., & Boone, D. (1991). Spouse attitudes toward the person with aphasia. *Journal of Speech and Hearing Research, 34,* 123–128.

Chapter 13

Treatment of Naming Impairment

Edith Chin Li

The effective remediation of naming disorders is a critical issue because of the prevalence of naming deficits in the aphasic population. Many techniques are currently available for the anomic patient, including various stimulation therapies and cueing procedures. For the clinician, the challenge lies in the choice of the most effective program for the individual patient. Researchers have long recognized that aphasic naming disorders do not represent a single impairment; the diversity and complexity of naming deficits among aphasic patients make designing effective remedial programs a formidable task.

However, advances in neurolinguistics afford new perspectives on the clinical management of naming deficits. Recent neurolinguistic models provide detailed information on the nature of underlying processes in naming deficits. These models are essential to the formulation of an effective treatment program. This chapter begins with an overview of both traditional and more recent models of naming deficits. These classification systems serve as the bases for discussing evaluation and treatment. Factors essential to evaluation are considered next. This section centers on naming contexts, stimulus characteristics, and documentation of errors during the evaluation. Lastly, the chapter addresses formulating effective treatment goals and procedures. This section relates effective remediation to the theoretical models and evaluation procedures discussed earlier.

CLASSIFICATION OF NAMING DISORDERS

Traditional Models

The first models of naming deficits emerged in the 1960s. Geschwind (1967) differentiated classical anomia (naming deficits across various modalities, coupled with intact object recognition) from disconnection anomia (impaired recognition and naming confined to a single modality). Luria (1966, 1970) elaborated on several types of aphasic naming deficits, whose characteristics were based on the loci of impairment. Canter, Trost, and Burns (1985) and Benson (1979, 1988) provided more comprehensive paradigms that relate the cognitive processes in naming to corresponding neurologic regions. In their models, the naming process essentially begins with a concept of the stimulus to be named. Stimulation arises from many primary and secondary sensory cortical areas (visual, somesthetic, auditory). Connections are then made with the angular gyrus of the parietal lobe, which acts as the crucial association region for the separate sensory areas. Next, an appropriate word/symbol corresponding to the nonverbal concept is selected from the "lexical repository." Benson (1979) suggested area 37, the temporal-occipital junction, as the location of the lexical repository. Pathways connect area 37 with the motor speech patterning area (Broca's area, area 44). At this point, specific motor commands needed to produce the target word are programmed. Finally, production of the actual name is achieved via motor pathways that innervate the appropriate peripheral structures. Table 13.1 illustrates the naming-process model.

Benson (1979, 1988) used this model to classify four types of aphasic anomia. The disconnection type is similar to Geschwind's (1967) disconnection anomia. The remaining three subtypes correspond to breakdowns at specific points of the naming model. Semantic anomia, associated with damage at the angular gyrus, was characterized by a deficit in object identification as well as in object naming. Word-selection anomia, associated with damage in area 37, affected the selection of the target name. In this disorder, the patient could recognize and describe an object but was unable to name it upon presentation. Finally, word-production anomias were classified into two subtypes. Articulatory initiation anomia with damage involving area 44 (Broca's area) was characterized by difficulty in initiating phonation. Patients with paraphasic anomia, involving damage to pathways such as the arcuate fasciculus, emitted fluent, paraphasic responses.

Recent Models

In a recent model of naming disorders, Lesser (1989a) parallels the stages in Benson's model, with a notable exception. In Lesser's model, the initial stage involving the stimulus concept is divided into two separate semantic systems: object and verbal. The object semantic system allows reaction to objects without involvement of the language system. The verbal semantic system is a pool of semantic features arranged associatively or hierarchically.

The notion of single versus separate modality-specific semantic systems remains an unresolved issue. Some authors agree with Lesser that independent semantic stores exist for different modalities (Morton, 1985; Shallice, 1987). Others, like Caramazza, Berndt, and Brownell (1982) propose a single system of semantic knowledge. Despite this lack of agreement, there is

TABLE 13.1   Naming-Process Model

Cognitive Process	Corresponding Neurologic Area
Stimulus concept	Primary/secondary cortical areas
Crossmodal associations	Angular gyrus
Lexical representation	Temporal-occipital junction
Motor speech programming	Broca's area
Production of target word	Primary motor area/peripheral motor pathways

Source: Modified from F. Benson. (1979). *Neurologic correlates of anomia.* In H. Whitaker, H. Whitaker (Eds.), *Studies in neurolinguistics,* Vol. 4. New York: Academic Press; F. Benson. (1988). Anomia in aphasia. *Aphasiology, 2,* 229–236; G. Canter, J. Trost, M. Burns. (1985). Contrasting speech patterns in apraxia of speech and phonemic paraphasia. *Brain and Language, 24,* 204–222.

widespread consensus for a two-stage model of lexical access, the first stage semantically organized and the second phonologically organized. Butterworth (1989) suggests a temporal relationship in these stages. In the first stage, the semantic lexicon takes a semantic code as input and yields a phonologic address as output. In the second stage, the phonologic address is used as input and the phonologic word form is delivered as output.

A number of authors focus on distinctions between semantic and phonologic deficits. Lesser (1989b), Kay and Ellis (1987), and Howard and Orchard-Lisle (1984) describe differential naming difficulties related to a semantic lexicon deficit in a patient who had difficulty making fine semantic discriminations on semantic comprehension tasks. Naming errors tended to consist of semantic paraphasias. In addition, the patient often made semantic naming errors if a therapist supplied the initial phoneme of a close associate of the target. For instance, given a picture of "shoe" and the cue "s", the patient would respond "sock." Howard and Orchard-Lisle (1984) also note the tendency to make semantic errors with the presentation of a related associate during auditory and written-word comprehension tasks. This disorder resembles the "semantic anomia" described by Benson (1979, 1988).

Difficulty in retrieving an item from the phonologic lexicon produces a different set of clinical signs (Lesser, 1989b; Kay & Ellis, 1987; Howard & Orchard-Lisle, 1984). These patients appear to have intact semantic representations for the target word, as evidenced by good performance on recognition tasks. Naming errors tend to consist of phonemic paraphasias and circumlocutions. The patient frequently exhibits partial awareness of phonologic characteristics of the word—"tip-of-the tongue" condition. This disorder parallels Benson's (1979, 1988) "word-selection" anomia.

Although recent investigations tend to focus on characteristics of semantic and phonologic-level disorders rather than on later word production, Lesser (1989b) also provides a description of "phonemic assembly" and "verbal praxis" naming deficits. Phonemic-assembly patients have difficulty in sequencing and organizing phonemic information. Predominant errors are target-oriented phonemic paraphasias. Benson (1979, 1988) classifies these patients as paraphasic anomics. Verbal praxic patients experience difficulty in organizing and programming articulation, exhibiting phoneme substitutions and difficulty in transition from one phoneme to another. Benson (1979, 1988) would consider these patients to be articulatory initiation anomics.

In summary, investigations of naming deficits indicate that the processes underlying naming are diverse and complex. The review of naming models focused on naming disorders commonly encountered in the aphasic population. These "classic" types of anomia included deficits at the semantic, phonologic, or articulatory programming levels.

The models have direct implications for the treatment of naming disorders. Different naming deficits logically require different types of remediation. To determine an effective treatment program, a comprehensive evaluation must be conducted. The following section covers recommended evaluation procedures.

EVALUATION OF NAMING DEFICITS

An accurate evaluation of naming deficits should provide comprehensive information on clinical naming behaviors in the patient. Inferences can then be drawn concerning the level of disruption in cognitive processing. The evaluation encompasses a series of controlled tasks across various modalities and verbal contexts. In addition, adequate documentation of specific error types is essential.

Oral Language Contexts

There is ample evidence that naming deficits vary across different contexts of naming. Barton, Maruszewski, and Urrea (1969) found sentence completion to be the most effective context for their group of aphasic subjects, followed by confrontation naming, and then naming to description. These three contexts should be included in the naming battery. A fourth task, verbal fluency, is frequently included on standardized batteries. Words within a category (e.g., animal names or words that start with a particular letter) are listed within a prescribed time limit. There is evidence that measures of verbal fluency provide useful information on lexical search strategies (Collins, McNeil, & Rosenbek, 1984; Grossman, 1978, 1981).

In addition to the more "traditional" tasks described above, recent studies reveal other contexts that affect the effectiveness of naming. In a series of studies (Williams, 1990; Williams & Canter, 1982, 1987), Williams and

Canter found three key variables that systematically influence naming performance: grammatical class (nouns versus verbs), situation context (confrontation naming compared to scene description), and presentation mode (line drawings versus videotaped presentation). The investigators discovered that with line-drawn stimuli, object-naming was superior to action-naming during both confrontation naming and picture-description tasks. However, when videotaped stimuli were used, object-naming exceeded action-naming performance during confrontation naming but not during scene description. The investigators suggested that naming live actions in drawings and videotape is more taxing to the semantic system than is naming real objects. However, when live actions were demonstrated within a semantically coherent context (i.e., scene description), naming performance was equivalent for nouns and verbs. The results of these studies indicate that the variables of grammatical class, situation context, and presentation play crucial roles in the effectiveness of naming. Thus the naming evaluation battery should include various grammatical classes such as nouns, verbs, and adjectives. In addition, sampling performance in context (picture description and conversational speech) as well as isolation is essential. Finally, Williams's (1990) study incorporating videotaped stimuli indicate that contexts that incorporate a more realistic mode of presentation can render different results from the traditional mode of line drawings.

Written Language Contexts

A thorough investigation of naming deficits requires examining written as well as oral language. For this, traditional notions of evaluating word retrieval—using clinical tests that focus solely on oral language—need to be expanded. A series of case studies (Caramazza & Hillis, 1990; Hillis, 1989; Hillis, Rapp, Romani, & Caramazza, 1990) illustrates the importance of including written as well as oral language tasks. In addition to oral naming tests, their studies used written naming, oral reading, writing to dictation, and printed-word picture matching tasks. Contrasts in error patterns across the various language tasks provided evidence that naming errors arose from different underlying deficits. For example, a patient in one reported case (Hillis, Rapp, Romani, & Caramazza, 1990) made errors in reading, writing, naming, and comprehension tests that were semantically related to the target word. This homogeneous pattern of semantic errors across modalities was interpreted as evidence for selective damage to a central semantic system, which was hypothesized to be modality-independent. On the other hand, two patients (Caramazza & Hillis, 1990) who exhibited frequent related-word errors in oral naming and oral reading displayed no semantic errors in comparable comprehension and written tasks. Their patterns of performance were interpreted as damage to the phonologic lexicon. The lack of semantic errors in comprehension and writing tasks suggests that the central semantic system was not affected.

Stimulus Characteristics

Aside from the use of various contexts for evaluation, key factors concerning the target stimulus should be controlled. The frequency of occurrence of the target word has proven to be a salient variable, with high-frequency words easier to retrieve than low-frequency (Newcombe, Oldfield, & Ratcliffe, 1971; Rochford & Williams, 1965). Word length should also be controlled; shorter words are named more easily (Barton, 1971).

The operativity (Gardner, 1973) and picturability (Goodglass, Hyde, & Blumstein, 1969) of the target stimulus also influence naming performance. Gardner (1973) found that operative items—objects that could be manipulated through a variety of actions and sensory modalities—were named more easily than were figurative items. For example, a *rock* was considered operative and a *cloud* was figurative. In the naming evaluation, both operative and figurative items should be examined across a variety of semantic categories.

Goodglass, Klein, Carey, and Jones (1966) demonstrated the importance of including diverse semantic categories. They found differential naming performance across five semantic categories—objects, letters, numbers, actions, and colors.

Documentation of Error Responses

Standardized naming tests (Goodglass & Kaplan, 1983; Kaplan, Goodglass, & Weintraub, 1983; Kertesz, 1982) routinely focus on quantitative levels of naming performance, such as percentage of correct responses. Although this information is necessary, recent studies and paradigms of naming demonstrate the need to assess not only the number but also the types of naming errors. Numerous categories and descriptions of aphasic error types are available. One system (Table 13.2) has provided sufficient detail and reliability in several clinical naming studies (Li & Williams, 1991a, 1991b).

In summary, a detailed evaluation of naming includes an investigation of types of errors emitted under various verbal and situational contexts. Such an investigation provides the framework for an effective remediation program.

REMEDIATION OF NAMING DISORDERS

Traditionally, remediation of naming disorders has focused on facilitating processes required for word retrieval. Shewan and Bandur (1986) note that naming efficiency can be reduced either through impaired access to the word-retrieval system or impaired functioning of the central language processes. The goal of therapy is to stimulate the processes to function

TABLE 13.2   Error Type Categories

Phonemic errors: approximations of the target word, with one or more erroneous phonemes ("bencil" for pencil).

Extended circumlocutions: extended utterances related to the target word ("You eat with it" for fork).

Related words: words semantically related to the target word ("bat" for ball).

Unrelated words: words that show no obvious phonologic or semantic resemblance to the target word ("log" for hand).

Indefinite terms: vague, general words substituted for the target word ("thing" for ball).

Neologisms: neither real words nor phonemic approximations of the target word ("barpo" for table).

Phonemic attempts: phonemic or syllabic attempts at the target word, either correct or incorrect ("bi . . . " for bicycle).

Semantic-phonemic errors: words that bear phonemic resemblance to the target word and are also real words themselves ("stair" for chair).

Multiple responses: two or more different responses from the patient.

Inadequate responses: instances in which the patient perseverates on a previous response, fails to respond, or states an inability to respond.

again, rather than to teach new words or responses. Toward this end, a number of procedures have been developed to stimulate target-word production.

The growing evidence that naming disorders do not represent a unitary disorder suggests that random application of stimulation may not be maximally effective. Rather, unique therapeutic approaches should be fashioned for each disorder. Hillis (1989, 1991) provides data demonstrating the efficacy of techniques designed to target specific processing components. In one study (1989), generalization and treatment effectiveness were shown to be dependent on the patients' underlying deficits. When using a cueing hierarchy to improve written naming responses, a patient with a central semantic deficit exhibited generalization across modalities and to untrained items. A patient with deficits in more peripheral processes improved on trained but not untrained items. Generalization apparently occurred only when a single semantic impairment was involved.

In a second study (1991), Hillis targeted two deficient levels in a chronically aphasic patient: the semantic system and the phonologic lexicon system. Results from a multiple-baseline study demonstrated the effectiveness of the separate intervention strategies. Differential effects were obtained for a phonemic retraining strategy targeting the phonologic level and for a semantic remediation strategy targeting the semantic system.

These studies suggest that targeting therapy approaches toward specific deficit processes are more effective than using these approaches randomly. Before discussing adapting approaches to deficit processes, several traditional stimulation approaches are reviewed below.

Schuell's Stimulation Therapy

Schuell, Jenkins, and Jimenez-Pabon (1964) recommended use of repeated multimodality stimulation to encourage language processes to function again. In a treatment program based on Schuell's principles, Wiegel-Crump and Koenigsknecht (1973) used target words from four superordinate categories: clothing, household items, living things, and action words. Each word was presented orally, both alone and in short sentences. In addition, confrontation naming tasks were used in conjunction with gestures, open-ended sentences, associations, and word-initial sounds. After 18 treatment sessions, naming of the treated target words improved, as did naming of untreated words within the same semantic categories. Improvement also extended to naming within an untreated semantic category (food).

Cueing Hierarchies

Aside from general stimulation, a number of clinical techniques incorporate specific cues. Several of these are based on a hierarchy of cues. Pease and Goodglass (1978) investigated the effectiveness of six types of cues: (1) the initial sound, (2) superordinate category, (3) environmental context or location, (4) rhyming word, (5) statement of function, and (6) sentence completion. Among these, the most effective was the initial-sound or phonemic cue, followed by sentence completion. There were no statistically significant differences among the remaining cues. Stimley and Noll (1991) suggest that phonemic cueing helped the semantic system activate the appropriate phonologic word forms.

In subsequent studies, the efficacy of phonemic cueing varied depending on the syndrome of aphasia and grammatical class of the target word. Li and Canter (1983, 1987) examined the effectiveness of the initial-sound cue following failure to name nouns. They found that Broca's aphasics were most responsive to phonemic cueing, followed by conduction, anomic, and then Wernicke's aphasias. Li and Williams (1990) examined phonemic and semantic cues in noun- and verb-naming tasks. They discovered that aphasic subgroups used phonemic cueing more effectively on nouns, but no significant difference between types of cues was seen on verbs. The authors suggested that the semantic cue was more useful in more abstract verb-naming, in which the patient frequently lacked the necessary semantic components for word retrieval.

Linebaugh (1990) and Linebaugh and Lehner (1977) have described a cueing hierarchy approach that can be adapted to a variety of tasks and patients. Cues are arranged according to increasing stimulus power and presented until the patient produces the target word. When the patient responds accurately, the cues are presented in the order of *decreasing* stimulus power until the patient again produces the correct response. A sample hierarchy follows:

Picture

Picture + gesture

Picture + sentence completion

Picture + sentence completion + phonemic cue

Picture + "Say_____."

This type of hierarchy has facilitated verbal or written naming abilities in several patients.

Semantic Facilitation Procedures

Howard, Patterson, Franklin, Orchard-Lisle, and Morton (1985a, 1985b) and Patterson, Purell, and Morton (1983) have found that tasks that require the patient to gain access to semantic representations have advantages over techniques that focus on phonologic forms. The facilitative effects of semantic therapy persisted for a longer period of time than those of phonologic therapy. Semantic tasks included printed and auditory word-to-picture matching, sorting words and pictures by semantic category, and making semantic judgments.

Long-term effects of semantically based techniques were also reported in a series of studies by Marshall, Pound, White-Thomson, and Pring (1990). Therapy procedures included reading printed words and matching words to pictures. The authors found higher naming accuracy on treated items when subjects were tested 2–4 weeks following treatment. When six of the seven original subjects were retested 1 year later, naming accuracy was also found to be higher in treated stimuli as compared to untreated control items (Pring, White-Thomson, Pound, Marshall, & Davis (1990).

Applying A Therapy Program to Naming Disorders

The techniques of general stimulation, cueing hierarchies, and semantic facilitation described above represent commonly used methods of remediating naming deficits. While studies have demonstrated the efficacy of each of these methods, the effectiveness of these methods might be increased if they were differentially applied, using available information on underlying cognitive processes.

The clinical behaviors and errors emitted during the type of comprehensive naming evaluation described earlier would provide evidence of the patient's level(s) of cognitive impairment. This analysis should serve as a framework for determining specific remediation goals and procedures. To illustrate differential therapy, the following sections compare therapy considerations for two main types of naming disorders: deficits at the semantic and phonologic levels of processing.

Semantic Naming Deficits

As discussed earlier, patients with a deficit at the semantic level are likely to exhibit semantic paraphasias and errors on semantic comprehension tasks. Recommended therapy for this patient includes semantic facilitation with an emphasis on gaining access to and clarifying word meaning. Procedures similar to those used by Howard et al. are useful (1985a, 1985b). Possible procedures include the following:

1. *Picture categorization.* The patient is asked to separate a mixture of picture cards into two semantic categories (e.g., wild versus domestic animals).

2. *Picture association.* When provided with a pictured stimulus, the patient chooses from a field of two or three pictures the target item associated with the stimulus. The stimulus and target items can be conceptually linked within the same semantic category (*cat* and *dog* as domestic animals) or the same functional context (*camel* lives in the *desert*). To increase the difficulty of this task, the distractor items could resemble the target item.

3. *Semantic judgments.* The patient can answer yes/no questions requiring access to semantic information on misnamed items. For example, a patient who cannot name *cow* could be asked "Does a cow live in a barn?"

4. *Lexical focus.* Linebaugh (1990) proposed that lexical focus therapy may be useful for the patient who has difficulty in retrieving a specific lexical entry from its semantic field. In this task, the client must retrieve lexical entries from progressively narrow semantic categories (defined as words closely related in meaning that are subsumed under a general term or superordinate category). The client is initially presented with a broad superordinate category and asked to name as many items in that category as possible. When patients experience difficulty, the clinician helps the patient find effective search strategies. This same procedure is carried out for progressively narrower categories. For example, the first-order category could consist of fruits and vegetables, the second order of fruits, and the third order of tropical fruits.

5. *Written tasks.* Although the previous tasks use verbal responses, Lesser (1989a) notes that it is not necessary to emphasize verbal productions during therapy. Since the central semantic system is implicated, any improvement in the semantic system is reflected in expressive naming. In her 1989 study, Hillis used written naming tasks to target a semantic system deficit in a patient. When a semantic paraphasia was produced, the target referent was illustrated, and contrasting features between the referent and the subject's erroneous response were discussed. For example, the perceptual differences (color, shape, taste) between the two items were emphasized.

Phonologic Naming Deficits

In contrast to semantic system deficits, the patient with phonologic lexicon problems exhibits good recognition of the target word. Naming errors frequently consist of phonemic paraphasias (e.g., sife/knife) and circumlocutions (e.g., you cut with it/knife). The problem may lie in using input from the semantic system to gain access to the appropriate entry from the phonologic system. Therapy for this patient should focus on linking items in the semantic lexicon to those in the phonologic lexicon. Lesser (1989b) suggests this could be accomplished by aiding retrieval of less-frequently used words. Frequently used words are likely to retain a high level of activation between phonologic and semantic systems, while lower-frequency words can achieve only decreased activation. Targeting retrieval of those lower frequency words that are most functional to the patient could improve access to the phonologic lexicon. Some recommended procedures follow.

1. *Determination of word pool.* The diagnostic procedures provide information on individual words that are difficult to retrieve in various contexts (e.g., confrontation naming, spontaneous speech, sentence completion). From this pool, lower-frequency words that are useful to the patient can be selected for therapy. It is likely that these words will be frequently misnamed by the patient.

2. *Procedures to improve phonologic access.* As mentioned earlier, therapy should focus on linking the semantic and phonologic systems. Patients with poor phonologic access need activities that simultaneously strengthen word associations and use these associations to gain access to the appropriate phonologic form. Rosenbek, LaPointe, and Wertz (1989) suggest that these therapy procedures can be based on the patient's existing behaviors. For example, the patient who uses sentence completion or descriptions is encouraged to perform these behaviors more effectively. The client and clinician jointly create a variety of vivid and effective cloze or sentence completion contexts for words. Target word images are visualized and strategies for pairing visualization with lexical recall/word production are reinforced through frequent practice. Later, as the patient learns to self-cue, analyze, and revise errors, therapy moves from clinician- to client-controlled activities. Procedures from both stimulation and cueing hierarchy approaches can be used in Rosenbek et al.'s program.

3. *Incorporation of prompts.* Despite the need to emphasize retrieval of word forms, it is not necessary to use phonemic cues exclusively. As reported earlier, Howard et al. (1985a, 1985b) showed that phonologic prompts alone do not produce lasting benefits. To facilitate linkage between semantic and phonologic systems, it would be more useful to incorporate both semantic and phonologic information. In a cueing hierarchy, the task continuum can begin with descriptions of target-word function or superordinate category and progressively add phonologic information on word shape.

CONCLUSIONS

This chapter emphasizes that an effective therapy program is based on understanding the patient's processing abilities. A comprehensive and detailed assessment of the patient's naming deficit must precede determination of therapy goals. Recent information regarding cognitive processes in word retrieval provides new insights for the diagnosis and management of naming deficits. However, empirical data on differential management of the aphasic patient based on type of disorder remains scarce. There is a need for research that focuses directly on differential therapy procedures useful in remediating deficient naming processes.

REFERENCES

Barton, M. (1971). Recall of generic properties of words in aphasic patients. *Cortex*, *7*, 73–82.

Barton, M., Maruszewski, M., & Urrea, D. (1969). Variations in stimulus context and its effect on word-finding ability in aphasics. *Cortex*, *5*, 351–365.

Benson, F. (1979). Neurologic correlates of anomia. In H. Whitaker & H. Whitaker (Eds.), *Studies in neurolinguistics* (Vol. 4, pp. 293–328). New York: Academic Press.

Benson, F. (1988). Anomia in aphasia. *Aphasiology, 2*, 229–236.

Butterworth, B. (1989). Lexical access in speech production. In W. Marslen-Wilson (Ed.), *Lexical representation and process* (pp. 108–135). Cambridge, MA: MIT Press.

Canter, G., Trost, J., & Burns, M. (1985). Contrasting speech patterns in apraxia of speech and phonemic paraphasia. *Brain and Language, 24*, 204–222.

Caramazza, A., Berndt, R., & Brownell, H. (1982). The semantic deficit hypothesis. *Brain and Language, 15*, 161–189.

Caramazza, A., & Hillis, A. (1990). Where do semantic errors come from? *Cortex, 26*, 95–122.

Collins, M., McNeil, M.R., & Rosenbek, J.C. (1984). Word fluency and aphasia: Some linguistic and not-so-linguistic considerations. In R. Brookshire (Ed.), *Clinical aphasiology conference proceedings* (pp. 78–84). Minneapolis: BRK Publishers.

Gardner, H. (1973). The contribution of operativity to naming capacity in aphasic patients. *Neuropsychologia, 11*, 213–220.

Geschwind, N. (1967). The varieties of naming errors. *Cortex, 3*, 97–112.

Goodglass, H., Hyde, M., & Blumstein, S. (1969). Frequency, picturability, and availability of nouns in aphasia. *Cortex, 5*, 104–119.

Goodglass, H., & Kaplan, E. (1983). *The assessment of aphasia and related disorders* (2nd ed.). Philadelphia: Lea and Febiger.

Goodglass, H., Klein, B., Carey, P., & Jones, K. (1966). Specific semantic word categories in aphasia. *Cortex, 2*, 74–89.

Grossman, M. (1978). The game of the name: An examination of linguistic reference after brain damage. *Brain and Language, 6*, 112–119.

Grossman, M. (1981). A bird is as bird is as bird: Making reference within and without superordinate categories. *Brain and Language, 12*, 313–331.

Hillis, A. (1989). Efficacy and generalization of treatment for aphasic naming errors. *Archives of Physical Medicine, 70*, 632–636.

Hillis, A. (1991). Effects of separate treatments for distinct impairments within the naming process. In T. Prescott (Ed.), *Clinical aphasiology* (Vol. 19, pp. 255–266). Austin, TX: PRO-ED.

Hillis, A., & Caramazza, A. (1991). Mechanisms for accessing lexical representations for output: Evidence from a category-specific semantic deficit. *Brain and Language, 40*, 106–144.

Hillis, A., Rapp, B., Romani, C., & Caramazza, A. (1990). Selective impairment of semantics in lexical processing. *Cognitive Neuropsychology, 7*, 191–243.

Howard, D., & Orchard-Lisle, V. (1984). On the origin of semantic errors in naming: Evidence from the case of a global aphasic. *Cognitive Neuropsychology 1*, 163–190.

Howard, D., Patterson, K., Franklin, S., Orchard-Lisle, V., & Morton, J. (1985a). The facilitation of picture naming in aphasia. *Cognitive Neuropsychology, 2*, 49–80.

Howard, D., Patterson, K., Franklin, S., Orchard-Lisle, V., & Morton, J. (1985b). Treatment of word retrieval deficits in aphasia: A comparison of two therapy methods. *Brain, 108*, 817–829.

Kaplan, E., Goodglass, H., & Weintraub, S. (1983). *Boston naming test.* Philadelphia: Lea & Febiger.

Kay, J., & Ellis, A. (1987). A cognitive neuropsychological case study of anomia. *Brain, 110*, 613–629.

Kertesz, A. (1982). *Western aphasia battery.* New York: Grune and Stratton.

Lesser, R. (1989a). Some issues in the neuropsychological rehabilitation of anomia. In X. Seron & G. Deloche (Eds.), *Cognitive approaches in neuropsychological rehabilitation* (pp.65–104). London: Lawrence Erlbaum Associates.

Lesser, R. (1989b). Aphasia: Theory-based intervention. In M. Leahy (Ed.), *Disorders of communication: The science of intervention* (pp. 185–205). London: Taylor & Francis.

Li, E., & Canter, G. (1983). Phonemic cueing: An investigation of subject variables. In R. Brookshire (Ed.), *Clinical aphasiology conference proceedings* (pp. 96–103). Minneapolis: BRK Publishers.

Li, E., & Canter, G. (1987). An investigation of Luria's hypothesis on prompting in aphasic naming disturbances. *Journal of Communication Disorders, 20*, 469–475.

Li, E., & Williams, S. (1990). The effects of grammatic class and cue type on cueing responsiveness in aphasia. *Brain and Language, 38*, 48–60.

Li, E., & Williams, S. (1991a). Varieties of errors produced by aphasic patients in phonemic cueing. *Aphasiology, 5*, 51–61.

Li, E., & Williams, S. (1991b). An investigation of naming errors following semantic and phonemic cueing. *Neuropsychologia, 29*, 1083–1093.

Linebaugh, C. (1990). Lexical retrieval problems: Anomia. In L. LaPointe (Ed.), *Aphasia and related neurogenic language disorders* (pp. 96–112). New York: Thieme Medical Publishers.

Linebaugh, C., & Lehner, L. (1977). Cueing hierarchies and word retrieval: A therapy program. In R. Brookshire (Ed.), *Clinical aphasiology conference proceedings* (pp. 19–31). Minneapolis: BRK Publishers.

Luria, A.R, (1966). *Higher cortical functions in man.* New York: Basic Books.

Luria, A.R. (1970). *Traumatic aphasia*. The Hague: Mouton.

Marshall, J., Pound, C., White-Thomson, M., & Pring, T. (1990). The use of picture/word matching tasks to assist word retrieval in aphasic patients. *Aphasiology, 4*, 167–184.

Morton, J. (1985). Naming. In S. Newman & R. Epstein (Eds.), *Current perspectives in dysphasia* (pp. 217–230). Edinburgh: Churchill Livingstone.

Newcombe, F., Oldfield, R., & Ratcliffe, G. (1971). Recognition and naming of object drawings by men with focal brain wounds. *Journal of Neurology, Neurosurgery, and Psychiatry, 34*, 329–430 .

Patterson, K., Purell, C., & Morton, J. (1983). The facilitation of word retrieval in aphasia. In C. Code & D. Muller (Eds.), *Aphasia therapy* (pp. 76–87). London: Edward Arnold.

Pease, D., & Goodglass, H. (1978). The effects of cueing on picture-naming in aphasia. *Cortex, 14*, 178–189.

Pring, T., White-Thomson, M., Pound, C., Marshall, J., & Davis, A. (1990). Picture/word matching tasks and word retrieval: Some follow-up data and second thoughts. *Aphasiology, 4*, 479–483.

Rochford, G., & Williams, M. (1965). Studies in the development and breakdown of the use of names, Part IV. *Journal of Neurology, Neurosurgery, and Psychiatry, 28*, 407–413.

Rosenbek, R., LaPointe, L., & Wertz, T. (1989). *Aphasia: A clinical approach*. Boston: College-Hill Press.

Schuell, H., Jenkins, J., & Jimenez-Pabon, E. (1964). *Aphasia in adults: Diagnosis, prognosis and therapy*. New York: Hoeber.

Shallice, T. (1987). Impairments of semantic processing: Multiple dissociations. In M. Coltheart, G. Sartori, & R. Job (Eds.), *The cognitive neuropsychology of language* (pp. 111–127). London: Lawrence Erlbaum Associates.

Shewan, C., & Bandur, D. (1986). *Treatment of aphasia: A language-oriented approach*. San Diego: College-Hill Press.

Stimley, M., & Noll, D. (1991). The effects of semantic and phonemic prestimulation cues on picture naming in aphasia. *Brain and Language, 41*, 496–509.

Wiegel-Crump, C., & Koenigsknecht, R. (1973). Tapping the lexical store of the adult aphasic: Analysis of the improvement made in word retrieval skills. *Cortex, 9*:,411–418.

Williams, S. (1990). The influence of situational context, grammatical class, cueing, and presentation mode on anomia. *FLASHA Journal* (December issue).

Williams, S., & Canter, G. (1982). The influence of situational context on naming performance in aphasic syndromes. *Brain and Language, 17*, 92–106.

Williams, S., & Canter, G. (1987). Action-naming performances in four syndromes of aphasia. *Brain and Language, 32*, 124–136.

Chapter 14

Treatment of Writing Impairment

Rick L. Bollinger

Writing is perhaps the least established of the primary psycholinguistic tasks—auditory comprehension, speech, reading, and writing. Reading and writing do not develop in humans without special exposure and instruction, and, of the two, reading skills and habits are frequently better developed than writing
(Caplan, 1987, p. 383).

THE RELATIONSHIP OF WRITING DISORDER TO APHASIA

Schuell's (1965) important premise advocating the unidimensionality of language disorder assumes that the writing performance of a given individual with aphasia is compatible with the generalized "reduction of available language." She wrote, "The writing of an aphasic patient often reflects reduction of language and nothing more" (p. 73). Similarly, Strub and Geschwind (1983) report, "The patient who is aphasic in speech . . . almost inevitably is agraphic and produces writing errors that are distinctly aphasic in nature" (p. 302).

While Schuell's model of language and language disorder now appears too general, writing deficits appear to be solidly linked with a number of aphasia diagnostic categories. Nonlanguage behaviors certainly affect writing output and may cause it to differ from spoken output. But different syndromes of aphasia—Broca's, Wernicke's, transcortical motor, transcortical sensory, mixed, global, and jargon—are appreciably different in linguistic performance, including writing (Kertesz, 1979).

Writing performance in aphasia, especially narrative writing, usually parallels the character of spoken language (Kaplan & Goodglass, 1981; Sgaramella, Willis, & Semenza, 1991). For example, individuals with Broca's aphasia demonstrate reduced written output that consists of a predominance of substantive words, verbs, a few simplistic attempts at sentence construction, unrelated word substitutions, and spelling errors. The motor output, via nondominant left hand, is slow and awkward. In general, the syntactic deficit that characterizes Broca's aphasia is seen both verbally and graphically.

In contrast, the writing of individuals with Wernicke's aphasia is characterized by at least the basic syntactic framework with a lack of substantives, and the appearance of neologisms, semantic paraphasias, and paragrammatism. This group usually accomplishes the mechanics of writing with relative ease. This ease of production parallels fluent speech. The empty character of verbal and written production is similar, though the patient's writing has "fewer runs of grammatically coherent words than does their speech" (Kaplan & Goodglass, 1981, p. 7).

Wapner and Gardner (1979) report that individuals with anterior and posterior aphasia have similar spelling performances on written and anagram arrangement tests (arranging letters to make words) but differ on the types of misspelled words and the types of other errors. In general, the errors of patients with posterior aphasia sounded like the target word ("sigeret" for cigarette). The errors of patients with anterior aphasia were visually similar to the target word ("cijrelle" for cigarette). Frederici, Schoenle, and Goodglass (1981) found similar patterns. In addition, they found that patients with anterior lesions present with two kinds of errors based on the relative preservation of oral or graphic naming. Individuals with aphasia due to anterior lesions who had better oral naming produced phonemically related spelling errors. Patients with anterior lesions and relatively better written than verbal naming presented more graphemically relevant (letter) errors. This pattern has significant implications for models and treatment of writing, both of which are discussed in this chapter.

NONAPHASIC AGRAPHIC DISORDERS

Strub and Geschwind (1983) describe three major types of agraphia: *aphasic* agraphia, *spatial* agraphia, and *apraxic* agraphia. In contrast to the language-based aphasic agraphia, spatial agraphia appears to be part of a more generalized impairment. Patients with spatial agraphia are unable to align letters and words on a page. They also write with marked distortion of letters and have significant difficulty copying words and sentences. Apraxic agraphia is a disorder of the ability to execute the voluntary learned movements for writing and does not involve language or visuoperceptual skills. Copying of printed or written words is relatively spared and drawing is better than writing. Spontaneous writing and writing to dictation show marked impairment (Roeltgen & Heilman, 1983). Apraxic agraphia occurs as a part of Gerstmann syndrome, which also includes finger agnosia, right-left disorientation, and acalculia (Kaplan & Goodglass, 1981).

Aphasic, apraxic, and spatial agraphias also may be early symptoms of generalized cognitive disorders such as dementia and are often present in closed head injury. The complex attentional, ideational, linguistic, visuospatial, and motoric integrations needed to write or draw are very sensitive to neurologic disorder. Horner, Lathrop, Fish, and Dawson (1987) and McNeil and Tseng (1990) describe writing as a critical test that provides valuable information for differential diagnosis and treatment development for neurogenic populations.

DESCRIPTIONS OF WRITING ERRORS IN APHASIA

Analysis of writing in aphasia is based on writing performances involving words and narrative. Early research in word-writing performance of individuals with aphasia demonstrated anticipation and perseveration errors (Pizzamiglio & Black, 1970), medial position errors (Frederici et al., 1981; Pizzamiglio & Black, 1970), greater errors with increased word length and decreased frequency of usage (Bricker, Schuell, & Jenkins, 1964; Pizzamiglio & Black, 1970), and more severe impairments in writing than in other modalities (Duffy & Ulrich, 1976). Impaired visual processing may add to the writing difficulty. When that occurs, a confusion of letters that are similar in appearance or distortion or reversal of letter forms may be present.

Narrative writing and word writing are markedly different tasks. While the two writing tasks have certain commonalities, narrative writing requires the application of written discourse rules, interpretive ability, and memory (Horner et al., 1987). In contrast to earlier studies of single-word writings, recent studies of aphasic narrative writing show patterns that are inconsistent with visuospatial or motor exacerbations of an underlying language disorder. Instead, they reflect a differential involvement of lexical unit (word) and grapheme (letter) retrieval (Hatfield, 1983; Hillis & Caramazza, 1987; Sgaramella et al., 1991).

Roeltgen and Heilman (1983) present a model of the normal writing process wherein an auditory word engram or image (reauditorization) is matched to visual word images for whole-word visualization, or to a phoneme-grapheme conversion process wherein the auditory word is analyzed for a sound-to-grapheme conversion. After either process, the image is then sent to a graphemic area responsible for guiding motor programming before it goes to the motor programming area for final graphic output. According to this model, writing disturbances characterized by semantic selection error could result in the writing of a related or unrelated word; a phoneme-grapheme conversion error could result in written-letter errors; a reduced storage time (phoneme buffer) could result in movement difficulties (accurate letters but in the wrong place); and finally combinations wherein an error word is retrieved from the lexicon and sent for phonemic analysis where errors in phoneme-to-grapheme conversion are made, with an unrelated, meaningless result. For example, if the target is "chair" and the word "table" is retrieved from the lexicon and the graphemes "t-e-f-u-l" are retrieved and written. In this example, the end product has no apparent relation to the target word.

Sgaramella et al. (1991) generated support for the primary features of the Roeltgen and Heilman (1983) model. They compared the quality and quantity of errors in essay writing by university students to the picture description writing errors by individuals with Broca's, Wernicke's, and conduction aphasia. The researchers distinguished selection errors (the misuse of language units that "imply central impairments to semantic, syntactic or lexical processes" [p. 36]) from movement errors (the misordering of words or letters in a sentence or word that may be anticipatory, perseverative, or reversals). Movement errors imply that letters or words are selected in advance, held in temporary storage, and then written at the incorrect location in a sequence of letters or words.

Subjects with aphasia made significantly more errors than did the non-aphasic individuals overall. They also made proportionately more word-selection errors (mostly omissions and substitutions) and fewer word-movement errors. Individuals with Broca's and conduction aphasia produced more unrelated, nonsemantic word substitutions than did the patients with Wernicke's aphasia, who made more semantic substitutions. These findings led to five conclusions: (1) individuals with Broca's and conduction aphasia have a reduced planning span that is clinically manifested as reduced syntactic planning; (2) individuals with Wernicke's aphasia make more related or semantic than unrelated substitutions or phonologic errors, a finding compatible with impairment of lexical-semantic processes; (3) patients with conduction and Broca's aphasia produce more nonsemantically related word substitutions than do patients with Wernicke's aphasia; (4) errors produced by individuals with conduction aphasia suggest a mislocation of graphemes in word sequences, even after the word has been retrieved; and (5) when neologisms occur in any syndrome, they may be the product of multiple error processes or errors of knowledge.

DEEP, PHONOLOGIC, AND SURFACE DYSGRAPHIA

To theoretically explain clinical syndromes, Hatfield (1983) presented a simplified version of a model of dysgraphia that was originally proposed by Beauvois and Derouesne (1981). The syndromes described are based on the disruption of two primary routes of translating heard or thought words into written words. For the lexical semantic (word meaning) route, the appropriate lexical unit (word) is retrieved as a whole. In the phonologic route, the phonemes (sounds) in words are converted to graphemes (letters) and retrieved according to rules of phoneme-grapheme conversion. Disruption of one or both of these routes may result in one of two primary syndromes of phonologic or deep dysgraphia. A third syndrome, surface dysgraphia, results from orthographic errors in the rules of spelling such as writing long and short vowels.

One way in which aphasic writing disorders are differentiated from nonaphasic writing disorders is by evaluating whether the patient can write dictated nonwords using orthographic rules. If dictated nonwords are relatively accurate, the phoneme-grapheme conversion process is assumed to be preserved, since sound analysis and matching sounds to graphemes can be accomplished without understanding word meaning. If nonwords are inaccurate but dictated regularly and irregularly spelled real words are accurate, then the lexical semantic retrieval process is presumed to be intact. Nonwords cannot be retrieved by the lexical process, since there is no referent. Nonwords can only be generated on the basis of "sounding out" or phoneme to grapheme conversion. Hatfield (1983) stresses the need for careful analysis of aphasic writing when he states "the two primary writing syndromes are clearly different and . . . it follows that their therapy (for patients with varying writing impairment) must differ fundamentally" (p. 164).

GENERAL ASSESSMENT OF WRITTEN LANGUAGE IN APHASIA

At its simplest, the process of writing begins with a concept—an idea or thing to be labeled that is then translated into graphemes. This process occurs because of a systematic set of activities, including reauditorization of the name, then retrieval of the graphemic representation (either via grapheme-to-phoneme correspondence or lexical whole-word retrieval), and finally motor processing so that the concept can be expressed in writing. If the language system is the only system that is impaired, then the person with aphasia writes with errors that parallel the nature and severity of the aphasic disorder. Because language is a complex cognitive skill, nonlanguage components may affect the final written product. Therefore, factors listed in Table 14.1 should be considered during the general assessment of the output.

Benson (1979) analyzes written language into several components, including the quality of handwriting (calligraphy), visual spatial attributes, spelling (orthography), and linguistic quality (word choice). He suggests that patients be evaluated across these domains according to a hierarchy of tasks of increasing complexity. According to Benson (1979), assessment should begin with an automatic writing task such as writing of a signature and other familiar information. This usually demonstrates the best motoric written response the patient can make either with the nondominant hand or preferred hand. The next level, copying words and sentences, provides an opportunity to observe visual spatial abilities without the complication of linguistic retrieval and formulation. The writing of letters, words, and sen-

TABLE 14.1   Considerations in the Evaluation of Writing Deficits

Compatibility of writing with the other characteristics of the language disorder (verbal output, reading level, aphasia diagnostic category)

Nature of writing errors (phonologic, deep, surface)

Physical or motor complications (weakness, incoordination)

Visual complications (hemianopsia, neglect, visual perceptual disturbance, acuity)

Nonlanguage cognitive features (perseveration, inattention, impulsive responding, lack of monitoring of output, disorientation, memory disorder(s), reduced general intelligence, increased latency of response)

Premorbid influences (education, learning disability, premorbid language use, personality)

Motivation

---

tences to dictation provides information regarding writing capability when retrieval of spelling and words is not a factor, though reductions in auditory processing may introduce a confounding factor. Finally, tasks involving narrative writing, where the patient is asked to describe an activity or event in writing, test a high level of language expression. Complex tasks of this nature generally reveal some level of impairment for all patients with aphasia, and if successfully completed "almost excludes significant language pathology" (p. 123).

Standardized Assessment of Writing in Aphasia

All current aphasia assessment batteries include examination of writing. To date, there is no standardized test that assesses only writing in aphasia, though McNeil and Tseng (1990) report preliminary work toward that end. The inclusion of writing in aphasia assessment is critical for determining the extent of language involvement, for identifying nonlanguage complicating factors, and for delineating modalities for the patient's functional use and for emphasis in treatment. Kertesz (1979) reports that the writing tasks on the Western Aphasia Battery (Kertesz, 1982) discriminate well between diagnostic groups with aphasia and normal controls.

Most tests of aphasia present graphic output tasks in a hierarchy of complexity, either in ascending or descending order, including narrative writing, word writing, writing to dictation, and copying. If no specific problems with visual motor construction are present, copying usually elicits the best mechanical performance and spontaneous writing the worst (Kertesz, 1979; Porch, 1981). The Porch Index of Communicative Ability (PICA) (Porch, 1981) begins with the most difficult task—generating written sentences; the Western Aphasia Battery (Kertesz, 1982) begins with the writing of a paragraph to describe a picture. In contrast, the Boston Diagnostic Aphasia Examination (Goodglass & Kaplan, 1983) begins with copying and progresses to more difficult tasks, as does the

Minnesota Test for Differential Diagnosis of Aphasia (Schuell, 1965), though the latter test administration may begin at whatever item the clinician judges to be appropriate.

Assessment tasks presented to the patient should provide sufficient information to determine whether writing is functional for communication and whether there is a pattern corresponding to the general features of impairment of phoneme-to-grapheme conversion, a broad impairment of lexical access and phoneme-grapheme conversion, or surface or spelling rule impairment. While the theoretical and practical reality of these three types of impairment is still under discussion, there is sufficient clinical data to suggest that differentiation into these major types of impairment is useful.

Not uncommonly, persons with aphasia cannot write with the preferred hand because of paralysis and must learn to write with the nondominant hand. While some do so with surprising ease, the majority present persisting impairment of fine movements in the nonparalyzed hand. However, the issue of post-stroke or neurologic-onset handedness has little bearing on the linguistic nature of writing in aphasia (Hansen, McNeil, & Vetter, 1986; Selinger, Prescott, & Katz, 1987).

INTERVENTION

Hillis and Caramazza (1987) stress the need for careful evaluation of the nature of the dysgraphia before planning treatment. This is particularly true when the aphasia is mild. Early studies of the effect of structured graphic-output programs on the writing ability and overall communication abilities of patients with aphasia demonstrated no significant benefit (Pizzamiglio & Roberts, 1967; Sarno, Silverman, & Sands, 1970; Schwartz, Nemeroff, & Reiss, 1964). Treatment described in these studies included the use of a specially designed typewriter-like teaching machine as well as programmed approaches. Two such studies used highly structured computer-based programs to determine the effect of treatment on spelling and overall communication for chronically aphasic patients (Rubin & Bollinger, 1983; Seron, Deloche, Moulard, & Rousselle, 1980). In both studies, improvement was noted for the treated spelling words, with limited carryover to nontreated words. However, neither study found any significant gain in overall communication as a result of the treatment.

Hatfield (1983) describes specific treatment for patients with chronic aphasia who were categorized as having one of the three types of dysgraphia (deep, phonologic, surface) described earlier. All treatment involved teaching cognitive linguistic strategies to retrieve the element or process required. For example, in retrieving properly spelled functors (prepositions, auxiliaries, and pronouns), a task of particular difficulty for patients with Broca's aphasia, patients were cued by writing a key word that contained elements of the word they were unable to retrieve. The key word served as a link to the target word, which would otherwise not be accessible due to disturbances in phoneme-to-grapheme processing. For example, one patient used the name "Don" to facilitate recognition and retrieval of the functor "on," and "history" to facilitate writing "his." Patients established and strengthened the association between a small number of linking words and target prepositions, auxiliaries, and pronouns through drill work in the clinic and at home. According to information provided by Hatfield (1983), specific spelling rules and patterns can be taught when the patient shows characteristics of surface dysgraphia, where writing shows poor application of orthographic rules. Hatfield suggests teaching rules of consonant doubling, which is used to maintain a short-vowel sound (e.g., stopping), and variations in rules for spelling long-vowel sounds (meat, meet, mete).

Trupe (1986) describes a treatment procedure for a woman with aphasia who was taught to spell phonetically, rather than orthographically (e.g., peetsa/pizza), in order to use a synthesized speech output system. The treatment consisted of training phoneme-to-grapheme correspondence via key words. With this technique, the patient retrieves a key word that has the desired phonetic representation in order to cue the appropriate sound for the phonetic spelling. This approach is similar to that of Hatfield (1983), described earlier.

Writing as Cognitive Retraining and Stimulation

Writing treatment, whether highly structured, general, clinician-presented, or completed independently by the patient with or without assistance by a family member, can enhance or at least maintain cognitive skills and specific levels of attention, retention, monitoring, visual-motor matching, and sequencing skills demanded by graphic-output tasks. Very few patients are neurologically impaired to the extent that they cannot match, copy, or complete words when the visual stimulus is present or when they are expected to complete these tasks using immediate memory (after the visual stimulus has been removed). Just as general language stimulation enhances written language output, treatment via writing enhances overall language processing.

Graphic output activities may serve as the core of a treatment program for acutely and chronically aphasic patients. Regardless of level of aphasia severity, graphic output tasks can be structured to enhance general language stimulation or to train the specific application of word-retrieval strategies or discrete syntactic and grammatical rules. Copying of letters and words may be the first successful activity accomplished by a severely aphasic patient. Such activities can be practiced on the ward, in the clinic, or at home. When pictures accompany the words to be copied, they reinforce the linguistic link between the referent and the graphemes.

For patients who are learning to write with the nondominant left hand, the writing paper should be placed on a clipboard and the clipboard angled diagonally across the writing field with the top to the right. Patients may write better by using a built-up pencil or marking pen.

Language Master activities or another audio-playback device can be structured to combine auditory and visual input with graphic output. Picture-word cards can be selected for content, frequency of occurrence, and number of letters (length). In addition, copying and writing tasks can be developed to meet the patient's specific level of ability. Appendix 1 to this chapter provides an example of task progression for structured treatment.

Treatment for Gain or Maintenance?

Writing performance generally improves as aphasia improves during the early months after the onset of a language disorder (Porch, 1981). Comparison of performances in different modalities—writing, speaking, reading, hearing—usually gives the best indication of the possibility for continued or additional change in any specific modality. The *Porch Index of Communicative Ability* (PICA) allows a clinician to compare a patient's performance in different modalities by providing percentile rankings by modality and subtest. A comparison of periodic test and retest scores for overall language performance and specific subtest performance should demonstrate when improvement in tested abilities has reached a plateau.

The PICA scores of some aphasia patients who are significantly past the acute period may suggest that further language performance improvement is possible. These patients usually demonstrate what is called a "negative HI-LO gap" of greater than 5 percentile points. This means that the percentile ranking of the mean score of the nine lowest PICA subtest performances is higher than the percentile rank of the nine highest subtest performances by greater than 5 percentile points. When this occurs, the patient's highest scores are not as high as expected, when compared with other patients' performance. This divergence is usually caused by nonlanguage confounds, including perseveration, impulsive responding, poor monitoring of output, and lack of attention to detail in reading and writing tasks. These are behaviors that can be modified when activities for improving the graphic output compose a major part of the treatment.

It is difficult to justify reinitiating treatment for individuals who are beyond a year after the onset of aphasia, particularly when they have been discharged from speech-language treatment. Any reinitiation of treatment should involve a significant amount of home treatment with visits to the speech-language pathologist as needed. The home treatment plan should include a daily routine of reading and writing drills using clinician-developed activities, published workbooks, recording and playback devices such as the Language Master, structured viewing of videotaped television programs, and social activities such as writing letters, writing shopping lists, and keeping a diary.

Structured Writing Activities at Home

Writing treatment for patients with severe aphasia serves primarily as a means of enhancing cognitive communication behaviors such as visual attention, vigilance and tracking, visual memory, sequencing, visual monitoring, and word recognition. It should be structured to combine discrete copying and writing tasks and functional pragmatic activities and events. It should be based on a patient's overall level of communication ability, and should consider specific strengths or weaknesses of writing. The focus is generally on sequenced copying, copying from memory, word/picture matching and copying, cloze activities that entail completing a stimulus item, word identification from newspapers and magazines, and attempted writing of key names and words for activities of daily living.

When a patient demonstrates that writing abilities are stabilized, the existing program can be modified for long-term home activity. It is a source of constant surprise that individuals with aphasia continue to perform simple and repetitive activities for many months. Whether such a routine provides measurable benefits for patients is not the issue. Many persons with aphasia appear to find satisfaction in the structure and routine of working with elements of language that once were automatic and that now require a significant amount of effort. Whenever possible, home activities should be structured to allow maximum success and independence. While many partners of individuals with aphasia enjoy the companionship of working together on language tasks, others appreciate the time to work independently.

There are many workbooks for home activity by individuals who have aphasia, though most cannot provide the quantity of work at the specific level required for each patient, particularly those who are chronically aphasic. The speech-language pathologist, spouse, or "significant other" at home can modify workbook exercises, changing the stimulus items. Workbooks that have a variety of activities and can be modified include *Therapy Guide for Language and Speech Disorders*, Volumes I, II, III, and IV, and Brubaker's *Workbook for Aphasia* and *Workbook for Language Skills* (see Appendix 2 to this chapter). The *Written Expression* volume from the Martinoff, Martinoff, & Stokke (1982) series in language rehabilitation is comprehensive and includes test probes to help establish a starting point (see Appendix 2).

For individuals with mild and moderate aphasia, home activities can be structured to incorporate modifications of many of the usual activities of daily life such as making lists of daily activities or grocery items or writing letters or diaries. Crossword puzzles and word-finding activities can be a pleasant language activity when a companion assists, and lists of words beginning with the same phoneme, containing a specific vowel or having a specified number of syllables encourage stimulation of phoneme rules and combinations. Writing category members can be structured for basic language stimulation or cognitive linguistic challenge. For the former, patients can generate and write the names of simple category items such as foods in the refrigerator or furniture in the house. For the latter, a more complex category activity is "branching." Higher level aphasic persons can work to develop increasingly refined subcategories of objects, events, or places. An example of category branching is the prime category "animal" and increasing refinements such as mammal/reptile/fish, carnivore/herbivore, domestic/wild, food source/work animal, and so on.

Tape-recorded television programs of specific interest can also serve as a meaningful activity for ongoing language stimulation as well as writing. For example, the individual with aphasia and his or her "significant other" might watch and tape a favorite situation comedy. While they watch the program, the significant other writes the names of the key characters and elements of the program as they occur, gauging the number and complexity of the words to the partner's language level. At the conclusion of the episode, the person with aphasia copies the written key elements. The episode is then replayed and the person with aphasia stops the tape each time one of the key elements occurs, copies the element, then resumes viewing. This activity can have a great or small amount of structure and complexity depending on the level of aphasic deficit and assistance available in completing the activity. It is remarkable how many times a single episode can be viewed and continue to be stimulating to the aphasic individuals.

SUMMARY

Writing disturbance is a part of aphasia. Except for individuals who have nonlanguage disturbances in speech output (e.g., apraxia and dysarthria), writing is not a primary modality of communication. However, the use of writing as a treatment modality can enhance and reinforce nonlanguage and language processes. Achieving maximal benefit from writing treatment in the clinic and at home necessitates careful analysis of the writing process and of breakdowns in writing; clear determination of the aphasic person's level of ability; and careful sequencing of the treatment stimulation and targets.

REFERENCES

Beauvois, M.F., & Derouesne, J. (1981). Lexical or orthographic agraphia. *Brain, 104,* 21–49.

Benson, A. (1979). *Aphasia, alexia, agraphia.* New York: Churchill Livingstone.

Bricker, A.L., Schuell, H., & Jenkins, J.J. (1964). Effect of word frequency and word length on aphasic spelling errors. *Journal of Speech and Hearing Research, 7,* 183–192.

Caplan, D. (1987). *Neurolinguistics and linguistic aphasiology. Cambridge studies in speech science and communication.* New York: Cambridge University Press.

Duffy, R.J., & Ulrich, S.R. (1976). A comparison of impairments in verbal comprehension, speech, reading, and writing in adult aphasics. *Journal of Speech and Hearing Disorders, 41,* 110–119.

Frederici, A.D., Schoenle, P.W., & Goodglass, H. (1981). Mechanisms underlying writing and speech in aphasia. *Brain and Language, 13,* 212–222.

Goodglass, H., & Kaplan, E. (1983). *The assessment of aphasia and related disorders.* Philadelphia: Lea & Febiger.

Hansen, A.M., McNeil, M.R., & Vetter, D.K. (1986). More differences between writing with the dominant and nondominant hand by normal geriatric subjects: Eight perceptual and eight computerized measures on a sentence dictation task. In R.H. Brookshire (Ed.), *Clinical aphasiology* (pp. 116–122). Minneapolis: BRK Publishers.

Hatfield, F.M. (1983). Aspects of acquired dysgraphia and implications for re-education. In C. Code & D. Muller (Eds.), *Aphasia therapy* (2nd ed., pp. 157–169). London: Edward Arnold.

Hillis, A.E., & Caramazza, A. (1987). Model-driven remediation of dysgraphia. In R.H. Brookshire (Ed.), *Clinical aphasiology* (pp. 84–99). Minneapolis: BRK Publishers.

Horner, J., Lathrop, D.L., Fish, A.M., & Dawson, D. (1987). Agraphia in left and right hemisphere stroke and Alzheimer dementia patients. In R.H. Brookshire (Ed.), *Clinical aphasiology* (pp. 61–75). Minneapolis: BRK Publishers.

Kaplan, E., & Goodglass, H. (1981). Aphasia-related disorders. In M.T. Taylor (Ed.), *Acquired aphasia* (pp. 303–325). New York: Academic Press.

Kertesz, A. (1979). *Aphasia and associated disorders, taxonomy, localization, and recovery.* New York: Grune & Stratton.

Kertesz, A. (1982). *Western aphasia battery.* New York: Grune & Stratton.

McNeil, M., & Tseng, C.H. (1990). Acquired neurogenic dysgraphias. In L.L. LaPointe (Ed.), *Aphasia and related neurogenic language disorders* (pp. 147–176). New York: Thieme Medical Publishers.

Pizzamiglio, L., & Black, J.W. (1970). Phonic trends in the writing of aphasic patients. *Journal of Speech and Hearing Research, 13,* 606–623.

Pizzamiglio, L., & Roberts, M. (1967). Writing in aphasia: A learning study. *Cortex, 3,* 250–257.

Porch, B.E. (1981). *Porch index of communicative ability* (2nd ed.). Palo Alto: Consulting Psychologists Press.

Roeltgen, D.P., & Heilman, K.M. (1983). Apractic agraphia in a patient with normal praxis. *Brain and Language, 18,* 35–46.

Rubin, C., & Bollinger, R. (1983). Aphasia: Treatment considerations, graphic output. *Topics in Language Disorders, 3,* 67–75.

Sarno, M.T., Silverman, M., & Sands, E. (1970). Speech therapy and language recovery in severe aphasia. *Journal of Speech and Hearing Research, 13,* 606–623.

Schuell, H. (1965). *The Minnesota test for differential diagnosis of aphasia.* Minneapolis: University of Minnesota Press.

Schwartz, L. Nemeroff, S., & Reiss, M. (1964). An investigation of writing therapy for the treatment of aphasic subjects with writing disorders. *Journal of Speech and Hearing Disorders, 1,* 344–367.

Selinger, M., Prescott, T.E., & Katz, R. (1987). Handwritten vs. computer responses on Porch index of communicative ability graphic subtests. In R.H. Brookshire (Ed.), *Clinical aphasiology* (pp. 136–142). Minneapolis: BRK Publishers.

Seron, X., Deloche, G., Moulard, G., & Rousselle, M.A. (1980). Computer-based therapy for the treatment of aphasic subjects with writing disorders. *Journal of Speech and Hearing Disorders, 45*, 45–58.

Sgaramella, T., Willis, A.W., & Semenza, C. (1991). Analysis of the spontaneous writing errors of normal and aphasic writers. *Cortex, 27*, 29–38.

Strub, R.L., & Geschwind, N. (1983). Localization in Gerstmann syndrome. In A. Kertesz (Ed.), *Localization in neuropsychology* (pp. 295–321). New York: Academic Press.

Trupe, E.H. (1986). Effectiveness of retraining phoneme to grapheme conversion. In R.H. Brookshire (Ed.), *Clinical aphasiology* (pp. 163–171). Minneapolis, BRK Publishers.

Wapner, W., & Gardner, H.A. (1979). A study of spelling in aphasia. *Brain and Language, 7*, 363–374.

Appendix 1

Sample Home Writing Treatment Program for Patients with Severe Aphasia

Set aside 1 hour each morning for a writing activity. Randomly select 20 word-picture cards to be used in activities described below. Have the patient complete each step of the program, progressing to subsequent steps as performance dictates.

1. Copy the alphabet.
2. Copy random letters.
3. Copy three- and four-letter noun words from the word-picture cards. Each word must be copied legibly without correction before moving on to the next step.
4. Copy the word from the word-picture card, then cover the last letter, copy the beginning letters, and complete the word from memory. Check for accuracy. If an error is noted, correct the error, then copy the complete word again. Repeat the target step. When accurate, move on to the next word.
5. Copy the word from the word-picture card. Then cover the last two letters. Copy the beginning letters, then complete the word from memory. Check and correct as above.
6. Continue the activity until the patient is able to copy the word from memory or until he or she reaches a plateau. If the patient has access to a Language Master, Language Master cards can be used for this activity. Use of the Language Master will enable the auditory stimulus to be combined with the visual presentation each time the patient attempts to copy the word. To increase the difficulty level, the patient can be asked to copy the word, cover the copied word, and cover the word on the card with a "sticky tab." The card is then played, after which time the patient is asked to write the word again. If errors are made at this point, the patient should return to the earlier step (using the printed word on the Language Master card). This same progressive copying and copying from memory can be carried out using pictures of real objects, events, and people in the individual's life. Photographs can be pasted on notebook

pages with the key word printed below. Additional pictures can be added as significant events occur. In addition to serving as a stimulus for graphic output, such a notebook may become an object of interest to visitors and family and in this way provide opportunities for the patient to participate in social interaction.

Appendix 2

Workbooks with Writing Activities for Patients with Aphasia

Brubaker, S.H. (1985). *Workbook for aphasia, revised edition: Exercises for the redevelopment of higher level language functioning.* Detroit: Wayne State University Press.

Brubaker, S.H. (1985). *Workbook for language skills: Exercises for written and verbal expression.* Detroit: Wayne State University Press.

Keith, R. (1977). *Speech and language rehabilitation: A workbook for the neurologically impaired* (Vol. 2). Springfield, IL: The Interstate Printers & Publishers.

Keith, R. (1987). *Speech and language rehabilitation: A workbook for the neurologically impaired and language delayed* (Vol. 1, 3rd ed.). Springfield, IL: The Interstate Printers & Publishers.

Kilpatrick, K. *Therapy guide for language and speech disorders: Volume I a selection of stimulus materials* (1980). *Volume II advanced stimulus materials* (1980). *Volume III working with words* (1980). *Volume IV putting the pieces together* (1985). Akron, OH: Visiting Nurse Service.

Lazzari, A.M. (1990). *Just for adults: An adult handbook for language rehabilitation.* East Moline, IL: LinguiSystems.

Martinoff, J.T., Martinoff, R., & Stokke, V. (1982). *Language rehabilitation: Written expression.* Tigard, OR: CC Publications.

Chapter 15

Augmentative and Alternative Communication: Applications to Treatment

Kathryn L. Garrett

Augmentative and alternative communication (AAC) refers broadly to an area of clinical practice and more narrowly to a collection of communication strategies that support individuals for whom writing or natural speech is not functional in one or more situations or environments (American Speech-Language-Hearing Association [ASHA], 1991; Garrett and Beukelman, 1992). Although many individuals with severe aphasia are non-speaking and therefore eligible for AAC interventions, the fields of AAC and aphasiology have not directed substantial, unified attention to severe aphasia in the past. The reasons for this historical dissociation are not well understood, although it is clear that the intricate language processing deficits in aphasia prevent a simple application of the AAC interventions developed for individuals with motor impairments.

Recent changes in the thinking of aphasiologists may pave the way for the incorporation of AAC strategies into treatment programs for persons with severe aphasia. Aphasiologists are shifting their focus from the treatment of specific deficits alone. They acknowledge that most patients with severe aphasia do not recover "normal" communication skills, and they are developing more realistic treatment goals and expectations (Marshall, 1987). The field of aphasiology is also increasingly aware that the integrity of the whole person is disrupted after the onset of aphasia; the life roles and needs of the whole person must be addressed in addition to his or her linguistic deficits.

The field of AAC is naturally attuned to thinking about the whole person. AAC is not a simple match of terminology to the specific physical and mental capabilities of the client; rather, it involves a fairly sophisticated assessment of the participation level and life-style needs of the person for whom speech or writing is not functional (Beukelman & Mirenda, 1987). Clinicians need extensive knowledge of the nonspeaking individual before choosing a communication system, selecting messages and vocabulary, and teaching the client to use the system in natural environments. This focus on the whole person has direct application to aphasia interventions.

This chapter sorts through information from the complementary areas of AAC and aphasiology. Principles of AAC are discussed and applied to aphasia treatment. An alternative to the traditional aphasia taxonomy for severe aphasia is presented. Each subcategory of severe aphasia in the new taxonomy is illustrated with examples of patient and partner treatment objectives. The unexplored role of technology in the treatment of aphasia, as well as service delivery issues, is discussed at the conclusion of this chapter.

EARLY INTERVENTIONS IN AAC AND APHASIA

Early AAC efforts with congenitally nonspeaking individuals (e.g., individuals with cerebral palsy) typically used a process or replacement approach to intervention. That is, alternative symbols replaced words, and alternative access (e.g., switches) replaced the complex motor movements associated with natural speech. Preliminary AAC interventions in aphasia were applied in much the same manner.

For example, Enderby and Hamilton (1983) used the SPLINK (Speech Link) system, an electronic word board containing 950 basic words, letters of the alphabet, numbers, common phrases, grammatical categories, and instruction controls, as a language intervention tool for persons with aphasia. An infrared hookup to a computer monitor allowed the person with aphasia to select individual words and then sequence them to construct messages. The researchers reported varying degrees of success: nine of the 37 subjects used the SPLINK system to communicate novel messages, although their output was telegraphic. An additional 12 subjects used the system in structured therapy sessions but not spontaneously. Three subjects demonstrated some initial success with the system, but family or staff support was lacking and the devices were not used in the home. Thirteen subjects demonstrated minimal ability to use the system.

Similarly, Glass, Gazaniga, and Premack (1975) trained seven adults with global aphasia to arrange word-equivalent paper symbols in sentence order. Two of their subjects could construct subject-verb-object strings by the end of the study; the other five subjects were more limited in their productions. The researchers presented no data on generalization to spontaneous communication situations. Bailey (1983) and Johannsen-Horbach, Cegla, Mager, and Schempp (1985) used Blissymbols with nonspeaking aphasic patients. Bailey's patient mastered a 200-word Blissymbol chart and then developed functional writing skills. The latter group of investigators also developed communication boards for four individuals with global aphasia; one subject reportedly used the board to communicate functionally in all situations, whereas others used it to enhance verbal expression, to respond in single words, or unsuccessfully. Steele, Weinrich, Wertz, Kleczewska, and Carlson (1989) developed a computerized version of a visual-symbol communication board, and a subject with global aphasia demonstrated some success in using it to communicate trained syntactic forms (Weinrich, Steele, Carlson, & Kleczewska, 1989).

Although some of these preliminary results showed promise for some persons with aphasia, other findings were more guarded. DeRuyter, Kennedy, and Doyle (1990) surveyed the long-term use patterns of aphasic communication board users and found that only 43% (24 of 56 subjects) were using communication boards as they had been designed 6 months after discharge from hospital settings. Thirty-nine percent of the aphasic patients had discarded them, and 17% were using the systems on a limited basis.

Bellaire, Georges, and Thompson's (1989) study echoed these limitations. Two of their nonspeaking and nonwriting aphasic subjects learned to request basic items (coffee and cookies) and to communicate personal information (name and occupation) by pointing to pictures on a communication board. Although the subjects completed the task with direct clinical instruction, they did not generalize this behavior to untrained messages until the twenty-third session. At that point, one subject did use his board to communicate personal information in a familiar social setting. Both subjects eventually used their boards to communicate five target messages after an additional period of naturalistic communication training. Neither of the subjects ever learned to communicate social responses such as "hi" or "thank you" with the board. Bellaire et al.'s study showed that carryover of the adaptive communication strategies is possible in severe aphasia, but it requires extensive time and message-specific training in the target natural context.

In summary, few researchers have been able to demonstrate that persons with severe aphasia could use "symbol substitution" AAC systems to generate a wide range of propositions in untrained contexts. As Kraat (1990) noted in her review of AAC interventions in aphasia, "it was as if the aphasic did not think to turn to these alternative forms, or could not shift strategies to use them, or somehow could not integrate them into real communication contexts" (p. 324).

There are many possible explanations for the insufficiency of a modality substitution approach for persons with acquired language disability. One possibility is that the disruption in the language system of an aphasic person is so great that symbol association skills, memory for sequencing, and judgment for using the right symbol at the right time are too impaired for generating language. Another possibility is that the moment-to-moment fluctuations typical of aphasic performance (McNeill, 1983) prevent the completion of the many sequential steps needed to convey a thought. A third possibility is that clinicians may be trying to apply techniques in a broad, indiscriminate manner rather than creating a "best fit" between patients and AAC techniques.

However, interpreting the above to mean that individuals with aphasia are unable to profit from AAC is too simplistic. An alternative perspective on aphasia and AAC is presented in the following sections.

PRINCIPLES OF AUGMENTATIVE COMMUNICATION THAT RELATE TO APHASIA

In recent years, the AAC field has developed a treatment philosophy that is interaction-based, sociocommunicative, and holistic. AAC typically emphasizes the communication process between all participating parties in a communication interaction. The following concepts, described elsewhere (Garrett & Beukelman, 1992), are restated and expanded below for the reader's convenience:

1. AAC interventions adopt a *holistic orientation* that considers the person, his or her lifestyle, family and partners, environment, needs and life goals, and societal restrictions and expectations. This principle influences many aspects of an AAC intervention, including vocabulary selection, family training, and goal-setting.

2. In contrast to focusing on communication products or subskills, one of the end goals of AAC interventions is the *enhanced participation* of the individual in important life activities. This philosophy creates some difference in treatment goals. In the case of the severely limited individual, the focus of treatment may shift from treating all language deficits in a clinical setting to increasing the person's ability to communicate in one important activity (e.g., saying family names over the phone). In the case of the individual with mild aphasia, it may be important to teach AAC strategies in specific community situations such as at the grocery store or the race track.

3. Another important goal of AAC interventions is the *communication of meaning and intent*. In short, an AAC therapist would probably emphasize the nonspeaking person's success in conveying a message to a partner more than the accuracy and method with which it was delivered.

4. A *decreased* emphasis is placed on *strengthening the subskills* of communication (e.g., improving motor movements, repeating words, following commands) in a hierarchical order using stimulus-response training paradigms. This viewpoint should not be interpreted to mean that AAC-oriented clinicians ignore underlying subskills and deficit patterns of a particular client. Rather, they acknowledge and incorporate this knowledge into each therapy activity holistically.

5. AAC interventions *emphasize the residual strengths* of the communication-impaired individual. This perspective evolved from interventions

for nonspeaking persons with congenital communication disorders who had to rely on residual skills as well as AAC systems to communicate. Clinicians can easily transfer this perspective to patients with aphasia, who also may retain many skills. Residual skills can occur in so-called deficit areas (e.g., patients with moderate to severe word-finding difficulties often do seize on the right word occasionally), or in an area of relative strength (e.g., the patient who can pantomime rather than tell a story verbally). This perspective is particularly useful when teaching patients that they can communicate immediately instead of waiting until speech returns.

6.   AAC interventions with nonspeaking persons emphasize *providing communication opportunities*. Clinicians and teachers have learned to adapt activities to increase the participation of nonspeaking children in normal school activities such as story hour and math class. They also learn to pause and provide enough time for the child to initiate thoughts or acknowledge a question at his or her own rate. Clinicians and partners can learn to provide similar kinds of communication opportunities with aphasic adults.

7.   The role of the *communication partner* is clearly important in an AAC treatment model. In AAC-aphasia interventions, partners are included in as many treatment sessions as possible. They participate in initial discussions about the client's lifestyle, supply lists of preferences and dislikes, construct photo albums of important life events, learn about aphasia, and practice new communication strategies.

8.   Practitioners recognize successful AAC interventions as a package of communication strategies rather than as a single device or technique. Communication is seen as a *multimodal* process, a collection of "whatever works" strategies and modes that can include gesturing for assistance, scrunching up the face to indicate displeasure, saying "hello," and pointing to words or symbols on a communication system. Nonspeaking persons also can use natural communication skills (writing and gestures) in conjunction with aided augmentative strategies (Yorkston & Dowden, 1983). Allowing persons with aphasia to choose the most effective communication modality helps them compensate for the variability of their performance and use the channel they are most competent with on a moment-by-moment basis. The challenge for clinicians implementing a multimodal AAC intervention is to teach the individual who has aphasia when and where to use a particular mode of communication.

9.   Communication is *individualistic and idiosyncratic*. Each individual with aphasia has a lifetime of acquired experiences and knowledge that must be acknowledged in daily interactions and incorporated into AAC-based treatment interventions and goals.

10.   It is important to understand the *purpose* of each communication interaction in AAC interventions. Janice Light (1988) proposed an eloquent model of communication interaction in which she made the critical point that humans do not always communicate to send and receive information.

Rather, they often communicate simply to socialize with one another. The communication activities of adults, particularly elderly adults, clearly illustrate this concept. For instance, discussions about the weather seldom transfer any new information but instead serve to establish a conversational meeting ground. Light's four functions of social interactions include the communication of wants and needs, the transfer of information, the development and maintenance of social closeness, and the maintenance of social etiquette. These communication functions are discussed in greater detail in the next section.

COMMUNICATION NEEDS IN APHASIA

The linguistic and nonlinguistic problems that accompany aphasia can obviously affect an individual's ability to maintain communicative competence in an unmodified social situation (Ryan, Giles, Bartolucci, & Henwood, 1986). These acquired problems interact with other behaviors that accompany each person as he or she grows older. Ryan et al.'s model of the *communication predicament of aging* depicts other factors that affect communication encounters with an older person: "old-age cues" consisting of physiologic, psychological, and sociocultural differences; stereotyped expectations of behavior; the partner's subsequently modified behavior; constrained opportunities for communication; and ultimately a loss of personal control and self-esteem as well as lessened social interaction. For the individual with aphasia, the combination of aphasia-related and age-related changes diminishes interaction quality, usually to a significant degree.

To better understand how the elements of interaction with the older adult are changed before and after the onset of aphasia, it is illustrative to return to Light's (1988) model of the four functions of communication interaction. These four functions (wants and needs, information transfer, social closeness, and social etiquette) can be applied to aphasia in two ways. First, persons with aphasia are seen as part of an "older" age cohort whose communication needs have often changed naturally even before the stroke (Beukelman & Garrett, 1992). While information transfer may have been a major component of the person's communication style when he or she was employed, it may have become somewhat less important following retirement. Instead, older adults may communicate primarily to be socially close to family or friends. Older adults continue to communicate wants and needs but do so on a limited basis while they are healthy and able to obtain items by themselves. They also communicate to maintain the rules of social etiquette.

Light's model can be applied a second time to the same older individuals who have become nonspeaking following a stroke. In this scenario, the proportional importance of each of the communication functions again changes, this time across the time frame of recovery stages (Beukelman &

Garrett, 1992). In the acute-care hospital, the family and nursing staff value the patient's ability to communicate pain or other physical needs. The patient may value opportunities to be close to family. It is probable, however, that communication of more abstract information (e.g., discussing world politics, making decisions about repairing the water heater) is not a priority in the first few days of acute-care treatment.

After the patient enters the rehabilitation setting, it may become important to communicate basic personal information such as his or her name, the names of family members, or his or her hometown. Social closeness becomes increasingly important. If the patient regains a reasonable level of physical competence, he or she can often meet an increasing number of physical needs independently. However, communication of physical needs does continue to be an issue for others.

Should a patient improve to the point of transferring to home, then communicating specific information becomes more important as he or she reenters the community. Families may express an interest in learning about ways to have a sincere conversation rather than being restricted to short exchanges about basic needs. On the other hand, patients who continue to require skilled nursing care may require a consistent means of gaining attention and managing needs for an extended period of time. It is interesting to observe that most aphasic individuals who are beyond the acute period of hospitalization manage the fourth area of interaction—social etiquette—very well with natural communication skills. A firm handshake or a slight nod of the head often convey social niceties and acknowledgment better than any clinician-designed strategy ever could.

AAC strategies do exist to address each of these areas: communication of wants and needs, establishment of social closeness, and communication of specific information. The strategies differ according to the strengths and problems of each patient. A classification system to assist in mapping techniques onto communication functions and patient types is proposed in the next section.

A REVISED CLASSIFICATION SYSTEM FOR APHASIA

To knit the above thoughts and concepts into a practical working system, Garrett and Beukelman (1992) proposed the following classification system for severe aphasia. The five groups of patients described in the system—the basic-choice communicator, the controlled-situation communicator, the comprehensive communicator, the specific-need communicator, and the augmented-input communicator—are based on the severity of the communication deficits that affect an individual's ability to meet needs and participate in communication exchanges. The groups are also distinguished by particular AAC strategies that have been demonstrated to work most effectively for that cluster of aphasic individuals. While the first three categories are roughly hierarchical in terms of severity (i.e., from most to least severe), the last two categories are based on communication needs alone.

The Basic-Choice Communicator

Some individuals with aphasia have sustained such massive injuries from one or more strokes that they have difficulty demonstrating basic environmental awareness, much less linguistic-level behaviors. These individuals present a clinical challenge in that most traditional evaluation and treatment tasks require a minimum level of language ability that they cannot demonstrate. Because these persons are so impaired, they generally progress slowly and are frequently viewed as poor candidates for rehabilitation programs. The speech-language pathologist may be involved primarily as a consultant in these cases or may treat the patient on a trial basis for a short time. The clinician often must answer difficult questions from the family about the prognosis for functional communication; in turn, the family learns rather quickly that ways of communicating and participating in life activities will be quite different than before.

Treatment techniques based on augmentative communication principles for this type of communicator emphasize choice-making at an object symbol level, partial participation in familiar routines, and elementary turn-taking and establishment of shared reference. For instance, a clinician might ask the patient to choose a piece of jewelry to wear by holding up the items and encouraging the client to look or point at the preferred item during an early-morning grooming and dressing routine. If the patient had severe limb apraxia, the clinician would physically help the client point to and put on the jewelry. The clinician would interpret all of the patient's behaviors during these activities, even if at first they were unintentional. For instance, if the person with severe aphasia moved toward one of the jewelry items non-purposefully, the clinician would interpret the movement as a request and respond by verbally labeling the action and providing the object. The clinician would also offer opportunities for the patient to confirm or reject a choice in an effort to build foundational skills for responding with a true yes or no signal.

The person with global aphasia would also be encouraged to participate in familiar interactive games, particularly those that are highly visual. For instance, he or she might be asked to make a mark on a tic-tac-toe grid or to add features to an outline drawing of a house. The clinician would also model turn-taking behaviors and would request that the client signal the beginning or end of a turn when appropriate.

Some basic-choice communicators may progress to higher levels of functioning. Others remain severely impaired for the long term. This profile of limited change requires clinicians to revise their primary focus of treatment and teach other partners new ways of interacting with the basic-choice communicator. Partners must learn to simplify their communication, enhance the patient's visual environment, incorporate choices into daily routines, and promote participation in meaningful activities to the greatest extent possible.

The Controlled-Situation Communicator

The controlled-situation communicator differs from the basic-choice communicator because the patient retains an acute awareness of the environment and a desire to communicate. This type of individual understands and participates in basic routines such as clearing the lapboard in anticipation of lunch or pointing to the clock to signal the end of a therapy session. The controlled-situation communicator makes frequent efforts to communicate, particularly to familiar people, though most of his or her attempts to convey linguistic information end in failure. Speech is often stereotypical or nonexistent. The controlled-situation communicator is frequently aware of the inadequacy of his or her communication efforts and often appears frustrated. Limb apraxia is a common characteristic, and self-initiated communicative gestures other than pointing are infrequent. Reading performance on standardized tests is poor, though reading ability is enhanced in contextual situations. Many of these individuals never overcome their linguistic deficits despite intensive or long-term treatment. Typical aphasia diagnoses can include global aphasia, or severe Wernicke's or Broca's aphasia.

Therapy goals derived from an augmentative communication approach attempt to take advantage of the individual's residual awareness and preserved linguistic and extralinguistic knowledge. However, because of their severe language limitations, it is difficult for controlled-situation communicators to independently link the many steps of the communication process—formulating the initial idea, gaining access to memory stores, semantically mapping the idea, executing the message via the motor speech system, and monitoring the partner's comprehension of the message. Therefore, support for the communication process is required at each of these steps. Because communication partners can often judge where communication breakdowns have occurred on a moment-by-moment basis, they may be particularly qualified to provide this support.

A conversational technique called *written choice conversation* can provide both clients and partners with an immediate means of communication (Garrett & Beukelman, 1992; Garrett & Beukelman, 1995). Briefly, this technique requires the person with aphasia to answer conversational questions by pointing to written word choices that are presented by a trained partner. The partner introduces possible topics and semantically scaffolds the controlled-situation communicator's response options on a turn-by-turn basis. If the aphasic communicator answers a question by pointing to the written word choice, then another question that predicates on the preceding question is asked. Every effort is made to ask questions that provide the client with sincere communication opportunities, such as offering opinions on presidential candidates or stating preferences with regard to paint colors or wallpaper during redecorating. While the partner does take the role of conversational initiator when using this technique, the aphasic person can partially participate in social interactions. A sample conversation is depicted below:

Partner:	What should I plant in my garden now that spring is almost over? [*Waits*]
Person with Aphasia (PWA):	[*No response*]
Partner:	[*Writes vertically on a sheet of paper in large block letters and says aloud*]: Petunias, asters, marigolds, daisies.
PWA:	[*Points to "asters" and nods.*]
Partner:	[*Circles "asters" and interprets.*] Oh, I should plant asters! What are the odds that they'll bloom by fall? [*Draws a 5-point scale with the endpoints marked "0%" and "100%" and verbalizes the endpoints aloud.*]
PWA:	[*Points to 25%*]
Partner:	[*Interprets*] Oh, you don't think my chances are that great . . . .
PWA:	[*Nods in agreement*]

Many individuals with severe Broca's aphasia or resolving global aphasia learn this communication technique very quickly, although some may need initial assistance to program the movements to point to or scan all of the word choices. Many individuals with minimal ability on standard reading comprehension batteries respond appropriately in this task to lists of words or phrases that are presented in conversational context; family members typically verify the patient's answers as 70–100% accurate (Garrett & Beukelman, 1995).

Engaging in partner-supported conversations may not have a lasting impact on the communication disability itself, but functional goals of increased social communication can be achieved. Specific training in other communication areas may also be beneficial. For example, the client might be taught to identify situations in which calling for assistance is necessary. The clinician provides a means for the client to call for assistance (e.g., bell, buzzer, hand signal) and helps the patient with severe aphasia practice this skill during actual attention-getting situations. Persons in this category can also practice interaction skills such as indicating their partner's turn or introducing themselves by pointing to a printed information card. Occasionally, individuals with this degree of aphasia may also learn to communicate some basic information (e.g., name, address, names of family members, favorite restaurants) by pointing to prestored messages in a communication notebook or system, though their ability to independently gain access to stored information is typically limited. Anecdotal reports of storing messages on a voice-output communication device so the person with severe aphasia can tell stories are also beginning to emerge (Fried-Oken, 1995; Stuart, 1994).

Goals for the partner include learning to identify interesting conversational topics, respond to and interpret all of the patient's communication attempts, provide written or graphic choices when natural communication modalities are insufficient, and schedule structured conversational opportunities on a regular basis.

Many controlled-situation communicators remain severely impaired. Their options for participating in life narrow because of physical limitations as well as ongoing communication difficulties. Helping partners to refocus their communication interactions and to include their communication-impaired friend or family member in personalized communication activities is clearly an essential part of the client's overall treatment program.

The Comprehensive Communicator

The individual with aphasia who naturally attempts to use a variety of modalities to communicate may be termed a comprehensive communicator (Beukelman & Garrett, 1988; Garrett & Beukelman, 1992). This type of aphasic client makes many efforts to communicate and often tries to persevere through multiple breakdowns until the partner understands the message. The patient may use limited speech, gestures, facial expression, and limited drawing and spelling to communicate. Unfortunately, many of these valiant efforts to communicate through residual channels are inefficient or ineffective, and the partner loses interest before the message is conveyed. At other times, the patient may "short-circuit" before a word is found or a thought is completed, and the communication effort collapses. This type of patient is often classified as having severe apraxia, Broca's aphasia, severe word-finding difficulties, or conduction aphasia. Many patients return to the community or live in supervised situations and face communication challenges many times a day.

The clinician's task is to reconcile the various strategies that the comprehensive communicator is already using in a fragmented manner into some type of cohesive, multiple-component communication system. For instance, the comprehensive communicator typically has difficulty communicating specific information because of severe word retrieval problems. To decrease the amount of search time and struggle for specific words, clinician and client may attempt to predict vocabulary that will be used in certain environments and store it ahead of time in a communication system. For example, a former client of the author's (Garrett, Beukelman, & Low, 1989) used a section of his communication notebook for the names of baseball teams and his predictions for the season. This section was used to participate in conversations with friends and family members during baseball season. Other specific-vocabulary sections of his communication notebook contained names of family members, horse racing terms, names of favorite restaurants, phrases used when traveling by taxi or bus, and a description of important life events. When they created this stored information component of the AAC system, the clinician and the client included only messages that required expedient delivery and linguistic accuracy, instead of compiling exhaustive vocabulary lists within each category.

Because comprehensive communicators also bring fragmented linguistic skills to communication situations, it is also important to provide them with more efficient methods for their expression. First, because these individuals often resort to searching for scraps of paper so they can write word fragments or draw when speech fails them, blank paper for writing should be incorporated into existing AAC systems. Second, if individuals with severe expressive aphasia produce frequent phonemic paraphasias, it is helpful to include an alphabet card in the system so that they can supplement their word production by pointing to the first letter of the word. Individuals with aphasia may not be able to retrieve the first letter of a target word on every occasion. But when they are successful, partners may receive sufficient information to guess the target word and circumvent a communication breakdown. This alphabet board word-cueing technique has been used similarly by individuals with severe dysarthria (Yorkston, Beukelman, & Bell, 1988). Third, gestural communication and pantomime are other natural communication modalities that often impart communicative intent quickly and accurately. Persons with aphasia may need instruction in using gestures or pantomime to convey information consistently and efficiently. These three means of communication serve to convey unique, unpredictable information, unlike the stored message components described earlier. The clinician should try to include strategies for unique message communication in AAC systems for comprehensive communicators, because novel messages can be expected to occur in most of their conversations.

The clinician's task, after the components of the system have been inventoried and assembled, is to teach clients to choose an appropriate modality to communicate their messages (e.g., using an alphabet card to express the first letter of a nearby town's name when speech is not quite clear enough to convey it perfectly; locating the name of a store in the "shopping" section of the notebook). The largest proportion of training time may be spent teaching clients to use strategies selectively in actual communication situations until the client can begin to use strategies spontaneously (Garrett et al., 1989). Some clients may even progress to the stage of resolving communication breakdowns by pointing to written phrases that re-establish conversational control (e.g., "You didn't understand me . . . I'll try again.").

Clinicians can also include communication partners in some treatment sessions. Partners may need to learn to allow their friend or family member enough time to communicate through the multimodal augmentative system. They may learn to encourage the communicator with aphasia to shift to another modality when the first one is not effective. They may also have to learn how and when to guess target messages when communication breaks down.

The Specific-Need Communicator

Individuals in this category have a specific communication need that transcends any description of severity or skills. The individual's lifestyle and personal choices may define the nature of the AAC system to a greater degree than deficits. In an example described in the technology section of this chapter, a person who was unable to speak as a result of aphasia demonstrated the need to communicate by phone with her family. Other individuals may have specific vocabulary needs for certain critical environments such as the bus or the bank, or at the racetrack. Still others may want a means to introduce themselves and to explain their communication disability in the community. A communication need may also be as simple as requiring a rubber stamp so that a signature can be executed legibly and quickly.

Clinical goals are varied and completely dependent on matching augmentative strategies to the individual's situation. In the first example in the preceding paragraph, the intervention to improve phone communication used a voice-output system with a limited number of messages (e.g., I'm fine; I need you; Come visit immediately). In the second case, a card containing the names of phrases for bus use (e.g., I want to be dropped off at _____; I need to buy _____ tokens), key bank transactions (e.g., I want to make a deposit; How much money is in my account?), and betting phrases (e.g., Trifecta, Exacta) may suffice. For the person who wants to introduce themselves to others, a laminated card containing essential information about the client and brief comments such as "Please speak a little slower—I don't understand all of your words" may be warranted.

Partners may also be included in the identification of specific-need situations, and in the development of messages and vocabulary. They may be required to learn skills related to the operation of a technical system, or may simply procure simple items to meet specific communication needs (e.g., buying a rubber signature stamp or a bell for calling attention). They may also have to learn specific interaction skills, such as learning to ask conversational questions in the same sequence when conversing with the person with aphasia by phone.

The Augmented-Input Communicator

The hallmark of the augmented-input communicator is a typically intermittent pattern of processing auditory information. He or she may be labeled as having Wernicke's or transcortical sensory aphasia. Frequently, however, patients from all of the preceding categories (basic-choice communicator, controlled-situation communicator, comprehensive communicator, specific-need communicator) experience breakdowns in auditory processing, and the strategies described below are often appropriate for them also. Characteristics of augmented input communicators include a puzzled facial expression when spoken to, frequent requests for the partner to repeat, continued conversation about an old topic, and a general air of confusion.

Many of these individuals appear to benefit from the use of supplemental graphic or gestural input. For example, when an individual with severe aphasia across modalities had difficulty understanding that the visitor at the door had come to design new window blinds, the partner supplemented her explanation by drawing a simple sketch of a window and the message was quickly understood. Another individual had tremendous difficulty conversing because he was unable to follow natural shifts in conversational topics. He was assisted when his partner learned to write down key words or topics on a notepad by his side. A third individual with mild to moderate aphasia preferred that his partners use a laptop computer to supplement the intermittent lapses in comprehension that he experienced throughout the day. He learned to signal these breakdowns by pointing to the computer at its permanent location by his desk.

The clinician's primary role in treating the augmented-input communicator is to teach the client to identify situations in which he or she has not understood a message. It is helpful to jointly identify a signal that the client can use to notify partners that a communication breakdown has occurred. The clinician should also encourage the client to carry a notebook with blank pages and a pen so that partners can jot down key words or topics. It may be helpful to provide a list of instructions for partners that can be taped to the cover (Garrett & Beukelman, 1992).

Therapy goals in this category place particular emphasis on the partner. In fact, no beneficial effect is seen if the partner chooses not to participate in the treatment strategy. Thus, the clinician's inclusion of the partner in treatment sessions is crucial. Partners may need assistance to identify the patient's communication breakdowns by observing facial expression or listening for unadjusted conversational output after topic changes. They may also need to practice the "written key word" strategy in actual communication situations.

THE ROLE OF TECHNOLOGY

Devising flexible, comprehensive, and efficient technological interventions for aphasic individuals is a difficult task. The capabilities of electronic message storage devices are constantly increasing, and they tempt clinicians to apply them to the significant number of aphasics with disordered message exchange skills. One of the major premises of this chapter is that any communication strategy, whether technical or nontechnical, must match the capabilities of the individual with aphasia. Many early efforts to provide aphasic clients with "high tech" AAC systems were implemented without a classification system to match individuals to the most appropriate techniques, which may have caused the mixed results cited earlier in this chapter.

Persons with aphasia who are dependent on partners to provide them with topical and semantic contexts so they can converse will probably not possess the skills to independently retrieve messages with a technological system. Clearly, basic-choice communicators and controlled-situation communicators would have tremendous difficulty using systems to initiate thoughts for the same reasons that success with their natural modalities eludes them; the succession of events that leads to the communication of a message breaks down somewhere. Difficulties can occur in reception, idea formulation, lexical mapping, phonemic encoding, or motor output, to name a few possibilities. When extralinguistic variables are added (e.g., performance with distractions, perseveration, fatigue, unfamiliarity with technology, lack of motivation, etc.), chances for success are further decreased. While good success with systems can be seen in structured exchanges in the clinical environment, patients rarely generalize to independent, natural situations. These patients clearly rely on partners for conversational or choice-making opportunities in which they are given very structured doses of information to process.

The third communicator type, the comprehensive communicator, uses technological interventions successfully on occasion. Beukelman, Yorkston, and Dowden (1985) report the case of Dallas, a 47-year-old man with severe verbal apraxia and moderately severe aphasia. He used a Handivoice 130 speech output device with a single programmable level to communicate whole messages related to his interior-design business. This patient required system portability, speech output, and rapid communication of specific messages so that clients could be interviewed. These messages were selected after an extensive interview with Dallas and his wife. Dallas practiced message retrieval in clinical situations as well as in natural contexts. He also learned to supplement the telegraphic output of the system with facial expression, gestures, and intonation to further clarify his message. The Handivoice 130 was also part of a more comprehensive system consisting of a written-word communication notebook (related to specific needs), a more general conversational photograph album, and gestures.

Clearly the personalization of his communication system helped Dallas communicate successfully using a technological system. Using idiosyncratic and environmentally specific vocabulary has long been an important factor in helping nonspeaking individuals with congenital disabilities to communicate and is more than likely a critical factor for adults with aphasia. It is important, then, that manufacturers develop programmable technological systems for adults with aphasia. Some comprehensive communicators, particularly those who are primarily apraxic, may be able to gain access to generically stored information. However, finding words stored in grammatical categories appears to demand greater processing than finding a personalized collection of messages and words related to a more holistic activity such as going to the bank or to a favorite restaurant. Research is needed to further investigate these issues.

Richard Steele and colleagues (1989, 1991) have developed a computer-based system called Lingraphica that provides a pictorial method of access to vocabulary. Using a mouse, the client selects categories or environments by dragging and then clicking the mouse to select a pictorial icon. The screen dynamically changes to reveal new vocabulary icons, and eliminates the need for changing paper overlays on other technical systems. Each message or vocabulary item is also spoken. Primary categories and environments include actors, actions, placement, modifiers, things, and other. Opening the "things" category allows the user to delve further into other levels, such as places > home > kitchen > food > individual food item. A unique feature of this system is that it represents some areas spatially. For example, when the "home" icon is selected, a floor plan of a typical house is represented. The user then clicks on the particular room that he or she is interested in and then has the option of seeing a room drawn in its entirety. After the level of individual symbols is selected, they can be sequenced on a "storyboard window" to create a unique message. This message can then be spoken in its entirety.

Clinical experience and anecdotal reports (Stuart, 1995; Fried-Oken, 1995; Garrett, 1995) suggest that other technological systems have been used intermittently in clinical interventions. For example, Garrett and Beukelman (1992) discussed a specific-need communicator who needed to communicate on the phone and used a limited-message digitized-speech output device (such as the Prentke Romich IntroTalker or Zygo Parrot) to say key messages such as "Come over now," and "This is _____. I need to make an appointment." The patient was able to imitate short messages, so her own voice was recorded on the device. The patient first learned to identify messages in rote recall situations, then to answer basic questions, and finally to initiate simple requests. Her family learned to ask questions in the same sequence, for any change in their delivery caused her to overload and process messages incorrectly. In this particular case, the patient used the system briefly but then stated that she was no longer interested in using the device, even though significant communication needs still existed.

Yorkston and Waugh (1989) also reported on the use of portable computers to generate the word choices used in the written-choice conversation technique for controlled-situation communicators. In this application, the partner types out the choices rather than writing them by hand. The client then responds by pointing to the appropriate choice on the computer display. This method is advantageous if either communicator wishes to keep a record of conversations, or if the partner's writing legibility is poor. Partners can also use a computer to generate key words and topics for the augmented-input communicator. It is intriguing to consider the potential usefulness of dual-screen computer displays in these applications (Beukelman & Garrett, 1988; Yorkston and Waugh, 1989).

The role of technology remains elusive—a combination of supportive research, clinical trials, and the development of successful user profiles will do much to encourage judicious applications of these systems.

RESEARCH NEEDS

The application of AAC strategies to aphasia will require extensive thought and investigation before a track record of consistent clinical effectiveness becomes a reality. The following list of research areas is offered as a starting point:

1. Conduct a demographic analysis of the aphasic population to determine whether the clinical groupings described above are valid.
2. Use case-study research paradigms to develop profiles of client and strategy successes with both low- and high-technology interventions.
3. Investigate the success of various strategies of message access for aphasics. For example, which do aphasics understand more readily—whole messages or single words? Are environmental, categorical, idiosyncratic, visual-spatial, or alphabetic storage strategies more effective? How does access to vocabulary items presented in pictorial environments differ from those stored as single words or pictures?
4. Determine how many sequential levels a comprehensive communicator can gain access to before he or she "short-circuits" without completing the message.
5. Determine the learning rates of different patient types across different strategies.
6. Focus on "success" studies. How satisfied are patients and partners with a particular system or strategy? How well did it meet their needs? How often do they use it? How did it change participation levels?
7. Follow up on how well comprehensive-communicator and specific-needs patients adapt to natural communication situations.
8. Determine which types of instructional methods work best for different types of patients, partners, and across which AAC techniques. Investigate how much time it takes to teach consolidated use of a multimodal system or specific-need system.

SUMMARY THOUGHTS ON SERVICE DELIVERY

Many of the techniques and approaches described above evolved from a need to serve aphasia-impaired clients in the most time-efficient yet effective manner. Clearly, matching clients to appropriate techniques is more efficient than attempting to teach all clients all skills. Written-choice conversation has become a tool that re-establishes immediate communication with individuals who would otherwise not have a mode for several months. This in turn allows patients to communicate with their families earlier in the recovery process. Likewise, clinicians and trained staff and family members can supplement the input of a patient with auditory processing problems almost immediately.

Often the comprehensive communicator can begin working on subskills of a multimodal communication system while still in the rehabilitation hospital; selecting messages and consolidating the system probably require more extensive time as an outpatient or participant in a university training clinic. Specific-need communicators often go home or back to work first; clear needs emerge in response to communication difficulties that cannot be predicted in advance. Understanding the goal of each strategy at each stage of recovery can also assist in obtaining third-party reimbursement, particularly if goals are stated in terms of impact on communication effectiveness and the meeting of needs.

In this AAC-oriented service delivery model for adults with severe aphasia, the target of the therapy process is expanded to the family and other significant communication partners. Many of the above strategies involve partners immediately following the medical episode. This early involvement in the treatment process can do much to alleviate the helplessness that the families often experience. Although partner training is not always successful, clinicians should strive to teach at least one key person how to manage efficient communication of needs or a basic social conversation with the client. This designation and training of key partners may have the most important impact on the life of an individual with severe aphasia.

Finally, most of the goals and objectives summarized above attempt to address the needs of the whole person. They acknowledge that each client has a rich history of experiences. This knowledge is a necessary part of developing interventions that allow individuals with severe aphasia to participate more fully in important life activities.

REFERENCES

American Speech-Language-Hearing Association (1991). Report: Augmentative and alternative communication. *ASHA*, *33*(Suppl. 5), 9–12.

Bailey, S. (1983). Blissymbolics and aphasia therapy: A case study. In C. Code & D. Muller (Eds.), *Aphasia therapy* (pp. 178–186). London: Edward Arnold.

Bellaire, K., Georges, J., & Thompson, C. (1989). *Establishing functional communication board use for non-verbal aphasia subjects.* Presented at the Clinical Aphasiology Conference, Lake Tahoe, Nevada.

Beukelman, D., & Garrett, K. (1988). Augmentative and alternative communication for adults with acquired severe communication disorders. *Augmentative and Alternative Communication, 4,* 104–121.

Beukelman, D., & Garrett, K. (1992). Adults with severe aphasia. In D. Beukelman and P. Mirenda (Eds). *Augmentative and alternative communication: Management of severe communication disorders in children and adults* (pp. 331–343). Baltimore: Paul H. Brookes.

Beukelman, D., & Mirenda, K. (1987). Communication options for persons who cannot speak: Assessment and evaluation. *Proceedings of the National Planners Conference of Assistive Device Service Delivery.* Columbus, OH: Great Lakes Area Regional Resource Center.

Beukelman, D., Yorkston, K., & Dowden, P. (1985). *Communication augmentation: A casebook of clinical management.* San Diego: College-Hill Press.

DeRuyter, F., Kennedy, M., & Doyle, M. (1990). *ACS outcomes: Do the data tell the whole story?* Presented at the International Society of Augmentative and Alternative Communication Biennial Conference, Stockholm, Sweden.

Di Simoni, F. (1986). Alternative communication systems for aphasic individuals. In R. Chapey (Ed.), *Language intervention in adult aphasia* (pp. 345–359). Baltimore: Williams & Wilkins.

Enderby, P., & Hamilton, G. (1983). Communication aid and therapeutic tools: A report on the clinical trial using SPLINK with aphasic individuals. In C. Code & D. Muller (Eds.), *Aphasia therapy* (pp. 187–193). London: Edward Arnold.

Fried-Oken, M. (1995). Story telling as an augmentative communication approach for a man with severe apraxia of speech and expressive aphasia. *ASHA AAC Special Interest Division Newsletter, 4,* 3–4.

Garrett, K. (1995). Expanding expressive communication options for a person wtih severe aphasia. *ASHA AAC Special Interest Division Newsletter, 4,* 5–7.

Garrett, K., & Beukelman, D. (1992). Augmentative communication approaches for persons with severe aphasia. In K. Yorkston (Ed.), *Augmentative communication in the medical setting* (pp. 245–338). Tucson, AZ: Communication Skill Builders.

Garrett, K., & Beukelman, D. (1995). Changes in the interaction patterns of an individual with severe aphasia given three types of partner support. *Clinical Aphasiology , 23,* 237–251.

Garrett, K., Beukelman, D., & Low, D. (1989). A comprehensive augmentative communication system for an adult with Broca's aphasia. *Augmentative and Alternative Communication, 5,* 55–61.

Glass, A., Gazaniga, M., & Premack, D. (1975). Artificial language training in global aphasics. *Neuropsychologia, 11,* 95–103.

Johannsen-Horbach, H., Cegla, B., Mager, V., & Schempp, B. (1985). Treatment of global aphasia with a nonverbal communication system. *Brain and Language, 24,* 74–82.

Kraat, A. (1990). Augmentative and alternative communication: Does it have a future in aphasia rehabilitation? *Aphasiology, 4,* 321–338.

Light, J. (1988). Interaction involving individuals using augmentative and alternative communication systems: State of the art and future directions. *Augmentative and Alternative Communication, 4*, 66–82.

Marshall, R. (1987). Reapportioning time for aphasia rehabilitation: A point of view. *Aphasiology, 1*, 59–73.

McNeill, M. (1983). Aphasia: Neurologic considerations. *Topics in Language Disorders, 3*, 1–19.

Ryan, E., Giles, H., Bartolucci, G., & Henwood, K. (1986). Linguistic and social psychological components of communication by and with the elderly. *Language and Communication, 6*, 1–24.

Steele, R., Weinrich, M., Wertz, R., Kleczewska, M., & Carlson, G. (1989). Computer-based visual communication in aphasia. *Neuropsychologia, 27*, 409–426.

Steele, R. (1991). *Lingraphica* [communication device]. Palo Alto, CA: Tolfa Corp.

Stuart, S. (1994). Assisted storytelling for an aphasic individual of Hispanic ancestry. Personal communication.

Weinrich, M., Steele, R., Carlson, G., & Kleczewska, M. (1989). Processing of visual syntax in a globally aphasic patient. *Brain and Language, 36*, 391–405.

Yorkston, K., Beukelman, D., & Bell, K. (1988). *Clinical management of dysarthric speakers.* Boston: College-Hill Press.

Yorkston, K., & Dowden, P. (1983). Nonspeech language and communication systems. In A. Holland (Ed.), *Language disorders in adults: Recent advances* (pp. 283-312). San Diego: College-Hill Press.

Yorkston, K., & Waugh, P. (1989). Use of augmentative communication devices with apractic individuals. In P. Square-Storer (Ed.), *Acquired apraxia of speech in aphasic adults* (pp. 267–283). New York: Taylor & Francis.

Chapter 16

Treatment Efficacy: Reflections and Projections

Betty Daggett Coleman and
Gloriajean L. Wallace

The outstanding ethical question surrounding the therapy enterprise is, of course, does it really "work"; do the effects of treatment really exceed those that might occur in its absence or by comparison with a credible placebo?
(Ingham, 1990, p. 22)

The issue of efficacy is both important and elusive. While it is important to know whether or not therapeutic efforts are helping an individual, it is not always clear how to select the best source of information for making judgments about recovery. Clinicians are simultaneously confronted with viewpoints of professionals, of the client, and of the client's family members and close associates, some of whom may criticize the therapeutic process.

This chapter discusses efficacy from each of those points of view. In addition, aspects of an ethnographic approach are described as useful methodologies for enhancing the perspective of persons with aphasia on the issue of treatment efficacy. A sampling of other current and future trends towards developing a deeper and broader understanding of what constitutes efficacious treatment for aphasia is also included.

VIEWPOINTS FROM PROFESSIONALS

History

Before speech-language pathology was established as a discipline in 1925, efficacy studies for aphasia treatment were few. Shewan (1986) noted two exceptions. One of the earliest was a 1904 study by Mills, who described a systematic training hierarchy for relearning lost speech in a patient with aphasia and outlined treatment methods that have survived to modern times. The second of these early studies was by Franz, who, 2 years later, expanded the concept of reeducation for individuals with aphasia by providing data on stimuli and number of trials and errors, hinting about the amount of treatment needed, and reporting continued improvement in performance with training for as long as 2 years after the onset of aphasia.

A number of confounding issues were identified early on. These included:

- Controlling for the tendency to self-treat (Weisenburg & McBride, 1935)
- Controlling for spontaneous recovery (Butfield & Zangwill, 1946)
- Including an acceptable no-treatment group, controlling for patient variables, and timing the start of treatment (Eisenson, 1949)

By the 1950s, researchers were using larger clinical populations and increasingly objective scientific measures to assess the effects of treatment (Wepman, 1951). McReynolds (1990) reported an upward swing in treatment efficacy research beginning in the 1970s.

Efficacy and Single-Subject Research Designs

Both group and single-subject research designs are important in assessing the efficacy of aphasia treatment. However, single-subject designs have done more to advance efficacy research because single-subject designs more readily lend themselves to investigation by practicing clinicians (Brookshire, 1985; Rosenbek, LaPointe, & Wertz, 1989; Wertz & Rosenbek, 1978).

While single-subject designs hold broad appeal for clinical researchers and practicing clinicians, they pose their own set of limitations. They are not glorified case studies. They must also be replicated across settings and across subjects. Davis (1978) observed that while single-case designs are appropriate for addressing a wide range of efficacy questions, confounding effects from numerous variables present the potential for false-positive conclusions. Kearns and Thompson (1991) warn against the lure of technology for its own sake in single-subject research.

Both group and single-case constructs involve quantifiable data. Later in this chapter, the promise of an ethnographic approach for filling the void left by such measures will be outlined.

Efficacy and Age

Since stroke is the most common cause of aphasia and the risk of stroke increases for older individuals (Tonkovich, 1988), it is no wonder that age has figured prominently in the general aphasia therapy enterprise.

Studies through the early 1970s (Darley, 1972) associated older age with poorer recovery and less improvement from treatment for aphasia. Later studies and reviews (Deal & Deal, 1978; Holland 1990; Wertz & Dronkers, 1990; Wertz, Weiss et al., 1986) concluded that age alone was an insufficient predictor of outcomes from aphasia treatment.

Efficacy and Time

The concept of time encompasses the initiation, intensity, and duration of treatment. Shewan (1986) reviewed 22 treatment studies and found that 3 hours of treatment weekly, involving three to five sessions per week lasting 45 minutes to 1 hour each, and durations of 6–12 months, were fairly typical.

Treatment initiated close to the time of onset of aphasia, generally within 1–3 months, has traditionally been considered optimal (Basso, Capitani, & Vignolo, 1979; Butfield & Zangwill, 1946; Deal & Deal, 1978; Vignolo, 1964). However, some very good evidence (Wertz, Weiss et al., 1986) showed no harm from delaying treatment.

The Naysayers

Many have disputed the value of aphasia treatment. As Benson ("Struggling with," 1969) suggested in a widely circulated article that appeared in *Medical World News*: "The classic aphasia patient comes in on a stretcher and isn't talking. When he leaves, he is walking but not talking" (p. 40). A more salient observation would have been to note whether or not the patient was communicating. Benson's 1969 remarks took on added significance when paired with findings by Taylor (1965) that severely aphasic patients made negligible recovery with communication skills despite intensive treatment efforts. Those two reports by such well-respected professionals in the field had a great impact on the medical rehabilitation community's perception of aphasia treatmnet efficacy during that time.

The most controversial of the negative-proof studies (Lincoln et al., 1984) concluded that speech therapy failed to demonstrate improvement in language beyond that of spontaneous recovery. Among the troubling aspects of the study were loose selection criteria, minimal treatment completed by very few patients, and failure to corroborate aphasia test results with medical data. Wertz, Deal, Holland, Kurtzke, and Weiss (1986) summarized the faults of this research succinctly when they wrote, "The results [of the Lincoln et al. study] indicate that when one does not treat patients who may or may not be aphasic, those patients do not improve" (p. 31). In general, while the negative-proof studies suggest that treatment for aphasia fails to demonstrate effectiveness beyond that to be expected from spontaneous recovery alone, conclusions drawn from those studies may be based on weak or inappropriate research design and questionable interpretations. A positive outcome of such studies may have been increased motivation for greater adherence to accepted scientific methodology; unfortunately, Holland and Wertz (1988) noted the persistence of the belief that therapy for aphasia is of little or no use.

Proof Positive

Greater adherence to natural science methodologies seems to have gone hand-in-glove with increased activity in aphasia treatment efficacy research. Using papers published in the *Clinical Aphasiology Conference Proceedings*, 1972–1988, as a barometer of such activity, Horner and Loverso (1991) confirmed a general trend in the direction of greater numbers of efficacy studies. Those selected for discussion below came from a variety of publications. All were considered pivotal in demonstrating that therapy for aphasia effected positive changes beyond spontaneous recovery alone. The nature of this research was consistent with the quantitative orientation of both group and single-subject designs referred to earlier. Later in the chapter, methodologies of a more qualitative subjective nature will be discussed.

A 1964 article by Vignolo may well have launched the modern era of treatment efficacy studies in aphasia by being the first to compare a control group of untreated cases with a treated group. Vignolo concluded that treatment, or reeducation, was effective if it was begun between 2 and 6 months post-onset and if it continued for longer than 6 months.

In a celebrated 1972 retrospective study, Darley suggested four fundamental design considerations: (1) assuring the presence of aphasia and defining its characteristics; (2) clarifying and accounting for spontaneous recovery, in particular, using a control group; (3) objectively measuring changes in language and related behaviors; and (4) defining the treatment provided by specifying procedures, materials, rationale, length of session, frequency, duration, and qualifications of the therapist.

Some time after Darley outlined these and other specifications, Basso et al. (1979) provided what some consider the most potent evidence up to that time of the efficacy of aphasia treatment. This evidence apparently convinced even Benson (who had characterized persons with aphasia as walking but still not talking by the end of therapy) that aphasia therapy caused improvement distinct from spontaneous recovery. Various post-onset initiation times, intensity, duration, and type of treatment were specified in this controlled study. Findings showed significant differences in improvement that favored treated patients and led the authors to recommend early initiation of treatment on a schedule of at least three individual sessions per week for 6 months or more.

The first Wertz et al. (1981) Veterans Administration (VA) cooperative study has been admired for careful control and rigid selection criteria, although the authors noted the absence of a control group and no specification of the type of aphasia. Significant positive outcomes in language measures were demonstrated for subjects who received group or individual treatment. Improvement occurred beyond a 6-month allowance for spontaneous recovery, indicating that the benefits resulted from treatment. This study was remarkable for its ambition, rigor, and insightful interpretation of results.

Finally, a second VA cooperative effort (Wertz, Weiss et al., 1986) replicated and expanded the tight subject-selection criteria of its predecessor. This time, the researchers included a control group, scrutinized the effects of both place of treatment (clinic or home) and of delaying treatment, identified aphasia type, and gave all subjects individual (as opposed to group) treatment. All groups showed significant improvement, though qualitative markers favored the treated groups. Most notably, the deferred-treatment group eventually caught up with the early-treatment groups.

The VA cooperative efforts probably represent the best-controlled aphasia efficacy studies in the literature. Follow-up data (Aten, Wertz, Simpson, Vogel, & Graner, 1991) on a select group of subjects from the second VA cooperative effort showed minimal change in test performance and maintenance of language improvement for many years after the termination of intensive treatment. The authors suggested that clinical investigators direct future attention towards deciding how much language treatment is sufficient, what to do after formal treatment ends, and when to do it.

Indeed, Davis (1986) had noted earlier that the basic question of whether or not aphasia treatment works was dull in comparison to the dozen or so viable efficacy-related questions that one might ask (such as what is the effect of a particular treatment technique on a specific type of verbal behavior?). Siegel (1987) went so far as to suggest that perhaps the question "Does therapy work?" was an inappropriate one for research.

VIEWPOINTS FROM INDIVIDUALS WITH APHASIA

Holland's (1975) observation made years ago that professionals talk a lot about aphasia but very little about persons with aphasia holds true today. That the voice of the aphasic person is the faintest is not surprising. Some aphasic people literally have no voice. Others are unlikely to squander the energy needed for functional communication on retrospective attempts at describing what worked and why. Not surprisingly, the most readily available accounts are from professional people who recovered well enough from their strokes to record their experiences. More time in these accounts is generally devoted to descriptions of aphasia symptomatology than to judgments of treatment. Many accounts hold a mixed, dim, or sometimes downright hostile view of the effectiveness of the treatment received or of specific speech-language therapists. The best therapists were characterized as projecting professional knowledge and displaying certain personal traits. In addition, many authors described significant language gains occurring well after the traditional 3- or even 6-month period of spontaneous recovery. Another interesting trend was the tendency to self-treat, which occurred in conjunction with descriptions of insight into the nature of the language disturbance.

Several particularly revelatory accounts are highlighted below. Although informative secondary accounts exist by playwrights Kopit ("Wings," 1979) and Yankowitz ("1991 Communication Awards," 1991) as well as by speech-language pathologists (Rolnick & Hoops, 1969; Skelly, 1975; Ulatowska, Haynes, Hildebrand, & Richardson, 1977), the present discussion covers only first-person accounts.

One of the first self-reports (Rose, 1948) of the effectiveness of aphasia treatment appeared in 1948 with a physician's discovery of fluency through singing, which he thought related to memorization. He noticed a substantial increase in speech facility after mastering several pieces of prose using a singing technique.

At least two personal accounts came from servicemen, both of whom acquired aphasia as one of the manifestations of non–combat-related closed head injuries. The first (Hall, 1961) reported relatively unfruitful experiences with speech therapy. It was Hall's impression that he might have benefited from speech therapy after first having undergone psychological counseling to facilitate adjustment postinjury. Information presented by Williams (see Chapter 17) supports this speculation.

In the second account (Sies & Butler, 1963), the greatest benefit from contact with a speech-language professional apparently came in the form of an opportunity to express thoughts, feelings, and perceptions of language function through interviews. The insight gained from that process was that dysphasia was not an isolated entity that existed apart from more intimate realms of the individual relating to feelings and reactions.

The unkindest cuts of all may have come from Buck (1963, 1968), a speech pathologist who acquired aphasia following a stroke in 1957. Buck stated flatly that commercial language drills, machines, and books were of no help to him. He found concentration on word-by-word expression antithetical to fluid communication. He preferred a therapeutic environment that fostered natural expression through greater automaticity and less deliberation. He could not tolerate the insult of elementary-level academics. By way of illustration, he noted that the phrase "build a house" meant nothing to his social survival. Requests for its repetition frequently led instead to outbursts of profanity.

An account by C. Scott Moss (1972), a professor of clinical psychology, deserves considerable attention for its erudite and detailed descriptions of the stroke event, aphasia symptomatology, and experiences with speech therapy and psychotherapy. Moss first enrolled in a course of speech therapy some 3 months after the onset of aphasia. Evaluation confirmed a high level of communicative functioning compared to other persons with aphasia but considerably less facility compared to his estimated prestroke level. Dr. Moss's recounting of his experiences in speech therapy presents a mixed bag of gratitude on the one hand and an opinion of inadequate management on the other. He expressed sympathy for the student clinicians assigned to his case, whom he believed were outclassed by their client in terms of education, vocational status, and experience. He suggested that he probably would have been better served had his language problems indicated the more severe disorders he assumed most therapists were better equipped to handle. He also suggested that therapy would have been more pertinent for him had it led to greater integration and organization of abstract-level verbal material through a series of reading-comprehension items.

Two additional reports are from professional women who focused on aspects of the speech-language pathologist's personality and skill level. In the first of these accounts (Post, 1983), a young speech-language pathologist was locked-in communicatively as a consequence of a stroke from a congenital arterial malformation at the base of her right cerebellum. After almost a year and a half of intensive therapy, she remained devoid of a communication mode, although cognitive skills were well-preserved. Speech spontaneously returned some 3 years later. She eventually told her story from a unique perspective afforded by her professional training and by the apparent absence of comprehension deficits common, at least initially, to many other authors of personal accounts. Post described bad therapy as the use of tasks whose purpose was never explained, which seemed meaningless and juvenile, and which frequently led to her feigning sleep as an avoidance tactic. Good therapy for her included the development of a functional communication system by a therapist who recognized and developed eye opening and closing as her most intact response mode.

Post also enumerated personal characteristics as markers of effective or ineffective clinicians. Patience, caring, empathy, knowledge of the disorder, good preparation, enthusiasm, and a sense of humor were listed as positive traits. Negative factors were failure to recognize the patient as a unique individual, lack of preparation, insufficient knowledge about the disorder, and clinicians "faking their therapy" (p. 25). The author closed with the observation that given her significant recovery and progress 3 years after the stroke and beyond, one should consider as essential long-range treatment goals.

Wender (1990), a professor of classics, made similar observations about the importance of the person behind the therapy in her perspective on treatment for the aphasia she acquired from a hemorrhagic stroke. With engaging good humor, she contrasted her experiences of bad therapy from a bad therapist with good therapy from a good therapist. She noted that her good therapist did not spend great amounts of time in testing, which had led her initially to feel stupid and to wonder if therapy was worth the investment. The good therapist addressed her as an intelligent adult, talked to her children about the condition, and planned therapeutic procedures based upon her areas of interest. She praised her good therapist's use of gentle correction and specific feedback. She recalled also how he lifted her out of silence and depression through a sincere request for information about the Greek gods, her area of specialty. In retrospect, she surmised that her good therapist taught her to teach herself. Some 2 years after the stroke, she realized that her own poststroke relearning resembled the multifaceted approach she used for helping her own students learn new words.

In what is probably the most lyrically written self-account of aphasia, Wulf (1973) devoted considerable space to discussions of speech therapy. The tone of those discussions is best exemplified by the title of Chapter 5, "My Life-Line To Sanity," and its subtitle, "The Marvels of Speech Therapy." Wulf found positive results from talking, reading, writing, figuring math problems, and participating in activities such as in-service training sessions. She cited as beneficial constant verbal practice, although at times she characterized her talking practice as correcting one error after another. She found her therapist's calm approach and a willingness to listen particularly gratifying.

First-person accounts of individuals with aphasia yield several instructive observations on the effectiveness of therapy. The most important criterion for therapeutic success might seem to be the personality of the aphasia clinician, at least at first glance. However, closer inspection reveals that authors couch their admiration of personal traits in terms that account for the clinician's projection of professional knowledge. In other words, a good personality alone is not enough to yield a judgment of good therapist. Juvenile and irrelevant materials are frequently criticized, while approaches that used personal and vocational interests are applauded. Initiating active participation in treatment later in the recovery process and for a longer time than has been customary are concepts advocated by many. Repetitive linguistically based, drill-like methods are appreciated by some and abhorred by others. Authors frequently mention the need to be treated from the very early stages on as a whole person, rather than as a language disorder, and to be included in decision making even when expression is severely limited. They also highlight the importance of the family, whose viewpoints are explored in the next section.

VIEWPOINTS FROM FAMILY MEMBERS

There is unanimous agreement about the importance of the family in dealing with aphasia. Indeed, Buck (1968) has characterized stroke as a family illness. In an early study, Turnblom and Myers (1952) set the stage for future investigations into the identification and management of the needs and role of family members in dealing with stroke and aphasia. Findings from their interviews led to conclusions about the need for speech pathologists to provide counseling programs for family members and to recognize the importance of the family in creating an atmosphere and promoting motivation for rehabilitation.

The voice of the family, both nuclear and extended, has been heard most commonly through questionnaires and interviews with spouses and, to a lesser degree, children of individuals who have become aphasic (Chwat, Chapey, Gurland, & Pieras, 1980). As is true with the voice of the individual with aphasia, the relationship of such information to issues surrounding treatment efficacy may not always be direct, but the insights gained are no less valuable.

Opinions, Roles, and Ratings

Group therapy has been applauded loudly by at least one author (Knox, 1971), who wrote a moving account of his wife's strokes. Reducing isolation and fear, providing healthy competition, and satisfying needs for socialization with and praise and understanding from peers were among the benefits he associated with the group experience. He even wondered if earlier exposure to group therapy might have made a crucial and positive difference in the course of his wife's recovery.

Spouses have been trained (Newhoff, Bugbee, & Ferreira, 1981) in specific techniques, such as "promoting aphasics' communicative effectiveness" (PACE) (Davis, 1980). Use of this approach, which primarily emphasizes the nonverbal domain, has been found to effect changes in verbal interactions.

Spousal perceptions about communication before and after the onset of aphasia in their partners have been elicited through methods such as the "critical incident technique" (Webster, Dans, & Saunders, 1982). Descriptive data about communicative interactions organized around specific events (critical incidents) reveal that patterns of interaction remained relatively unchanged after the onset of aphasia and suggest that such information might be helpful in directing intervention procedures. Obtaining this type of descriptive data is promoted later in the section on ethnography.

Similarly, ratings by spouses of communication near and during the time of treatment have been gathered (Helmick, Watamori, & Palmer, 1976) through instruments such as the Functional Communication Profile (FCP) (Taylor, 1965). Findings showed that FCP ratings by spouses suggested less impairment than those of ratings by speech pathologists. The authors concluded that spouses' impressions of communicative functioning in their aphasic partners were unrealistically inflated. However, they failed to recommend further investigation into the disparity between professional and spousal ratings, or to suggest that the judgments of the spouses might be truer representations of actual communication than were those of the speech pathologists. In a letter questioning the interpretations of the findings from this study, Holland (1977) voted for the spouses.

Indeed, a study by Furbacher and Wertz (1983) served to corroborate the accuracy of spousal perceptions. Wives of husbands with aphasia who were asked to simulate their spouse's communication deficits while responding to the test items on the Porch Index of Communicative Ability (PICA) did so well enough to generate test profiles consistent with aphasia.

Other authors have confirmed that ratings of aphasia made by family members typically indicate higher communicative functioning than ratings determined by speech-language pathologists. One wife suggested that she understood her husband with greater ease than others because she was better able to understand his inflections and gestures (Alice, pp. 34–35, in Ewing & Pfalzgraf, 1990). Likewise, Linebaugh and Young-Charles (1981) recommended that speech-language clinicians elicit from family members examples of communication successes and failures of their relatives with aphasia, and that clinical ratings be tempered with those of family members.

In addition to spouses, significant others may be useful in planning and then assessing the efficacy of treatment. In a study by Florance (1979), benefits of this involvement included the identification of focal points of interaction and the discovery of productive strategies, such as interview tactics, to promote "effective circumlocution."

Counseling Needs

The scope of a speech-language pathologist's practice is further broadened when the educational and emotional counseling needs of family members are considered. How well those needs are addressed is a vital consideration in assessing the efficacy of aphasia treatment. The line between emotional and educational counseling needs is often blurred and sometimes contradictory. Those needs often arise directly from family members' uncertain or mixed feelings, beliefs, and attitudes about aphasia.

Guilt is a typical feeling expressed by family members of relatives with aphasia. For example, a family member may feel guilty about resenting the illness and the attention it demands (Cathy, p. 61, in Ewing & Pfalzgraf, 1990).

Investigations of feelings quite naturally lead to adaptations of techniques from the field of psychology. For example, Q-sort methodology (Zraick & Boone, 1991) and transactional analysis (Porter & Dabul, 1977) have been borrowed from that field to help rank perceptions of characteristics of the spouse with aphasia, and to identify recurring themes and nonproductive mind games used by partners of aphasic spouses. Revelations of negative attitudes and of guilt from cards containing descriptive adjectives (multiple Q-sorting) might be applied to improve therapeutic intervention by clarifying attitudes and exploring options for change. Adapted transactional analysis is thought to have helped wives appreciate a spouse with aphasia as he is rather than as he is believed to be.

Feelings that arise from dealing with the consequences of stroke and aphasia are related to attitudes and beliefs, which in turn signal the need to provide or to clarify information. For example, deficits in auditory comprehension are particularly vulnerable to misunderstanding and are perceived to be especially difficult to manage. In one study (Czvik, 1977), some family members likened auditory processing disorders to mental retardation.

That belief failed to change even after auditory deficits and procedures for their remediation were presented in a demonstration session. Better acceptance of that aspect of aphasia was called for as a way to maximize treatment results and to promote understanding of failure to regain speech through treatment.

Families often call for additional information about stroke and aphasia, and professionals likewise believe that distributing more of such information could only be better. Linebaugh and Young-Charles (1978) found that 50% or more of their respondents had been provided with reading materials on stroke and aphasia. However, many spouses found such materials inadequate and pointed to a need for additional reading. Discussion of prognostications, even unfavorable ones, stood out almost unanimously as one point of information that should be shared.

Other family members find little value in receiving more information. Newhoff and Davis (1978) cite a report that spouses of aphasic persons declared information about terminology and causes of stroke of little importance since an understanding of facts failed to alter the course of recovery. Along those same lines, the mother of a stroke patient recalled her reluctance to obtain additional information during the course of her son's therapy for fear of discovering how bad the situation might really be (Tom's mother, p. 61, in Ewing & Pfalzgraf, 1990). In summary, investigating how the offerings of both professionals and family members might promote effective treatment for aphasia is more productive than debating whose perceptions are correct. Lack of agreement about the amount and type of counseling that is appropriate cannot obscure the importance of families to the process of treatment for aphasia and to the evaluation of the efficacy of that treatment.

AN ETHNOGRAPHIC APPROACH: A NATURAL SETTING, AN ACTIVE VOICE

A great deal of information exists on the efficacy of treatment for aphasia, particularly in the form of quantitative data from group studies. The research methodologies used in those studies were derived largely from the physical sciences. Voices of individuals with aphasia have been only weakly integrated into that data. Qualitative research through an ethnographic approach may help strengthen those voices by focusing more directly on the recipient of our therapeutic efforts in his or her day-to-day home environment. Darley (1991) seems to have spoken to that very sentiment when he reminded us that aphasia is not a thing but an individual who must be defined within the context of many personal relationships.

Others writing in the field of communication disorders have also called for the inclusion of information that may be considered more subjective in nature. Such a stand was made by an impressive group of researchers cited by Kovarsky and Crago in their paper on the ethnography of communication (1991). The contradictions inherent in practices that abstract language from its context and in models of inquiry that quantify language without regard to real-world usage were among the significant observations made. Abkarian (1977) wrote a lengthy piece in the *Journal of Speech and Hearing Disorders* that addressed the importance of "romantic" factors thought by some to contaminate pure scientific inquiry. Further, Thompson and Kearns (1991) suggested to a gathering of clinical aphasiologists that use of controlled experimental studies does not necessarily represent better science. They exhorted researchers to devote increased efforts towards validating laboratory procedures ecologically.

Practicing clinicians would be well served by joining Beukelman (cited in Holland & Wertz, 1988) in defining disability in relation to an individual's participation in normal societal roles. The fulfillment of those roles comes about within a natural environment and through personal contacts. Contextual setting and interpersonal relationships should be accounted for if we are to appreciate more fully the nature of aphasia and if we are to develop meaningful treatments for its remediation. An ethnographic approach may provide the canvas for this larger landscape.

A Definition

Ethnography is "the process of documenting and interpreting human action and social life in writing (-graphy) in its cultural context (ethno-)" (Kovarsky & Crago, 1991, p. 12). The approach, identified more than a century ago by Hoffman (cited in Maxwell, 1990), encompasses qualitative research and field observation and is associated most closely with anthropology. An ethnographic approach may help our field address the relationship between functionality and therapy, because it illuminates "how people interpret behavior within the real-world contexts of their daily lives" (Kovarsky & Crago, 1991, p. 27).

Precedents and New Directions

Use of terminology and specific approaches of an ethnographic nature are relatively new in our field. Inquiries into child language and its disorders currently represent the most direct application of ethnographic principles. However, an ethnographic perspective has also been documented in the form of opinions expressed by prominent aphasiologists and in the development of various assessment and treatment procedures for aphasia.

Real People, Real Settings

Wepman (1951, 1972) advocated that professionals actively consider those who are significant others in the life of the individual with aphasia. That

sage advice ran against the prevailing practice of treating persons with aphasia in the sterile environment created by therapist-patient, stimulus-
response boundaries. He reminded us that a patient with aphasia is not
merely a person with impaired communication, but a living, changing
organism who requires an appropriate climate for growth. Similarly, Helm-
Estabrooks (1983) said that, "aphasia rehabilitation should take place wher-
ever the aphasic individual finds himself" (p. 236). Practicing clinicians
may find that matters of cost effectiveness and practicality work against following that advice if it means moving treatment to off-site locations.
However, the growth in home health delivery systems holds promise for an
increased pairing of cost-effective service and a natural setting. In addition,
"communication partners," who are community volunteers, might be
recruited as liaisons in facilitating functional communication in real-life situations, as suggested by Lyon (1992) (see Chapter 8).

Simulations

A number of creative attempts have also been made to simulate natural
environments and contexts while retaining the convenience and efficiency
of clinic-based treatment. Simmons (1989) suggested applying a marketing
and fund-raising tool called "Easy Street Environments." She provided
examples of communication attempts that failed in traditional treatment
paradigms but succeeded in a familiar setting afforded by the replica of a
typical community environment.

Commercially produced simulated environments are likely to be luxu-
ries beyond the means of most clinics and rehabilitation centers. However,
readily available materials and procedures have been used to promote naturalistic simulations in the clinic setting. Aten, Caligiuri, and Holland
(1982) promoted functionality through group therapy focused on everyday
interactions made realistic by role-playing materials such as menus, calen-
dars, and grocery items. Communication Abilities in Daily Living (CADL)
(Holland, 1980) test scores revealed significant gains both immediately
after treatment stopped and 6 weeks later. Another approach that simulates
the give-and-take of natural communication within the convenience of the
clinic is PACE, developed by Davis and Wilcox (Davis, 1980) and mentioned earlier as part of a study that involved training spouses. The give-
and-take of message transmission and receipt is facilitated by the use of
stimulus materials—for example, pictured actions. Positive reinforcement
comes about as the natural consequence of successful message transmission. In this way, modeling and reinforcement evolve within the natural
context of communication.

Thompson and Byrne (1984) made yet another attempt at structuring the
training environment to approximate more closely a natural setting. This
method, an application of an approach termed "loose training," allows for
variations in responses, stimuli, and feedback. Thompson and Byrne's adap-

tation involved helping persons with aphasia learn specific social conventions in a progression from imitation to more naturalistic role-playing. Findings suggested that a loose training approach was effective in facilitating generalized use of social conventions.

Client Centering

An additional loose training procedure was developed in part from principles of incidental teaching used in child language intervention. Response elaboration training (RET) was designed by Kearns (1985) to encourage self-initiated rather than clinician-selected responses in patients with aphasia. The clinician fosters responses through modeling and reinforcement based on any patient utterance relevant to the given stimulus item of a photo or line drawing depicting actions. An initial single-word verbing response might result in an elaboration through expansion, modeling, reinforcing, and cuing. For example, the clinician instructs and presents a stimulus, and the patient offers the word "crying." Through positive verbal reinforcement, Wh cuing, and modeling, the elaborations, "hit head," and ultimately, "hit head . . . crying," emerge. Holland (1980) suggests that good treatment is typified by more responses, in general, and refinement of responses, in particular. RET demonstrated positive effects by encouraging elaboration on responses, by increasing the number of content words used, and by fostering moderate degrees of generalization.

Assessment

Generalization, or carry-over, is a measure of the extent to which useful improvement in language function carries over beyond the clinical setting to the environment where change is needed most (Davis, 1983). Thus, generalization is tied to functional assessment of outcome. In a review of generalization research in aphasia, Thompson (1989) noted that conditions for measuring generalization, generalization criteria, and the frequency of measurement vary across studies. Further, only three of the 35 studies Thompson reviewed measured generalization to the natural environment.

Holland (1982) warned that no test reveals the aphasic person's real capabilities in actual everyday communication. Poor performance on tests does not necessarily mean lack of improvement. For example, results of the Aten et al. study (1982) showed that the more functional assessment afforded by CADL testing yielded significant gains not observed through PICA testing for patients with chronic aphasia who had received group functional therapy. Similarly, less tangible benefits of treatment, such as improved confidence, deserve inclusion in outcome assessment, which has traditionally focused on linguistic performance (Green, 1984).

The value of ethnography in assessing a person at the onset of treatment for aphasia becomes clear when one realizes the flaws in traditional assessment techniques. Many years ago, Martin (1974) questioned the use of those test scores that issue primarily from an interrogative format. Similarly, Holland (1975) noted that procedures that essentially command someone to talk are probably among the least productive ways to gather samples of language. Green (1984) suggested filling the gap left by traditional aphasia testing with general observation schedules, spontaneous speech samples, and behavioral checklists afforded within a naturalistic communication therapy model.

Given the constraints of traditional methods, a number of appraisal methodologies speak to an ethnographic model. Three such methodologies are phonologic analysis, pragmatic analysis, and discourse analysis. For example, one area of controversy is the distinction between articulatory errors in aphasia and those that are related to apraxia of speech. Rosenbek et al. (1989) have summarized research that suggests that phonological process analysis may serve to differentiate between language and motor speech disorders.

In that same publication, those authors also summarized work on pragmatic analysis (analysis of the use of language in context). For example, applications of the communication profile and of the pragmatic protocol provide windows into interactions with a variety of communication partners and into the verbal, paralinguistic, and nonverbal aspects of language. Pragmatic sampling may yield important information not revealed by more traditional measures of aphasia. The richness of pragmatic information that can be obtained by using an ethnographic approach is also highlighted by Simmons (1993). Simmons' research, which represents the first comprehensive ethnographic study of aphasia, provides a more accurate and complete description of the use of compensatory strategies and message transmission by aphasics than has to date been reported.

With regard to discourse analysis, Rosenbek et al. (1989) applauded the inclusion of this aspect of appraisal, which is not readily available through other measures. Such analysis may permit an assessment of the effect of context and may be applied to writing and gesturing, as well as to speaking. Two of the four types of discourse enumerated seem most pertinent to the present discussion. Narrative discourse (describing, retelling) has been widely used in aphasia research, and conversational discourse is particularly well suited for emphasizing pragmatic considerations and natural context.

Rao (1990) suggested that the components of a modern functional assessment should include (1) information from patients and significant others, gathered in a pre-interview questionnaire; (2) an interview and case history, complete with recordings of observations within and outside the clinic setting; and (3) attitudinal scales.

Models from Child Language

Findings from even the very best and most inclusive assessment procedures ring hollow in the absence of normative data. Holland (1990) noted that examples of such data were far more prominent in child-, as compared to geriatric-language research endeavors. Indeed, Green (1984) has said that studies both of language development and of disorders in children were among the main sources from which the aphasia clinician of that time had to extrapolate relevant information.

Similarly, qualitatively based treatment approaches and inquiries into normal and disordered childhood communication may indeed have pre-dated those in the area of adult communication. The prominence of this lag in aphasia treatment research may relate to the tenacity of a symptom-oriented and cure-focused medical model (Holland, 1975; Holland & Wertz, 1988; Kearns & Thompson, 1991) despite a decades-old interest in language pragmatics with regard to adult communication disorders. Some examples that do exist in the adult aphasia literature—for instance, the loose training and incidental teaching procedures described earlier—have been borrowed from child-language intervention.

That ethnography as a specifically identified approach has been more apparent in inquiries of child rather than adult language is exemplified by the fact that an entire issue (Damico, Maxwell, & Kovarsky, 1990) of the *Journal of Childhood Communication Disorders* (*JCCD*) was devoted to that topic.

Some aphasia efficacy studies that fit the ethnographic spirit call for the inclusion of information obtained through observation and accounts of find-ings from multiple sources, but most still tend to use preset categories and close-ended questions. The ethnographically focused issue of *JCCD* was filled with attempts by researchers to develop themes or trends (categories) based on analysis of various stages of field observation, rather than on enter-ing the study with those themes predetermined. In addition, interview for-mats were geared toward helping respondents paint pictures of events and interactions, rather than on making decisions based on forced choices. Pleas have been made to include observation of communicative interactions in context and with a variety of partners, as well as to include measures that permit descriptions of greater variety and depth in both initial and treat-ment-outcome appraisals of individuals with aphasia.

Deeper Description

While many authors have called for greater use of observation, few studies incorporate observational methodologies. The statement that there are "lit-erally no data on aphasics as communicators in their natural environment" (Holland, 1975, p. 152) has remained relatively constant over the past two decades. Of 54 efficacy studies, Davis (1986) found only four instances of explicit observation of natural communication. Holland (1982), once again addressing the topic, remarked on the systematic use of field observation by social and behavioral scientists, in particular, during investigations related to language acquisition. However, she noted that such observation is used far less in the study of language problems and even less in the study of disordered language and communication use in natural settings. Such informa-tion typically comes instead from the manipulation of experimental condi-tions, formalized testing, treatment, personal written accounts, and discus-sions with patients and families. She wisely offered an opinion that no test can match the potential richness afforded by observation, which she charac-terized as a qualitative means of getting to know the aphasic person better. Holland believes that such knowledge has the potential for increasing immeasurably the clinician's effectiveness. She went on to suggest guide-lines for observing persons with aphasia in their natural environments.

However, the conduct of field observation presents a constant challenge within the ethnographic mode of inquiry. Davis (1978) no doubt represents the ongoing sentiments of many when he expresses concern about the con-founding factor that the very act of observation may pose.

The nature of an ethnographer's description of a person with aphasia stems in part from field observations. However, as Patton (1980) points out, no one can observe feelings, thoughts, intentions, prior behaviors, or situations. In short, we cannot observe everything. A need to gather information from multi-ple sources, a process called *triangulation*, is as central to the ethnographer's qualitative methodologies as reliability and validity are to quantitative approaches (Kovarsky, 1989). More specifically, observing, interviewing, and gathering data from sources such as artifacts (e.g., diaries, objects) represents a desirable three-pronged approach. The point was made previously that research on the efficacy of aphasia treatment has been relatively longer on procedures such as interviews and questionnaires and shorter on direct field observation.

Data sources for triangulation from the aphasia literature include ques-tionnaires such as those mentioned earlier, or as in the questionnaire devel-oped by Swindell, Pashek, and Holland (1982) as a tool in helping to deter-mine prognosis for recovery from aphasia. It is important to remember that the ratings of other people may not be representative of the self-perceptions of our clients with aphasia. Once again, what remains elusive is the "native's" point of view, that point of view that ethnography hopes to capture (Spradley, 1979, 1980).

People with aphasia who live in institutionalized settings present an even greater challenge. Their situation illustrates dramatically the need for nontradi-tional and numerous avenues of information gathering during assessment, inter-vention, and evaluation of treatment efficacy. Consideration of factors such as multihandicaps (Lubinski, 1988) and the effects of an unfamiliar environment (Rao, 1990) are essential for fair and meaningful initial and outcome assess-ments of communication for older adults in extended-care settings. While repeated discussions and observations of interactions with staff fit nicely into an ethnographic approach, such time-consuming tactics fly in the face of many funding-source regulations. Modifications in such settings might include using questions that focus on broad aspects of communication problems, profiling the motivational status of both the residents and their primary communication part-ners, and determining environmental opportunities and barriers.

The concept of *thick description* represents another basic principle of ethnography applicable to the study of aphasia treatment efficacy. Throughout the process of collecting and analyzing multisourced data, description is built progressively. Geertz in 1973 (cited in Kovarsky & Crago, 1991) used the term *thick description* to include richness of detail, meaning, and interpretation. Thick descriptions are constructed by adding layered interpretations of behavior to the thin descriptions represented by the mere recording of behavioral responses. In his seminal 1972 challenge to the profession regarding language rehabilitation in aphasia, Darley implored researchers to recognize the complexity of the issues involved in designing studies and selecting subjects such that "a richness of description" (p. 20) might be introduced into future inquiries into issues of efficacy. Thompson and Kearns (1991) suggest that what is needed now is really no different than what was needed before—that is, deeper investigation of underpinnings and an accumulation of layers of information about the types and amount of treatment needed. The pot of gold represented by Darley's plea for such description is still beyond our reach. However, trends in efficacy research are promising indicators of change, which may constitute "the Midas touch" (p. 52) alluded to by Thompson and Kearns (1991).

FUTURE TRENDS

Mention was made earlier in this chapter of Siegel's concern that the question, "Does therapy work?" may be inappropriate for research (1987). Wertz (1993) replies to that concern with a resounding "yes" and goes on to cite Kent, who believes that additional crucial answers to that ongoing question will come from clinicians.

Greater inclusion of clinicians in the treatment efficacy research enterprise is a future trend launched in part by a model research mentoring process (Wofford, Boysen, & Riding, 1991).

In addition, the collection of normative adult language data (e.g., Wambaugh, Thompson, Doyle, & Camarata, 1991) is a move towards adding that richer, thicker layer of support to the treatment efficacy endeavor.

Finally, we might consider along with Darley (1991) the formation of bonds with pharmacologists, neurologists, and psychologists. Renewed interest in the use of pharmacologic agents (e.g., Mimura, Albert, & McNamara, 1995; Helm-Estabrooks & Albert, 1991; McLennan, Nicholas, Morley, & Brookshire, 1991; Walker-Batson, Devous, Curtis, Unwin, & Greenlee, 1991) and of procedures such as hypnosis and memory training further expands the boundaries of efficacious treatment for aphasia.

CONCLUSION

The 1970s spawned significant efforts in aphasia efficacy research, a topic that has interested clinicians since before speech-language pathology was a recognized discipline. At the same time, the use of single-case experimental designs facilitated greater clinical applications. Yet the body of evidence demonstrating that therapy for aphasia works still leaves many questions unanswered. Richness of description, a phrase that relates to a goal of the ethnographic model, is still needed in efficacy literature. Qualitative methodologies such as those associated with ethnography provide potential for building a deeper and more authentic core of efficacy data.

REFERENCES

Abkarian, G.G. (1977). The changing face of our discipline: Isn't it "romantic"? *Journal of Speech and Hearing Disorders, 42*, 422–435.

Aten, J.L., Caligiuri, M.P., & Holland, A.L. (1982). The efficacy of functional communication therapy for chronic aphasic patients. *Journal of Speech and Hearing Disorders, 47*, 93–96.

Aten, J., Wertz, R.T., Simpson, M., Vogel, D., & Graner, D. (1991). A long-term follow-up of aphasic patients after intensive treatment. In T.E. Prescott (Ed.), *Clinical aphasiology* (Vol. 20, pp. 299-306). Austin, TX: PRO-ED.

Basso, A., Capitani, E., & Vignolo, L. (1979). Influence of rehabilitation of language skills in aphasic patients: A controlled study. *Archives of Neurology, 36*, 190–196.

Brookshire, R.H. (1985). Clinical research in aphasiology. In R.H. Brookshire (Ed.), *Proceedings of the Conference on Clinical Aphasiology* (pp. 9–14). Minneapolis: BRK Publishers.

Buck, M. (1963). The language disorders. *Journal of Rehabilitation, 24*, 37–38.

Buck, M. (1968). *Dysphasia: Professional guidance for family and patient.* Englewood Cliffs, NJ: Prentice-Hall.

Butfield, E., & Zangwill, O. (1946). Re-education in aphasia: A review of 70 cases. *Journal of Neurology, Neurosurgery, and Psychiatry, 9*, 75–79.

Chwat, S., Chapey, R., Gurland, G., & Pieras, G. (1980). Environmental impact of aphasia: The child's perspective. In R.H. Brookshire (Ed.), *Proceedings of the Conference on Clinical Aphasiology* (pp. 127–138). Minneapolis: BRK Publishers.

Czvik, P.S. (1977). Assessment of family attitudes toward aphasic patients with severe auditory processing disorders. In R.H. Brookshire (Ed.), *Proceedings of the Conference on Clinical Aphasiology* (pp. 160–165). Minneapolis: BRK Publishers.

Damico, J.S., Maxwell, M.M., & Kovarsky, D. (Eds.), (1990). Ethnographic inquiries into communication sciences and disorders [Special issue]. *Journal of Childhood Communication Disorders, 13* (1).

Darley, F.L. (1972). The efficacy of language rehabilitation in aphasia. *Journal of Speech and Hearing Disorders, 37*, 3–21.

Darley, F.L. (1991). I think it begins with an "A." In T.E. Prescott (Ed.), *Clinical aphasiology* (Vol. 20, pp. 9-20). Austin, TX: PRO-ED.

Davis, G.A. (1978). Discussion: "Our data, not our word." In R.H. Brookshire (Ed.), *Proceedings of the Conference on Clinical Aphasiology* (pp. 37–39). Minneapolis: BRK Publishers.

Davis, G.A. (1980). A critical look at PACE therapy. In R.H. Brookshire (Ed.),

Proceedings of the Conference on Clinical Aphasiology (pp. 248–257). Minneapolis: BRK Publishers.

Davis, G.A. (1983). *A survey of adult aphasia.* Englewood Cliffs, NJ: Prentice-Hall.

Davis, G.A. (1986). Questions of efficacy in clinical aphasiology. In R.H. Brookshire (Ed.), *Clinical aphasiology* (Vol. 16, pp. 154–162). Minneapolis: BRK Publishers.

Deal, J.L., & Deal, L.A. (1978). Efficacy of aphasia rehabilitation: Preliminary results. In R.H. Brookshire (Ed.), *Proceedings of the Conference on Clinical Aphasiology* (pp. 66–77). Minneapolis: BRK Publishers.

Eisenson, J. (1949). Prognostic factors relating to language rehabilitation in aphasic patients. *Journal of Speech and Hearing Disorders, 14,* 262–264.

Ewing, S.A., & Pfalzgraf, B. (1990). *Pathways: Moving beyond stroke and aphasia.* Detroit: Wayne State University Press.

Florance, C.L. (1979). The aphasic's significant other: Training and counseling, a round table discussion. In R.H. Brookshire (Ed.), *Proceedings of the Conference on Clinical Aphasiology* (pp. 295–299). Minneapolis: BRK Publishers.

Furbacher, E.A., & Wertz, R.T. (1983). Simulation of aphasia by wives of aphasic patients. In R.H. Brookshire (Ed.), *Proceedings of the Conference on Clinical Aphasiology* (pp. 227–232). Minneapolis: BRK Publishers.

Green, G. (1984). Communication in aphasia therapy: Some of the procedures and issues involved. *British Journal of Disorders of Communication, 19,* 35–46.

Hall, W.A. (1961). Return from silence: A personal experience. *Journal of Speech and Hearing Disorders, 26,* 174–176.

Helm-Estabrooks, N. (1983). Language intervention for adults: Environmental considerations. In J. Miller, R. Schiefelbusch, & D. Yoder (Eds.), *Contemporary issues in language intervention* (ASHA Reports 12, pp. 229–238). Rockville, MD: American Speech-Language-Hearing Association.

Helm-Estabrooks, N., & Albert M.L. (1991). Pharmacotherapy for aphasia. In N. Helm-Estabrooks & M.L. Albert (Eds.), *Manual of aphasia therapy* (pp. 245–249). Austin, TX: PRO-ED.

Helmick, J.W., Watamori, T.S., & Palmer, J.M. (1976). Spouses' understanding of the communication disabilities of aphasic patients. *Journal of Speech and Hearing Disorders, 41,* 238–243.

Holland, A.L. (1975). The effectiveness of treatment in aphasia. In R.H. Brookshire (Ed.), *Clinical aphasiology (Collected Proceedings, 1972–1976,* pp. 145–156). Minneapolis: BRK Publishers. (1978).

Holland, A.L. (1977). Comment on "Spouses' understanding of the communication disabilities of aphasic patients." *Journal of Speech and Hearing Disorders, 42,* 307–308.

Holland, A.L. (1980). The usefulness of treatment for aphasia: A serendipitous study. In R.H. Brookshire (Ed.), *Proceedings of the Conference on Clinical Aphasiology* (pp. 240–247). Minneapolis: BRK Publishers.

Holland, A.L. (1982). Observing functional communication of aphasic adults. *Journal of Speech and Hearing Disorders, 47,* 50–56.

Holland, A.L. (1990). Research methodology: I. Implications for speech-language pathology. In E. Cherow (Ed.), *Proceedings of the Research Symposium on Communication Sciences and Disorders and Aging* (ASHA Reports 19, pp. 35–39). Rockville, MD: American Speech-Language-Hearing Association.

Holland, A.L., & Wertz, R.T. (1988). Measuring aphasia treatment effects: Large-group, small-group, and single-subject studies. In F. Plum (Ed.), *Language, communication, and the brain* (pp. 276–273). New York: Raven Press.

Horner, J., & Loverso, F.L. (1991). Models of aphasia treatment in Clinical Aphasiology, 1972-1988. In T.E. Prescott (Ed.), *Clinical aphasiology* (Vol. 20, pp. 61–75). Austin, TX: PRO-ED.

Ingham, R.J. (1990). Theoretical, methodological, and ethical issues in treatment efficacy research: Stuttering therapy as a case study. In L. Olswang, C.Thompson, S. Warren, & N. Minghetti (Eds.), *Treatment efficacy research in communication disorders* (pp. 15–29). Rockville, MD: American Speech-Language-Hearing Foundation.

Kearns, K.P. (1985). Response elaboration training for patient initiated utterances. In R.H. Brookshire (Ed.), *Proceedings of the Conference on Clinical Aphasiology* (pp. 196–204). Minneapolis: BRK Publishers.

Kearns, K.P., & Thompson, C.K. (1991). Technical drift and conceptual myopia: The Merlin effect. In T.E. Prescott (Ed.), *Clinical aphasiology* (Vol. 19, pp. 31–40). Austin, TX: PRO-ED.

Knox, D. (1971). *Portrait of aphasia.* Detroit: Wayne State University Press.

Kovarsky, D. (1989). The contribution of ethnography to assessment, intervention and research methods in speech-language pathology. *The Journal of the Kansas Speech-Language-Hearing Association, 29,* 17–24.

Kovarsky, D., & Crago, M. (1991). Toward the ethnography of communication disorders. *NSSLHA Journal, 18,* 44–55.

Linebaugh, C.W., & Young-Charles, H.Y. (1978). The counseling needs of the families of aphasic patients. In R.H. Brookshire (Ed.), *Proceedings of the Conference on Clinical Aphasiology* (pp. 304–313). Minneapolis: BRK Publishers.

Linebaugh, C.W., & Young-Charles, H.Y. (1981). Confidence in ratings of aphasic patients' functional communication: Spouses and speech-language pathologists. In R.H. Brookshire (Ed.), *Proceedings of the Conference on Clinical Aphasiology* (pp. 226–233). Minneapolis: BRK Publishers.

Lincoln, N.B., McGuik, E., Mulley, G.P., Lendrem, W., Jones, A.C., & Mitchell, J.R.A. (1984). Effectiveness of speech therapy for aphasic stroke patients: A randomized controlled trial. *Lancet, 1,* 1197–1200.

Lubinski, R. (1988). A model for intervention: Communication skills, effectiveness, and opportunity. In B. Shadden (Ed.), *Communication behavior and aging: A sourcebook for clinicians* (pp. 294–308). Baltimore: Williams & Wilkins.

Lyon, J.G. (1992). Communication use and participation in life for adults with aphasia in natural settings: The scope of the problem. *American Journal of Speech-Language Pathology, 1,* 7–14.

Martin, A.D. (1974). A proposed rationale for aphasia therapy. In R.H. Brookshire (Ed.), *Collected Proceedings, 1972–1976, of the Conference on Clinical Aphasiology* (pp. 60–70). Minneapolis: BRK Publishers (1978).

Maxwell, M.M. (1990). The authenticity of ethnographic research. *Journal of Childhood Communication Disorders, 13,* 1–12.

McLennan, D.L., Nicholas, L.E., Morley, G.K., & Brookshire, R.H. (1991). The effects of bromocriptine on speech and language function in a man with transcortical motor aphasia. In T.E. Prescott (Ed.), *Clinical aphasiology* (Vol. 20, pp. 145–156). Austin, TX: PRO-ED.

McReynolds, L.V. (1990). Historical perspective of treatment efficacy research. In L. Olswang, C. Thompson, S. Warren, & N. Minghetti (Eds.), *Treatment efficacy research in communication disorders* (pp. 5–14). Rockville, MD: American Speech-Language-Hearing Foundation.

Mimura, M., Albert, M.L., & McNamara, P. (1995). Toward a pharmacotherapy for aphasia. In H.S. Kirschner (Ed.), *Handbook of neurological speech and language disorders* (pp. 465–482). New York: Marcel Dekker.

Moss, C.S. (1972). *Recovery with aphasia: The aftermath of my stroke.* Urbana, IL: University of Illinois Press.

Newhoff, M., Bugbee, J.K., & Ferreira, A. (1981). A change of PACE: Spouses as treatment targets In R.H. Brookshire (Ed.), *Proceedings of the Conference on Clinical Aphasiology* (pp. 234–235) Minneapolis: BRK Publishers.

Newhoff, M., & Davis, G.A. (1978) A spouse intervention program: Planning, implementation, and problems of evaluation. In R.H. Brookshire (Ed.), *Proceedings of the Conference on Clinical Aphasiology* (pp. 318–326). Minneapolis: BRK Publishers.

1991 Communication Awards. (1991, August). *ASHA, 33*, 34–37.

Patton, M.Q. (1980). *Qualitative evaluation methods.* Beverly Hills, CA: Sage.

Porter, J., & Dabul, B. (1977). The application of transactional analysis to therapy with wives of adult aphasic patients. *ASHA, 19*, 244–248.

Post, J.G., with Leith, W.R. (1983, April). I'd rather tell a story than be one. *ASHA, 25*, 23–26.

Rao, P. (1990). Functional communication assessment of the elderly. In E. Cherow (Ed.), *Proceedings of the Research Symposium on Communication Sciences and Disorders and Aging* (ASHA Reports 19, pp. 28–34). Rockville, MD: American Speech-Language-Hearing Association.

Rolnick, M., & Hoops, H.R. (1969). Aphasia as seen by the aphasic. *Journal of Speech and Hearing Disorders, 34*, 48–53.

Rose, R.H. (1948). A physician's account of his own aphasia. *Journal of Speech and Hearing Disorders, 13*, 294–305.

Rosenbek, J.C., LaPointe, L.L., & Wertz, R.T. (1989). Aphasia treatment: Its efficacy. In *Aphasia: A clinical approach* (pp. 104–130). Boston: Little, Brown.

Shewan, C.M. (1986). The history and efficacy of aphasia treatment. In R. Chapey (Ed.), *Intervention strategies in adult aphasia* (2nd ed., pp. 28–43). Baltimore: Williams & Wilkins.

Siegel, G.M. (1987). The limits of science in communication disorders. *Journal of Speech and Hearing Disorders, 52*, 306–312.

Sies, L.F., & Butler, B. (1963). A personal account of dysphasia. *Journal of Speech and Hearing Disorders, 28*, 261–266.

Simmons, N.N. (1989). A trip down easy street. In T.E. Prescott (Ed.), *Clinical aphasiology* (pp. 19–30). Austin, TX: PRO-ED.

Simmons, N.N. (1993). *An ethnographic investigation of compensatory strategies in aphasia.* (Vols. 1 and 2). Dissertation, Dept. of Communication Sciences and Disorders, Louisiana State University and Agricultural and Mechanical College.

Skelly, M. (1975). Aphasic patients talk back. *American Journal of Nursing, 75*, 1140–1142.

Spradley, J.P. (1979). *The ethnographic interview.* New York: Holt, Rinehart, & Winston.

Spradley, J.P. (1980). *Participant observation.* New York: Holt, Rinehart, & Winston.

Struggling with aphasia. (1969, March 21). *Medical World News, 10*, 37–40.

Swindell, C.S., Pashek, G.V., & Holland, A.L. (1982). A questionnaire for surveying personal and communicative style. In R.H. Brookshire (Ed.), *Proceedings of the Conference on Clinical Aphasiology* (pp. 50–63). Minneapolis: BRK Publishers.

Taylor, M.L. (1965). A measurement of functional communication in aphasia. *Archives of Physical Medicine and Rehabilitation, 46,* 101–107.

Thompson, C.K. (1989). Generalization research in aphasia: A review of the literature. In T.E. Prescott (Ed.), *Clinical aphasiology* (pp. 195–222). Austin, TX: PRO-ED.

Thompson, C.K., & Byrne, M.E. (1984). Across setting generalization of social conventions in aphasia: An experimental analysis of "loose training." In R.H. Brookshire (Ed.), *Proceedings of the Conference on Clinical Aphasiology* (pp. 132–144). Minneapolis: BRK Publishers.

Thompson, C.K., & Kearns, K. (1991). Analytical and technical directions in applied aphasia analysis: The Midas touch. In T.E. Prescott (Ed.), *Clinical aphasiology* (Vol. 19, pp. 41–54). Austin, TX: PRO-ED.

Tonkovich, J.D. (1988). Communication disorders in the elderly. In B.B. Shadden (Ed.), *Communication behavior and aging: A sourcebook for clinicians* (pp. 197–215). Baltimore: Williams & Wilkins.

Turnblom, M., & Myers, J.S. (1952). A group discussion with families of aphasic patients. *Journal of Speech and Hearing Disorders, 17,* 393–396.

Ulatowska, H.K., Haynes, S.M., Hildebrand, B.H., & Richardson, S.M. (1977). The aphasic individual: A speaker and a listener, not a patient. In R.H. Brookshire (Ed.), *Proceedings of the Conference on Clinical Aphasiology* (pp. 198–213). Minneapolis: BRK Publishers.

Vignolo, L. (1964). Evolution of aphasia and language rehabilitation: A retrospective exploratory study. *Cortex, 1,* 344–367.

Walker-Batson, D., Devous, Sr., M.D., Curtis, S.S., Unwin, D.H., & Greenlee, R.G. (1991). Response to amphetamine to facilitate recovery from aphasic subsequent to stroke. In T.E. Prescott (Ed.), *Clinical aphasiology* (Vol. 20, pp. 137–143). Austin, TX: PRO-ED.

Wambaugh, J.L., Thompson, C.K., Doyle, P.J., & Camarata, S. (1991). Conversational discourse of aphasic and normal adults: An analysis of communicative functions. In T.E. Prescott (Ed.), *Clinical aphasiology* (Vol. 20, pp. 343–353). Austin, TX: PRO-ED.

Webster, E.J., Dans, J.C., Saunders, P.T. (1982). Descriptions of husband-wife communication pre- and post-aphasia. In R.H. Brookshire (Ed.), *Proceedings of the Conference on Clinical Aphasiology* (pp. 64–74). Minneapolis: BRK Publishers.

Weisenberg, T., & McBride, K.E. (1935). *Aphasia: A clinical and psychological study.* New York: Commonwealth Fund.

Wender, D. (1990, January). Quality: A personal perspective. *ASHA, 32,* 41–44.

Wepman, J.M. (1951). *Recovery from aphasia.* New York: Ronald Press.

Wepman, J.M. (1972). Aphasia therapy: Some relative comments and some purely personal prejudices. In M.T. Sarno (Ed.), *Aphasia: Selected readings* (pp. 436–444). Englewood Cliffs, NJ: Prentice-Hall.

Wertz, R.T. (1993, January). Adult onset disorders. *ASHA, 35,* 38–39.

Wertz, R.T., Collins, M.J., Weiss, D., Kurtzke, J.F., Friden, T., Brookshire, R.H., Pierce, J., Holtzapple, P.L., Hubbard, D.J., Porch, B.E., West, J.A., Davis, L., Matovitch, V., Morley, G.K., & Resurrecion, E. (1981). Veterans Administration cooperative study on aphasia: A comparison of individual and group treatment. *Journal of Speech and Hearing Research, 24,* 580–594.

Wertz, R.T., Deal, J.L., Holland, A.L., Kurtzke, J.F., & Weiss, D.G. (1986, January). Comments on an uncontrolled aphasia no treatment trial. *ASHA, 28,* 31.

Wertz, R.T., & Dronkers, N.F. (1990). Effects of age on aphasia. In E. Cherow (Ed.), *Proceedings of the Research Symposium on Communication Sciences and Disorders and Aging* (ASHA Reports 19, pp. 88–98). Rockville, MD: American Speech-Language-Hearing Association.

Wertz, R.T., & Rosenbek, J.C. (1978). Group designs for the study of aphasia. In R.H. Brookshire (Ed.), *Proceedings of the Conference on Clinical Aphasiology* (pp. 1–10). Minneapolis: BRK Publishers.

Wertz, R.T., Weiss, D.G., Aten, J.L., Brookshire, R.H., Garcia-Bunuel, L., Holland, A.L., Kurtzke, J.F., LaPointe, L.L., Milanti, F.J., Brannegan, R., Greenbaum, H., Marshall, R.C., Vogel, D., Carter, J., Barnes, N.S., & Goodman, R. (1986). Comparison of clinic, home, and deferred language treatment for aphasia: A Veterans Administration cooperative study. *Archives of Neurology, 43,* 653–658.

Wings. (1979, August). *ASHA, 21,* 552–561.

Wofford, M., Boysen, A., & Riding, L. (1991, September). A research mentoring process. *ASHA, 33,* 39–42.

Wulf, H.H. (1973). *Aphasia, my world alone.* Detroit: Wayne State University Press.

Zraick, R.I., & Boone, D.R. (1991). Spouse attitudes toward the person with aphasia. *Journal of Speech and Hearing Research, 34,* 123–128.

Chapter 17

Psychological Adjustment Following Stroke

Sarah E. Williams

Observers have long recognized that mood disorders are a frequent and sometimes serious consequence of stroke. However, compared to such disorders as aphasia or sensorimotor impairment, the emotional consequences of stroke have received little attention in the literature. Empirical evaluations of mood changes following insult to the brain began in the late 1960s (Gainotti, 1972). Since then, a number of investigations have confirmed the occurrence of psychological changes after stroke and their effects on recovery. This chapter reviews these psychological changes in stroke patients and their families. Strategies designed to enhance psychological well-being following stroke are also summarized. The primary purpose of the chapter is to increase awareness of the psychological devastation that can occur after stroke, in hopes that students and clinicians alike will focus more on the entire patient, rather than just on one specific consequence of stroke.

PATTERNS OF EMOTIONAL RESPONSE

In his landmark study, Gainotti (1972) examined the emotional reactions displayed by stroke patients with right- versus left-hemisphere damage. Three types of emotional reactions were described: (1) catastrophic reaction (anxiety, tears, aggressive behavior, swears, displacements, refusals, renouncements, and compensatory boasting); (2) more elaborate expressions of anxiety and depression (discouragement, anticipation, statements of incapacity); and (3) indifference toward the disability, and even euphoria. Catastrophic reaction was more prevalent in left-hemisphere–damaged patients, while indifference was found more often in patients with right-hemisphere damage. These differences in emotional response have since been confirmed by Robinson (1986) and by Sackeim and Greenberg (1982), who suggested that they may reflect asymmetries in the content of, or response to, particular neurotransmitters in the two hemispheres.

In their descriptive study, House, Dennis, Hawton, and Warlow (1989) estimated that 15% of 128 patients reported emotionalism 1 month after a stroke, 21% at 6 months, and 11% at 12 months. Psychiatric assessment revealed that patients with emotionalism had high scores on measures of mood disorder and more apparent psychiatric disorders. Larger brain lesions were documented in the patients who displayed emotionalism; these patients also showed more intellectual impairment. Left frontal and temporal lesions were especially associated with emotionalism.

In an attempt to explain their findings, House and colleagues described poststroke emotionalism as a form of disinhibition in which the ability to suppress an emotional response at low levels of stimulation is compromised. Although patients described their emotionalism as distressing and socially disabling, none had received treatment for their symptoms and no patient had been referred to a psychologist or psychiatrist.

PSYCHOSOCIAL REACTIONS

The psychosocial complications from stroke become crucial during rehabilitation (Mesulam, 1985). In fact, social reintegration of stroke patients is possibly the most difficult and problematic phase of rehabilitation (Folstein, Mailbeger, & McHugh, 1977; Hyman, 1971).

Labi, Phillips, and Gresham (1980) examined the extent to which stroke patients continued to display psychosocial disabilities, despite regaining independence in self-care and mobility. Stroke survivors displayed a significant decrease in socialization in and outside of the home, and decreased involvement with hobbies and other interests. This observation was noted for many of the subjects regardless of level of independence in physical activity and self care. The authors reasoned that sensitivity to stigma may cause the stroke patient to avoid interactions with people who were once social equals. Interestingly, individuals with the most education had more of a reduction in outside socialization than did those who were less educated.

This investigation also indicated that patients who live alone and have a friend outside the home are less likely than those who live with their families to decrease outside socialization. Thus, while ongoing support and encouragement from families is essential, overprotective families may actually deter long-term recovery of socialization.

Leisure activities suffer after a stroke as well. Sjogren (1982) found marked decreases in all leisure activities for hemiplegic poststroke patients. Feibel and Springer (1982) confirmed this and other findings (Labi et al., 1980; Sjorgen, 1982) regarding leisure activities after stroke. Moreover, they found the reduction in socialization and leisure activities strongly related to depression. Depressed patients disengaged from 67% of prestroke social activities, while nondepressed patients showed a 43% reduction in such activities.

Significant others also experience psychosocial problems following stroke in their partners. These include decreased opportunities for social activity, feelings of isolation, lack of companionship, role changes, and lack of time for self (Artes & Hoops, 1976; Coughlan & Humphrey, 1982; Holbrook, 1982; Kinsella & Duffy, 1978; Kinsella & Duffy, 1979; Webster & Newhoff, 1981). Stroke with aphasia appears to have an even greater impact on a spouse's adjustment. Spouses of individuals who have incurred stroke and aphasia report greater feelings of loneliness than do spouses of patients who have incurred stroke but not aphasia (Kinsella & Duffy, 1979). Tompkins, Schultz, and Rauk (1988) found that support persons who were at the greatest risk for depression were those who named the fewest number of people in their social networks.

Stroke often causes significant change in interpersonal relationships. Lawrence and Christie (1979) found that the extent of physical disability after a stroke was directly related to the degree of deterioration in interpersonal relationships. As early as 1957, Biorn-Hansen (1957) noted that the most common change in relationships among 30 stroke patients was role change. Wives had to assume a more dominant role; many wives had to work outside the home. Rollin (1987) also emphasized that adjustment to stroke typically involves role changes within the family, with the most significant change affecting the unimpaired spouse. Role changes experienced by spouses of patients who have aphasia seem to be greater than those experienced by spouses of patients who do not have aphasia (Christensen & Anderson, 1989). At the same time the family is assuming new roles, the patient may be rejecting his or her new handicapped status (Lubinski, 1981).

Satisfaction with marriage has been the topic of numerous investigations. Kinsella and Duffy (1979) found that marital relationships were greatly affected by stroke, with decreased or complete loss in sexual activity, reticence, friction, and loss of partnership. Not surprisingly, spouses of patients with aphasia experienced more marital difficulties than did spouses of patients who had incurred stroke but who did not have aphasia. Williams and Freer (1986) found that while marital satisfaction declined after a stroke, the change was unrelated to either spousal knowledge about aphasia or the severity of aphasia.

DEPRESSION

Prevalence

By far the most common mood disorder after a stroke is depression. Robinson (1986) found major depression in approximately one-fourth to one-third of a group of patients followed for 2 years poststroke. Symptoms of minor (dysthymic) depression were also common, occurring in up to one-fourth of all stroke patients. Interestingly, Robinson found that one-third of patients who did not develop depression immediately following the stroke did so between 3 months and 2 years poststroke.

More recently, Starkstein and Robinson (1989) and Robinson and Starkstein (1990) have summarized the prevalence of poststroke depression in both inpatient and outpatient populations. Thirty percent of 103 consecutive outpatients were found to be depressed. This is consistent with findings of Feibel and Springer (1982). Among 103 acute stroke patients, 27% displayed major depression while 20% showed minor depression. These figures are somewhat higher than those of Wade, Legh-Smith, and Hewer (1987), who found that 3 weeks after stroke, 22% of the patients were depressed, while an additional 11% were probably depressed. Prevalence figures reported by Ebrahim, Baer, and Nouri (1987) for patients with acute stroke admitted to a general hospital were 23% each for mild-to-moderate depression and for severe depression.

Thus, prevalence studies indicate that 40–50% of stroke patients may develop depression during the acute period, and an additional 30% may develop depression at some time during the first 2 years. Since depression is found in only 15% of normal elderly living at home (Gurland & Copeland, 1983; Kay, Beamish, & Roth, 1964; Murphy, 1982), it appears that the incidence of depression following stroke is at least twice as high as in the normal elderly.

Definition and Symptomatology

Diagnosis of depression in stroke patients requires a standardized approach to defining the disorder. Robinson and Starkstein (1990) and others use the symptom criteria for major affective disorder and dysthymic disorder from the *Diagnostic and Statistical Manual of Mental Disorders, Third Edition* (DSM-III) (American Psychiatric Association, 1980) and the terminology from the *Research Diagnostic Criteria* (Spitzer, Endicott, & Robins, 1975) for major and minor depression (dysthymic disorder) in their definition and subsequent diagnosis. According to the DSM-III:

> the essential feature of a major depressive episode is either a dysphoric mood, usually depression or loss of interest or pleasure in all or almost all usual activities and pastimes. This disturbance is prominent, relatively persistent, and associated with other symptoms of the depressive syndrome. These symptoms include appetite disturbance, change in weight, sleep disturbance, psychomotor agitation or retardation, decreased energy, feelings of worthlessness or guilt, difficulty concentrating or thinking, and thought of death or suicide or suicidal attempts. (p. 210)

Other features commonly associated with major depression include depressed appearance, tearfulness, anxiety, fear, irritability, phobias, panic attacks, and an obsessive concern with health.

Dysthymic disorder, or minor depression, is characterized by the same symptoms as major depression, but of a lesser severity. The depressed mood may be either fairly persistent or intermittent. If a normal mood is apparent, it may last only a few days to a few weeks, but no more than a few months at a time. During the depressive periods, at least three of the following symptoms are present: (1) insomnia or hypersomnia; (2) low energy level or chronic tiredness; (3) feelings of inadequacy, loss of self-esteem, or self-deprecation; (4) decreased effectiveness or productivity at school, work, or home; (5) decreased attention, concentration, or ability to think clearly; (6) social withdrawal; (7) loss of interest in or enjoyment of pleasurable activities; (8) irritability or excessive anger (in children, expressed toward parents or caretakers); (9) inability to respond with apparent pleasure to praise or rewards; (10) less activity or talkativity than usual, or feelings of being slowed down or restless; (11) pessimistic attitude toward the future, brooding about past events, or feeling sorry for self; (12) tearfulness or crying; (13) recurrent thoughts of death or suicide.

Robinson and colleagues (Robinson, Bolduc, & Price, 1987; Robinson, Starkstein, & Price, 1988; Starkstein & Robinson, 1989; Robinson & Starkstein, 1990) have presented data that support the distinction between major and minor depression following stroke. First, these two forms of depression differ in the location of the associated brain lesion. In addition, the evolution and resolution of major depression differ from that of minor depression, and major depression has been associated with a significant intellectual decline. Finally, patients with major depression have shown a different response to the administration of dexamethasone during the dexamethasone suppression test than have patients with minor depression.

Robinson and Starkstein (1990) feel that when diagnosing poststroke depression, it may be important to consider whether the medical condition itself produces symptoms, such as loss of appetite, that may lead to an incorrect diagnosis of depression (false-positives), or whether the medical condition actually masks symptoms of depression, which would result in failure to diagnose a true depression (false-negatives). These investigators find that stroke does not appear to create significant numbers of false positive or false negative diagnoses, and that patients who deny feelings of depression usually have one vegetative (unconscious) depressive symptom.

Lipsey, Spenser, Robins, and Robinson (1986) compared symptoms of poststroke depression with symptoms of functional depression in persons with no known neuropathology. While the great majority of symptoms were identical in the two groups, two symptoms were different: (1) slowness, which was more frequent in poststroke depression than in functional depression; and (2) loss of interest and concentration, which was more frequent in functional depression than in poststroke depression.

Underlying Mechanisms

Although poststroke depression historically has been viewed as a normal reaction to a serious sudden disability, recent evidence suggests that this mood disorder reflects a more direct response to the brain injury itself. The precise mechanisms underlying poststroke depression are not known. Nonetheless, a number of theories have been advanced to explain its etiology. Swindell and Hammons (1991) name and summarize three such theories: the neuropharmacology model, the neuroendocrine model, and the neuroanatomical model. These models are briefly described below.

Neuropharmacology Model

The most commonly discussed agent in terms of the neuropharmacology model is the neurotransmitter catecholamine norepinephrine. Basically, the model suggests that a depletion of norepinephrine at functionally important adrenergic receptor sites results in depression.

This theory is supported by the association of major poststroke depression with lesions having close proximity to the frontal pole. Specifically, Morrison, Molliver, and Grzanna (1979) and Pickel, Segal, and Bloom (1974) have demonstrated that noradrenergic cell bodies sending main axonal tracts to terminal, downstream fibers, originate in the brainstem and project through the median forebrain bundle to the frontal cortex. The axons then arc posteriorly and run longitudinally through the deep cortical layers. Lesions disrupting these pathways in the frontal cortex or basal ganglia are likely to affect terminal fibers. More posterior lesions would disrupt fewer downstream fibers, resulting in a less marked depletion of norepinephrine than more anterior cortical lesions.

Neuroendocrine Model

The metabolism of hormones along the hypothalamic-pituitary-adrenal (HPA) axis and the pituitary-thyroid axis is not normal in depressed patients. In a normally functioning system, the hypothalamus reacts to stress by secreting corticotropin-releasing factor (CRF). The presence of CRF then stimulates the pituitary gland to release adrenocorticotropic hormone (ACTH), which then stimulates the adrenal glands to release glucocorticoids, of which cortisol is the primary hormone. Cortisol inhibits further release of CRF and ACTH in an attempt to reduce the physiologic effects of stress. In a circular way, therefore, elevated levels of cortisol inhibits its subsequent production. When stress is no longer present, cortisol levels normalize.

In a large percentage of depressed patients, cortisol levels are elevated. In major depression, cortisol levels do not diminish when challenged by an exogenous cortisol, dexamethasone. This procedure, wherein dexamethasone is administered to the patient, is called the dexamethasone suppression test (DST). Results of the DST support the neuroendocrine model, which proposes that in depression, there is a breakdown in the circular feedback system that regulates cortisol production.

Neuroanatomical Model

The neuroanatomical model focuses on the brain structures responsible for mediating emotions. According to Silverman and Weingartner (1986), three basic processes are involved in the recognition and regulation of emotion: intrahemispheric activation, contralateral inhibition, and interhemispheric coupling. The left and right cerebral hemispheres appear to regulate different emotions intrahemispherically (i.e., positive emotions by the left hemisphere; negative emotions by the right hemisphere). The stability of moods, however, depends on contralateral inhibition and interhemispheric coupling. Using this theory, it becomes easy to understand how an individual with a unilateral lesion loses the inhibition normally provided by the involved hemisphere. Thus, the explanation for the depression resulting from a left-hemisphere lesion is that the right hemisphere is now uninhibited or deregulated and continues to mediate negative emotions. In contrast, the finding that right-hemisphere lesions frequently cause lack of interest, joking, and euphoria is based on the lack of inhibition of the left hemisphere's positive emotional mediation.

Diagnosis and Assessment of Depression

Depression is diagnosed and assessed primarily through the use of rating scales completed either by the patient or by a clinician or nurse. In addition, the DST has been found useful in certain situations. These methods, as well as clinical guidelines for identifying depressed patients, are briefly described below.

Self-Rating Scales

There are a number of self-rating scales for assessing depression. The three most commonly reported in the literature are the Geriatric Depression Scale (GDS) (Rapp, Parisi, Walsh, & Wallace, 1988; Weiss, Nagel, & Aronson, 1986), the Zung Self-Rating Depression Scale (SDS) (Zung, 1965), and the Beck Depression Inventory (BDI) (Beck, Ward, Mandelson, Mock, & Erbaugh, 1961).

The GDS, which consists of 30 items in a yes-no format, has demonstrated strong internal reliability and test-retest reliability. Importantly, the GDS has proved equally successful with subjects displaying symptoms of cognitive impairment (Parmallei, Lawton, & Katz, 1989). The SDS consists of 20 items requiring patients to indicate the frequency with which they experience a particular symptom or feeling. An index score for the SDS determines whether significant depression is present, and if so, the level of severity. The BDI is a questionnaire to be completed during an interview format. It is composed of 21 categories of symptoms and moods. For each item, patients must listen to several statements and select the one that best describes themselves at that time.

Generally, the reliability and validity of depression ratings used with stroke patients are questionable. Self- or clinician-assisted evaluation is difficult, particularly when aphasia is present. House, Dennis, Hawton, and Warlow (1989) suggest two main drawbacks of using self-report methods to identify poststroke depression: low response rates and relative inaccuracy as a method of individual case detection. Hence, they recommend that these tools should be used with caution and in combination with other assessment information.

Clinician-Administered Scale and Clinical Guidelines

The standard tool used by clinicians to rate depression is the Hamilton Rating Scale for Depression (Hamilton, 1960). This scale was designed to rate the degree of symptoms displayed by patients already diagnosed as depressed. To accomplish this, 17 symptoms are rated by the clinicians on either a three- or a five-point scale.

Because of the difficulties in using rating scales with brain-damaged patients, Ross and Rush (1981) have outlined a number of clinical guidelines that may first signal depression in such patients: (1) poor or erratic recovery; (2) failure to cooperate in rehabilitation; (3) difficulty in general "management" of the patient; and (4) deterioration from a previously stable neurologic condition. Ross and Rush state that in questionable cases of depression, both the patient and the family should be interviewed. Moreover, since patients may deny symptoms of depression, special attention must be given to vegetative signs.

Dexamethasone Suppression Test

The DST is a laboratory test designed to determine whether cortisol production is suppressed (as in normals) following the administration of dexamethasone. Patients with major depression typically do not show this normal pattern of cortisol suppression, while patients with minor depression follow the normal pattern (Robinson, 1986). Thus, the DST may serve as an important discriminator between these two types of depression, particularly when mood evaluation is complicated by aphasia (Agarwal, Nag, Kar, Agarwal, & Chowdhury, 1987). However, Price (1990) cautions that with large strokes, DST results may be abnormal, even when the patient is not clinically depressed.

Depression and Lesion Location

Starkstein and Robinson (1989) and Robinson and Starkstein (1990) have consistently found a strong relationship between lesion location and major depression after stroke. Left-hemisphere lesions, primarily in the frontal cortex or basal ganglia, are strongly linked to poststroke depression. When depression is associated with anxiety disorders, the lesion is typically cortical, whereas depression without anxiety is more frequently associated with a subcortical lesion in the basal ganglia. Further, according to these investigators, for both cortical and subcortical lesions, the closer the lesion is to the frontal pole, the more severe is the depression. This finding has been substantiated by Eastwood, Rifat, Nobbs, and Ruderman (1989). Although depression stemming from left-hemisphere lesions is infrequent, it is possible. The lesion in such cases is most frequently found in the white matter of the parietal lobe (Starkstein et al., 1989).

Support for the findings of Robinson and his colleagues has not been entirely consistent. Sinyor et al. (1986) and Smith (1989), for example, have neither documented hemispheric differences with depression, nor been able to replicate the relationship between severity of depression and proximity of the lesion to the frontal pole. Such discrepancies in findings may stem from methodological differences. For example, testing patients in the acute versus chronic state, or testing outpatients versus patients residing in a rehabilitation facility, may affect results. Robinson and Starkstein (1990) suggest that other confounding variables that may account for discrepancies in findings include the amount of time elapsed after the stroke, intrahemispheric site of lesion, history of mood disorder, and possible occurrence of a previous brain insult.

Aphasia and Depression

The question of whether the presence of aphasia increases the risk of poststroke depression has been addressed. Starkstein and Robinson (1989) found that 53% of patients with aphasia, but only 44% of patients without aphasia, were depressed following their strokes. This difference was not statistically significant. Hence, the authors reasoned that aphasia, per se, does not seem to produce depression. Rather, aphasia and depression are likely to coexist, given the presence of brain damage.

Robinson and Benson (1981) examined the frequency of depression in patients with nonfluent, fluent, and global aphasia. Depression was both more frequent and more severe in patients with nonfluent aphasia, as compared with patients with fluent aphasia and global aphasia. The investigators stated that the combination of an anterior site of lesion and intact "awareness" in the nonfluent patients contributed to these findings.

Cognitive Impairment and Depression

Robinson and colleagues (Robinson, Bolla-Wilson, Kaplan, Lipsey, & Price, 1986) examined the relationship between intellectual deficit and poststroke depression. All patients with major depression and single left-hemisphere lesions were found to have intellectual impairment. Only 40% of the nondepressed patients with single, left-hemisphere lesions were found to have intellectual impairment. Interestingly, over a 6-month follow-up period, nondepressed patients showed improvement in intellectual status, while depressed patients showed either no change or a slight decline in intellectual status.

Parikh, Lipsey, Robinson, and Price (1987) followed patients with poststroke depression at 3 months, 6 months, 1 year, and 2 years after stroke. At the first two follow-up evaluations, the most severe intellectual impairments were associated with the most severe depression. However, at the 1- and 2-year follow-ups, this relationship was no longer present.

Evolution of Poststroke Depression

Robinson and colleagues have published a series of reports regarding the average duration and evolution of poststroke depression. In their first report, Robinson and Price (1982) stated that the average duration of untreated depression from the time of diagnosis is 8–9 months. In addition, patients are more likely to develop depression during the first 2 years following stroke than they are 3–10 years after the stroke.

Robinson et al. (1987) differentiated the evolution of major and minor depression during the first 2 years after a stroke. Patients with major depression improved significantly between years 1 and 2. In contrast, patients with minor depression did not demonstrate such improvement; some of these patients actually developed major depression by the 2-year follow-up evaluation. Hence, major depression appears to have a natural course of approximately 1 year, while minor depression frequently has a longer course.

In an attempt to identify variables associated with rapid spontaneous recovery, Starkstein, Robinson, and Price (1988) compared patients who had recovered from their depression by 6 months post-onset with those who had not recovered. Nonrecovered patients had cortical lesions in the distribution of the middle cerebral artery. No patient in this group had purely subcortical damage or damage in the distribution of the posterior cerebral artery. Patients who did not recover from their depression also had a greater degree of physical impairment than did patients who spontaneously recovered. In contrast to the nonrecovered group, patients who had recovered from depression at 6 months poststroke had predominantly subcortical lesions and lesions in the distribution of the posterior cerebral artery. These were also the patients who were less physically impaired than the recovered group.

Parikh, Lipsey, Robinson, and Price (1988) have acknowledged the importance of lesion location and extent of physical impairment to the evolution and duration of poststroke depression. These investigators suggest that although lesion location is the strongest predictor of subsequent depression, there appears to be a reciprocal relationship between depression and physical impairment. That is to say, once depression develops, it is sustained by severe physical impairment, and severe physical impairment is sustained by depression.

The Effects of Psychological Status on Rehabilitation

As early as 1971, Hyman (1971) demonstrated that when patients feel stigmatized at the start of a stroke rehabilitation program, their motivation and functional improvement during the program are impaired. In addition, these feelings reduce the likelihood that patients will return to their prestroke level of functioning even a number of months after discharge.

A number of investigators have since supported the notion that depression has a significant impact on rehabilitation outcome (Ebrahim et al., 1987; Parikh et al., 1990; Sinyor et al., 1986). Sinyor et al. (1986) found that depression affected long-term (6 weeks postdischarge) but not short-term rehabilitation of stroke patients. Parikh et al. (1990) have documented similar long-term effects of both major and minor depression. Interestingly, in patients with major depression, delayed recovery was apparent even after the depression had lessened in severity. This finding suggests that, when depression reduces the initial impetus for physical recovery, optimal levels of recovery may not be achieved, even after the depression has improved.

Therapeutic Intervention to Improve Poststroke Depression

Unfortunately, despite the high incidence of poststroke depression, few patients receive treatment for it. In a series of patients evaluated by Feibel and Springer (1982) 6 months after stroke, less than 5% had received treatment.

Different theories regarding the cause of poststroke depression tend to dictate different forms of treatment. For example, theories that explain depression as organic and as a direct result of the lesion tend to dictate treatment with antidepressant medication. In contrast, theories that explain poststroke depression as a normal reaction to the unpleasant events that have transpired tend to recommend psychotherapy. Psychotherapy may also be recommended if antidepressant medication has proved to be nonbeneficial.

Different treatment strategies for patients with poststroke depression are reviewed below. These must be carefully selected according to the specific needs of each patient, and not all patients respond similarly to a given method. In addition, the methods involve a variety of different professionals.

Pharmacotherapy

Robinson and colleagues (1984, 1986, 1990) and others (Finklestein et al., 1987; Reding et al., 1986) emphasize that antidepressants appear to be indicated for both major and minor poststroke depressive disorders. The more commonly prescribed tricyclic antidepressants function to prolong the effects of pertinent neurotransmitters (i.e., norepinephrine, serotonin, and dopamine) at the neuronal synapse. Robinson (1986) cautions that antidepressants are contraindicated in some patients, particularly the elderly, and may be associated with serious side effects.

Electroconvulsive Therapy

Electroconvulsive therapy (ECT) has been found effective in treating patients with poststroke depression (Robinson & Starkstein, 1990). Although transient memory disturbances may occur following ECT (Fink, 1982, 1984; Murry, Shea, & Conn, 1987), no neurologic deterioration has been noted (Murry et al., 1987). ECT is typically prescribed when antidepressant therapy is not successful.

Psychotherapies

Family Systems Therapy.   Sudden disability is neither minor, nor anticipated. A stroke sends "emotional shockwaves" (Bowen, 1978), which result in serious disruption of a family's equilibrium. Because this disruption is likely to hurt psychological well-being as well as rehabilitation, a number of investigators stress the importance of including the family in treatment (Overs & Belknap, 1967; Rollin, 1987; Wahrborg, 1989; Wahrborg & Borenstein, 1989). While traditional family counseling excludes direct participation of the patient who has incurred a stroke, family systems therapy includes all members of the family (including the patient).

Family systems therapy is a systematic and interactional approach wherein family members help each other re-establish family equilibrium. Wahrborg and Borenstein (1989) use a family systems therapy technique based on systems theory, communication theory, and process theory. Cooperation is emphasized and attitudes are reinforced accordingly. Wahrborg and Borenstein (1989) found that family systems therapy benefited both aphasic patients and their family members. For the patients, notable changes were made in tendency toward depression, emotional isolation, impatience, social isolation, and dependency. For family members, improvement was noted in level of irritation and quality and quantity of communication.

Social Support Intervention Therapy.   Social support leads an individual to believe that she or he is cared for and loved, esteemed, and a member of a network of mutual obligations. There is evidence that supportive interactions among people protect against the consequences of life stress, such as depression (Cobb, 1976). Nussbaum, Thompson, and Robinson (1989) state that social support is particularly important in the elderly, the age group of most stroke patients.

Friedland and McColl (1987) studied patients during the first 2 years after a stroke to determine aspects of social support that offer a protective effect. Four aspects were revealed: (1) satisfaction with social support; (2) the single most significant relationship in the individual's life; (3) close friends and family; and (4) community (neighbors, friends, work colleagues, and service people).

Based on these findings, Friedland and McColl (1989) developed an intervention program designed to capitalize on the buffering effects of social support. Their program consists of eight to 12 sessions attended by a specially trained occupational therapist, the stroke patient, and his or her support system. With the therapist and the client working as collaborators, the support system is developed and mobilized to enhance its involvement with the client. Change is expected in the support system—not in the client. The combination of different sources of support (i.e., personal, friend, and community) ensures that any one source is not relied on excessively. Should a patient not have a "natural" social network, volunteers, community leaders, or mutual self-support groups can devise one (Turkat, 1980).

Pet-Facilitated Therapy.   Pets have both psychological and physiologic impacts on individuals with whom they interact (Carmack, 1991). Pet-facilitated therapy involves introducing a pet to a patient after carefully considering both personalities. Patients are allowed to bond and interact with a given pet over time, either as a live-in or through temporary pet visitation. Pet therapy is a nontraditional, yet safe treatment that is cost-effective, yet beneficial.

Corson and Corson and colleagues (1975, 1977, 1978) were among the first researchers to evaluate the use of pets as a treatment modality. They introduced dogs to psychiatric patients who had not responded to traditional forms of therapy such as drugs and ECT. Through pet therapy, previously uncommunicative patients who had been confined to their rooms began to communicate and care for themselves so well that they became candidates for discharge. Similarly, Francis (1991), who implemented pet therapy in residential homes for adults discharged from psychiatric facilities, found improvement in seven of nine indicators of quality of life.

Calvert (1989) found that pet therapy decreases loneliness experienced by nursing home patients. Since the association between loneliness and depression is clear and consistent (Mullins & Dugan, 1980), Calvert's results might lend support for using pet therapy with depressed patients. Likewise, data from Garrity, Stallones, Marx, and Johnson (1989) show that pet attachment is inversely related to depression as measured by a scale of symptoms.

Although the usefulness of pet therapy in brief, controlled experimental settings has been well-documented, the question of its long-term usefulness remains. Some support in this regard comes from programs that have operated successfully for at least a decade. For example, Ross (1991) reports that emotionally disturbed children enrolled in a 40-year-old pet therapy program at Green Chimneys (Brewster, New York) "overcome their depression immediately."

Another noteworthy program has operated since 1975 at Lima State Hospital, which treats convicts with severe mental illnesses. Pet therapy has improved scores on the Minnesota Multiphasic Personality Inventory and led to a 50% reduction in psychotropic medications needed on wards where pets are present, a marked reduction in violence on these wards, and a zero incidence of suicides on wards with pets.

Cognitive Therapy.   Cognitive therapy is an active, direct, time-limited, structured approach that can be used to treat a variety of psychiatric disorders, including depression (Beck, Rush, Shaw, & Emery, 1979). The theory underlying this approach is that an individual's affect and behavior are largely determined by the way in which she or he structures the world.

The therapy implements highly specific learning techniques designed to identify, reality-test, and correct distorted conceptualizations and the dysfunctional beliefs that underlie them. Behavioral rather than verbal techniques are used with more severely depressed patients or patients who would have difficulty engaging in introspection (for example, individuals with aphasia). The therapist, who must be trained in the cognitive model of psychotherapy, helps the individual think and behave more realistically and adaptively about his or her psychological problems. This, in turn, tends to reduce depressive symptoms. Therapy typically consists of 15–25 weekly sessions with follow-up treatment recommended three to four times during the year following termination of formal therapy.

A number of systematic studies of cognitive therapy in the treatment of depression are promising. However, its effectiveness has not been demonstrated for the treatment of poststroke depression. Because of its cognitive orientation, this approach would seem to be useful only for those patients who can fully participate in its techniques, meaning those who are not severely compromised in terms of cognition or language functioning.

Laughter and Humor.   As early as 1928, Walsh wrote, "there is nothing which means so much for the lifting of mental depression . . . as good hearty laughter" (p. 125). A number of investigators have found that laughter and a sense of humor reduce stress (Cousins, 1979; Dugan, 1989; Martin & Lefcourt, 1983), discomfort levels, and depression (Cogan, Cogan, Waltz, & McCue, 1987; Cousins, 1979; Peter & Dana, 1982).

Dixon (1980) suggests that the beneficial effects of humor are produced through the cognitive shifts it entails and the changes in affective quality that accompany it. O'Connell (1976) believes that the capacity to rapidly shift perceptual frames of reference allows humorists to distance themselves from the immediate threat of a problem, thereby reducing feelings of anxiety and helplessness. Humor that results in laughter may actually interrupt a downward psychological spiral that, if left unresolved, may result in depression (Schmitt, 1990). Martin and Lefcourt (1983) found that subjects with high scores on humor measures had a lower association between life events and moods than did those with low scores on humor measures. More important, for those subjects reporting many negative life occurrences, lower mean mood disturbance scores were found for those with higher scores on the humor measures than for those with lower scores.

Humor can be introduced to patients and families in "humor groups" (Ljungdahl, 1989) or individually (Schmitt, 1990) through jokes, videotapes and films, television, and comic books.

Group Therapy. One of the primary objectives of group therapy is to provide psychological support through socialization; motivation from peers rather than from an unimpaired therapist; and an opportunity to ventilate feelings and air grievances, hence improving psychological adjustment (Eisenson, 1984). Providing information and facilitating coping strategies are also frequent group goals (Rice, Paul, & Muller, 1986). These may apply to both stroke patients and their spouses or significant others (Bardach, 1969; D'Afflitti & Wertz, 1974; Rice et al., 1986; Singler, 1975).

Rice et al. (1986) found that spouses of stroke patients who consistently attended the group meetings showed significant improvement on tests of social dysfunction, somatic symptoms, anxiety, and a general measure of psychological well-being. Some functional improvement in the partners of the good attenders was also noted.

Borenstein, Linell, and Wahrborg (1987) developed a 5-day residential therapeutic program for aphasic stroke patients and their families. The aims of the program were to provide information regarding etiology, treatment, and prognosis; to address personal and interpersonal problems through psychological counseling; and to provide intensive stimulation to improve language functioning. One year after the course ended, the participants reported having learned how to better identify and constructively deal with their psychological problems.

FUTURE DIRECTIONS

In most patients, poststroke depression can be improved through treatment. To ensure that treatment is prescribed, however, physicians and other health care professionals must be educated regarding the prevalence of depression in the stroke population. Moreover, these professionals must understand that poststroke depression is not necessarily a "normal" reaction to an unfortunate set of circumstances.

An interdisciplinary approach is critical in diagnosing and treating poststroke depression. In fact, Wahrborg and Borenstein (1990) state that one of the most important goals for the twenty-first century should be to develop theories that integrate information from a number of different disciplines, such as neuropsychology, neuroendocrinology, and neurolinguistics. Particularly in the area of aphasia, this concept would seem beneficial since a number of recent findings emphasize the interconnections between the brain lesion, the psychological reaction to it, language impairment, and resultant social changes.

Cross-cultural investigation of psychological adjustment following stroke would also seem to provide insight into the management of poststroke patients. For example, individuals from cultures in which extended families live together may react differently to their family member who has incurred a stroke than might an individual from a culture that does not foster close extended-family relationships. Such differences could have implications for the choice of therapy.

Finally, Robinson and Starkstein (1990) feel that future investigations need to provide insight into the mechanism underlying the development of poststroke mood disorders. They state that only through a better understanding of this mechanism will it be possible to develop more specific, effective treatments.

REFERENCES

Agarwal, A., Nag, D., Kar, A.M., Agarwal, A.K., & Chowdhury, S.R. (1987). Dexamethasone suppression test and post stroke depression. *Indian Journal of Medical Research, 85,* 297–301.

American Psychiatric Association. (1980). *Diagnostic and statistical manual of mental disorders* (3rd ed.). Washington, D.C.: American Psychiatric Press.

Artes, R., & Hoops, R. (1976). Problems of aphasic and nonaphasic stroke patients as identified and evaluated by patients' wives. In Y. Lebrun & R. Hoops (Eds.), *Recovery in aphasics.* Amsterdam: Swets & Zeitlinger.

Bardach, J.L. (1969). Group sessions with wives of aphasic patients. *International Journal of Group Psychotherapy, 19,* 361–365.

Beck, A., Rush, A., Shaw, B., & Emery, G. (1979). *Cognitive therapy of depression..* New York: Guilford Press.

Beck, A.T., Ward, C.H., Mandelson, M., Mock, J., & Erbaugh, J. (1961). An inventory for measuring depression. *American Journal of Psychiatry, 146,* 627–634.

Biorn-Hansen, V. (1957). Social and emotional aspects of aphasia. *Journal of Speech and Hearing Disorders, 22,* 53–59.

Borenstein, P., Linell, S., & Wahrborg, P. (1987). An innovative therapeutic program for aphasia patients and their relatives. *Scandinavian Journal of Rehabilitative Medicine, 19,* 51–56.

Bowen, M. (1978). *Family therapy in clinical practice.* New York: Jason Aronson.

Calvert, M. (1989). Human pet interaction and loneliness: A test of concept from Roy's adaptation model. *Nursing Science Quarterly, 2,* 194-202.

Carmack, B. (1991). The role of companion animals for persons with AIDS/HIV. *Holistic Nursing Practices, 5,* 24–31.

Christensen, J., & Anderson, J. (1989). Spouse adjustment to stroke: Aphasic versus nonaphasic partners. *Journal of Communication Disorders, 22,* 225–231.

Cobb, S. (1976). Social support as a moderator of life stress. *Psychosomatic Medicine, 38* (No. 5, September–October), 300–314.

Cogan, R., Cogan, D., Waltz, W., & McCue, M. (1987). Effects of laughter and relaxation on discomfort thresholds. *Journal of Behavioral Medicine, 10,* 139–144.

Corson, S., & Corson, E. (1978). Pets as mediators of therapy. In H. Masserman (Ed.), *Current psychiatric therapies* (pp. 195–205). New York: Grune & Stratton.

Corson, S., Corson, E., & Gwynne, P. (1975). Pet facilitated psychotherapy in a hospital setting. In H.J. Masserman (Ed.), *Current psychiatric therapies* (pp. 277–286). Philadelphia: Grune & Stratton.

Corson, S., Corson, E., Gwynne, P., & Arnold, L. (1977). Pet dogs as nonverbal communication links in hospital psychiatry. *Comprehensive Psychiatry, 18,* 61–72.

Coughlan, G.W., & Humphrey, M. (1982). Presenile stroke: Long term outcome for patients and their families. *Rehabilitation, 21,* 115–122.

Cousins, N. (1979). *Anatomy of an illness.* New York: W.W. Norton.

D'Afflitti, J.G., & Wertz, G. (1974). Rehabilitating the stroke patient through patient family groups. *National Journal of Group Psychotherapy, Psychodrama, and Sociometry 24,* 323–332.

Dixon, N.F. (1980). A cognitive alternative to stress? In I.G. Sarason & C.D. Spielberger (Eds.), *Stress and anxiety* (pp. 281–288). Washington, D.C.: Hemisphere.

Dugan, D. (1989). Laughter and tears: Best medicine for stress. *Nursing Forum, XXIV,* 18–26.

Eastwood, M.R., Rifat, S.L., Nobbs, H., & Ruderman, J. (1989). Mood disorder following cerebrovascular accident. *British Journal of Psychiatry, 154,* 195–200.

Ebrahim, S., Baer, D., & Nouri, F. (1987). Affective illness after stroke. *British Journal of Psychiatry, 151,* 56–57.

Eisenson, J. (1984). *Adult aphasia.* Englewood Cliffs, NJ: Prentice-Hall.

Feibel, J.H., & Springer, C.J. (1982). Depression and failure to resume social activities after stroke. *Archives of Physical Medicine and Rehabilitation, 63,* 276–278.

Fink, M. (1982). Convulsive therapy: A risk-benefit analysis. *Psychopharmacology Bulletin, 18,* 110–116.

Fink, M. (1984). Neuroendocrine aspects of the relief of melancholia by induced seizures (electroconvulsive treatment). *Advances in Biochemical Psychopharmacology 39,* 345–357.

Finklestein, S., Weintraub, R., Davar, G., Karmouz, N., Asklnazl, C., & Baldessarini, R. (1987). Antidepressant drug treatment of post-stroke depression: Retrospective study. *Archives of Physical Medicine and Rehabilitation, 68,* 772–776.

Folstein, M.F., Mailberger, R., & McHugh, P.R. (1977). Mood disorder as a specific complication of stroke. *Journal of Neurology, Neurosurgery, and Psychiatry, 40,* 1018–1020.

Francis, G. (1991). Here come the puppies: The power of the human/animal bond. *Holistic Nursing Practice, 5,* 11–15.

Friedland, J., & McColl, M.A. (1987). Social support and psychosocial dysfunction after stroke: Buffering Effects in a community sample. *Archives of Physical Medicine and Rehabilitation, 68,* 475–480.

Friedland, J., & McColl, M.A. (1989). Social support for stroke survivors: Development and evaluation of an intervention program. *Physical and Occupational Therapy in Geriatrics, 7,* 55–69.

Gainotti, G. (1972). Emotional behavior and hemispheric side of the lesion. *Cortex, 8,* 41–55.

Garrity, T., Stallones, L., Marx, M., & Johnson, T. (1989). Pet ownership and attachment as supportive factors in the health of the elderly. *Anthrozoos, 3,* 35–44.

Gurland, B.J., & Copeland, J. (1983). *The mind and mood of aging.* New York: Croom Helm.

Hamilton, M. (1960). A rating scale for depression. *Journal of Neurology, Neurosurgery, and Psychiatry, 12,* 189–198.

Holbrook, S.E. (1982). Stroke: Social and emotional outcome. *Journal of the Royal College of Physicians of London, 16,* 100–104.

House, A., Dennis, M., Hawton, K., & Warlow, C. (1989). Method of identifying mood disorders in stroke patients: Experience in the Oxfordshire community stroke project. *Age and Aging, 18,* 371–379.

House, A., Dennis, M., Molyneux, A., Warlow, C., & Hawton, K. (1989). Emotionalism after stroke. *British Medical Journal, 298,* 991–994.

Hyman, M. (1971). The stigma of stroke, its effects on performance during and after rehabilitation. *Geriatrics, 26,* 132–141.

Kay, D.W.K., Beamish, P., & Roth, M. (1964). Old age mental disorders in Newcastle upon Tyne. *British Journal of Psychiatry, 110,* 668–682.

Kinsella, G., & Duffy, F. (1978). The spouse of the aphasic patient. In Y. Lebrun (Ed.), *The management of aphasia.* Amsterdam & Lisse: Swets & Zeitlinger.

Kinsella, G., & Duffy, F. (1979). Psychosocial readjustments in the spouses of aphasic patients. *Scandinavian Journal of Rehabilitative Medicine, 11,* 129–132.

Labi, M., Phillips, T., & Gresham, G. (1980). Psychosocial disability in physically restored long-term stroke survivors. *Archives of Physical Medicine and Rehabilitation, 61,* 561–565.

Lawrence, L., & Christie, D. (1979). Quality of life after stroke: A three year follow-up. *Age and Aging, 8,* 167–172.

Lipsey, J.R., Spenser, W.C., Robins, P.V., & Robinson, R.G. (1986). Phenomenological comparison of post-stroke depression and functional depression. *American Journal of Psychiatry, 143,* 527–529.

Ljungdahl, L. (1989). Laugh if this is a joke. *Journal of the American Medical Association, 261,* 558.

Lubinski, R. (1981). Languages and aging: An environmental approach to intervention. *Topics in Language Disorders, 1,* 89–97.

Martin, R.A., & Lefcourt, H.M. (1983). Sense of humor as a moderator of the relation between stressors and moods. *Journal of Personality and Social Psychology, 45,* 1313–1324.

Mesulam, M.M. (1985). *Principles of behavioral neurology.* Philadelphia: F.A. Davis.

Morrison, J.H., Molliver, M.E., & Grzanna, R. (1979). Noradrenergic innervation of the cerebral cortex: Widespread effects of local cortical lesions. *Science, 205,* 313–316.

Mullins, L., & Dugan, E. (1980). The influence of depression and family and friendship relations on residents' loneliness in congregate housing. *The Gerontologist, 30,* 293–307.

Murphy, E. (1982). Social origins of depression in old age. *British Journal of Psychiatry, 141,* 135–142.

Murry, G.B., Shea, V., & Conn, D.K. (1987). Electroconvulsive therapy for post-stroke depression. *Journal of Clinical Psychiatry, 47,* 258–260.

O'Connell, W.E. (1976). The eupsychia of everyday life. In A.J. Chapman & H. Foot (Eds.), *Humor and laughter: Theory, research and applications.* London: Wiley.

Overs, R., & Belknap, E. (1967). Educating stroke patient families. *Journal of Chronic Disorders, 20,* 45–51.

Nussbaum, J., Thompson, T., & Robinson, J. (1989). *Communication and aging.* New York: Harper & Row.

Parikh, R.M., Lipsey, J.R., Robinson, R.G., & Price, T.R. (1987). Two-year longitudinal study of post-stroke mood disorders: Dynamic changes in correlates of depression at one and two years. *Stroke, 18,* 579–584.

Parikh, R.M., Lipsey, J.R., Robinson, R.G., & Price, T.R. (1988). A two year longitudinal study of post-stroke mood disorders: Prognostic factors related to outcome. *International Journal of Psychiatry in Medicine, 18,* 45–56.

Parikh, R.M., Robinson, R.G., Lipsey, J.R., Starkstein, S.E., Fedoroff, J.P., & Price, T.R. (1990). The impact of post-stroke depression on recovery in activities of daily living over a 2-year follow-up. *Archives of Neurology, 47,* 485–789.

Parmallei, P., Lawton, M., & Katz, I. (1989). Psychometric properties of the geriatric depression scale among the institutionalized aged. *Psychological Assessment, 4,* 331–338.

Peter, L.J., & Dana, B. (1982). *The laughter prescription.* Toronto: Dana Corwin Enterprises.

Pickel, V.M., Segal, M., & Bloom, F.E. (1974). A radioautographic study of the different pathways of the nucleus locus coeruleus. *Journal of Comparative Neurology, 155,* 15–42.

Price, T. (1990). Affective disorders after stroke. *Stroke, 21*(Suppl II), 12–13.

Rapp, S., Parisi, A., Walsh, D., & Wallace, C. (1988). Detecting depression in elderly medical patients. *Journal of Consulting and Clinical Psychology, 56,* 509–513.

Reding, M.J., Orto, L.A., Winter, S.W., Fortune, I.M., Ponte, P.D., & McDowell, F. (1986). Antidepressant therapy after stroke. *Archives of Neurology, 43,* 763–765.

Rice, B., Paul, A., & Muller, D.J. (1986). An evaluation of a social support group for spouses of aphasic partners. *Aphasiology, 1,* 247–256.

Robinson, R.G. (1986). Post-stroke mood disorders. *Hospital Practice, 21,* 83–89.

Robinson, R.G., & Benson, D.F. (1981). Depression in aphasic patients: Frequency, severity, and clinical-pathological correlations. *Brain and Language, 14,* 282–291.

Robinson, R.G., Bolduc, P.L., & Price, T.R. (1987). Two-year longitudinal study of post-stroke mood disorders: Diagnosis and outcome at one and two years. *Stroke, 18,* 837–843.

Robinson, R.G., Bolla-Wilson, K., Kaplan, E., Lipsey, J.R., & Price, T.R. (1986). Depression influences intellectual impairment in stroke patients. *British Journal of Psychiatry, 148,* 541–547.

Robinson, R.G., & Price, T.R. (1982). Post-stroke depressive disorders: A follow-up study of 103 patients. *Stroke, 13,* 635–641.

Robinson, R.G., & Starkstein, S.E. (1990). Current research in affective disorders following stroke. *Journal of Neuropsychiatry, 2,* 1–14.

Robinson, R.G., Starkstein, S.E., & Price, T.R. (1988). Post-stroke depression and lesion location. *Stroke, 19*, 125–126.

Robinson, R.G., Starr, L.B., & Price, T.R. (1984). A two-year longitudinal study of mood disorder following stroke: Prevalence and duration at six months follow-up. *British Journal of Psychiatry, 144*, 256–262.

Rollin, W.J. (1987). *The psychology of communication disorders.* Englewood Cliffs, NJ: Prentice-Hall.

Ross, E.D., & Rush, A.J. (1981). Diagnosis and neuroanatomical correlates of depression in brain damaged patients. *Archives of General Psychiatry, 38*, 1344–1354.

Ross, S. (1991). Personal communication. Green Chimneys Children's Services, Inc. Brewster, NY.

Sackeim, H.A., & Greenberg, M.S. (1982). Hemispheric asymmetry in the expression of positive and negative emotions: Neurological evidence. *Archives of Neurology, 39*, 210–218.

Schmitt, N. (1990). Patients' perception of laughter in a rehabilitation hospital. *Rehabilitation Nursing, 15*, 143–146.

Silverman, E.K., & Weingartner, H. (1986). Hemispheric lateralization of functions related to emotion. *Brain and Cognition, 5*, 322–353.

Singler, J. (1975). Group work with hospitalized stroke patients. *Social Casework, 56*, 348–354.

Sinyor, D., Jacques, P., Kaloupek, D.G., Becker, R., Goldenbert, M., & Coopersmith, H. (1986). Post-stroke depression and lesion location: An attempted replication. *Brain, 109*, 537–546.

Sjogren, K. (1982). Leisure after stroke. *International Rehabilitation Medicine, 4*, 80–87.

Smith, G.E. (1989). *Patterns of self-reported symptomatology in post-stroke depression.* Presented at the 97th Annual Meeting of the American Psychological Association, New Orleans.

Spitzer, R., Endicott, J., & Robins, E. (1975). *Research Diagnostic Criteria (RDC) for a group of functional disorders.* New York: Biometrics Research Division, New York Psychiatric Institute.

Starkstein, S., & Robinson, R. (1989). Affective disorders and cerebral vascular disease. *British Journal of Psychiatry, 154*, 170–182.

Starkstein, S.E., Robinson, R.G., Honig, M.A., Parikh, R.M., Joselyn, J., & Price, T.R. (1989). Mood changes after right-hemisphere lesions. *British Journal of Psychiatry, 155*, 79–85.

Starkstein, S.E., Robinson, R.G., & Price, T.R. (1988). Comparison of patients with and without post-stroke major depression matched for size and location of lesion. *Archives of General Psychiatry, 45*, 247–252.

Swindell, C.S., & Hammons, J.A. (1991). Poststroke depression: Neurologic, physiologic, diagnostic and treatment implications. *Journal of Speech and Hearing Research, 34*, 325–333.

Tompkins, C.A., Schultz, K., & Rauk, M.T. (1988). Post-stroke depression in primary support persons: Predicting those at risk. *Journal of Consulting and Clinical Psychology, 56*, 502–506.

Turkat, D. (1980). Social networks: Theory and practice. *Journal of Community Psychology, 8*, 99–109.

Wade, D.T., Legh-Smith, J., & Hewer, R.A. (1987). Depressed mood after stroke: A community study of its frequency. *British Journal of Psychiatry, 151*, 200–205.

Wahrborg, P. (1989). Aphasia and family therapy. *Aphasiology, 3*, 479–482.

Wahrborg, P., & Borenstein, P. (1989). Family therapy in families with an aphasic member. *Aphasiology, 3*, 93–98.

Wahrborg, P., & Borenstein, P. (1990) Depression after stroke: Some nosological considerations. In R. Simon & J. Stark (Eds.), *The First European Conference on Aphasiology.* The Austrian Workers Compensation Board.

Walsh, J.J. (1928). *Laughter and health.* New York/London: D. Appleton and Company.

Webster, E.J., & Newhoff, M. (1981). Intervention with families of communicatively impaired adults. In D.S. Beasley & G.A. Davis (Eds.), *Aging communication process and disorders.* New York: Grune & Stratton.

Weiss, I., Nagel, C., & Aronson, M. (1986). Applicability of depression scales to the old old person. *Journal of the American Geriatrics Society, 34*, 215–218.

Williams, S.E., & Freer, C.A. (1986). Aphasia: Its effect on marital relationships. *Archives of Physical Medicine and Rehabilitation, 67*, 250–252.

Zung, W.W.K. (1965). A self-rating depression scale. *Archives of General Psychiatry, 12*, 63–70.

Chapter 18

Planning Rehabilitation Services for Rural and Remote Communities

Daniel D. Anderson, Maureen H. Fitzgerald, Herbert K. M. Yee, and Gloriajean L. Wallace

Large urban centers, especially in the developed world, have well-established systems for providing health and rehabilitation services. Indeed, most service providers are located in large urban centers. However, most of the world's population resides in rural and often remote communities. For this segment of the population, medical services are not as accessible, and rehabilitation services are practically nonexistent (Elling, 1980).

Rural and remote communities present special challenges for the development of rehabilitation service delivery systems (Lazarus, Page, & Barcome, 1984; Schneider, Leland, & Ferritor, 1986). These communities rarely have the physical, economic, and personnel resources that are available in large urban centers. The number of individuals requiring rehabilitation services in a given community may be small, and the distances between them great. Each community presents unique needs, mix of resources, and challenges to service delivery. Thus, information obtained for one community may not be transferable to others (Doezema, Skler, Roth, Rodolico, & Key, 1991; Maretzki, 1990).

No single service delivery model can address the rehabilitation needs of every rural community. However, several factors increase the likelihood of establishing an effective program. These include (1) a supportive context (understanding and support from community leaders); (2) community involvement in assessing needs and planning services; (3) a well-developed plan of implementation; and (4) the commitment of adequate resources, including well-trained personnel. Although programs must be tailored to each community's needs and resources, the process of planning service delivery programs is much the same for all communities. In fact, in many respects, program planning at the community level parallels a process that the reader may find familiar: planning for the individual client.

This chapter presents a framework for planning rehabilitation services for individuals, compares that framework to a model for planning service programs in rural and remote communities, and presents two examples of rehabilitation program development (one general and one specific to speech-language pathology) from our experiences in the Pacific Basin.

PLANNING REHABILITATION SERVICES FOR THE INDIVIDUAL

A service provider generally follows a series of logical steps when planning services for an individual client. The provider obtains background information about the client's capabilities, suspected service needs, cultural background, and available resources. This information provides a foundation of general knowledge for constructing an assessment plan. The assessment of specific service needs (e.g., speech-language pathology) often uses a "performance deficit" model (Scriven & Roth, 1990) to determine whether the client has impaired performance that affects functioning in day-to-day home, school, or employment activities. A word of caution when using a "performance deficit" model for assessment planning—Sue, Arredondo, and McDavis (1992) remind us that the deficit model can be harmful if it is used to portray an individual or group as inferior (i.e., "disadvantaged" or "deprived"). Assessments should emphasize strengths as well as limitations.

Service objectives that reflect the desired behavior can be stated, and procedures designed to help the client reach specific objectives can be implemented and evaluated. These steps in the rehabilitation planning process are listed in Table 18.1. At each step along the way, the clinician ensures that decisions are guided by information provided collectively by the client, the client's family, assessment data obtained by the clinician, and information from other service providers.

Those planning rehabilitation services in a rural community can use a step-by-step process similar to the one used in planning individualized services. Steps in the process of planning community services are listed in Table 18.1 and are described below.

BACKGROUND

Information from community members needs to be considered to obtain a comprehensive profile of likely program needs. This general description of service needs may also be called a "service deficit" (Roth, 1990; Scriven & Roth, 1990), a term that parallels the concept of "performance deficit," described in the previous section on planning for the individual client.

Service deficit refers to the discrepancy between the services desired by the community and the services actually available (Roth, 1990; Scriven &

TABLE 18.1 Steps in Planning Rehabilitation for the Individual and for Communities

I. Individual
   A. Background Information
      1. Suspected services needed
      2. Cultural background
      3. Resources
   B. Assessment plan
   C. Developing treatment objectives
   D. Developing treatment procedures and treatment implementation
   E. Treatment evaluation
II. Community
   A. Background information
      1. Suspected program needs
      2. Community context
      3. Organizational context
      4. Target population
      5. Economic resources
   B. Needs assessment
   C. Developing program objectives
   D. Program planning and implementation
   E. Program evaluation

Roth, 1990). A service deficit approach to planning has been used with communities in the Pacific Basin. For example, in the early 1980s, a rehabilitation technician program was developed in the U.S.-affiliated Pacific Islands in response to concern that six of nine jurisdictions offered no rehabilitation services (i.e., no physical therapy, occupational therapy, or speech-language and hearing services). The health directors for these regions specified that each of the nine rural, remote island communities should have a minimum of one rehabilitation technician. This individual would serve a transdisciplinary role by providing basic yet comprehensive rehabilitation services.

Community participation and input is also necessary in the collection of other background and planning information regarding community context, organizational context, target population, and economic resources.

Community Context

Our concern with community context is based on the fact that a program and its environment are interdependent. Therefore, general knowledge of the community context is essential for effective program planning. New service programs are often located within existing community organizations. Thus, knowledge of a program's potential or existing organizational environment is also essential and will be discussed below.

Planners might begin a context assessment with a set of general questions related to community conditions. Those questions may include the following: How large is the general population? Is the community homogeneous or culturally, socially, and economically diverse? How large a geographic area will be served? Are there reasonable, reliable, economical, and readily available means of transportation and communication? What is the social and political structure of the community? Is the community in general and target population in particular, individual- or family-oriented? Are people comfortable using resources outside of the family network? Will traditional beliefs about social relationships, health, or health and human services affect the use of new services?

Organizational Context

General information about a community serves as a foundation for more specific questions about organizations through which services may be provided. Sample questions might include: What is the current organizational structure for delivering rehabilitation or similar services? Who is being (or can be) served by the organizations? What organizational factors (e.g., personnel and fiscal resources, service policies and procedures) affect service delivery? How does the organization that may house a new program respond to change? Will organizational employees be threatened or invigorated by the prospect of change? Who, in addition to persons from the target population, are the key stakeholders (e.g., employers, unions, professional organizations) in the services being planned? Who are the key decision makers?

Target Population

Given some knowledge of the community and the population in general, a service planner can then focus on the target population. Among the questions to consider: What segment(s) of the general population are to be addressed and included in planning? How might that target population be described (by size, age groups, locations, etc.)? Can all persons in the target population be served? Is the target population likely to increase (if, for example, more cases are likely to be identified) or decrease (if, for example, the proposed program or other programs will address causative factors) in the future?

Economic Resources

The availability of funding influences service delivery regardless of the needs of the target population, program objectives, or the availability of other resources (such as trained personnel). The following questions may help assess the availability of financial resources: What are the potential sources of funding (e.g., consumers, service agency, third-party, etc.) for the program being planned? Will services be subsidized (as in a government-supported program or sponsorship by a philanthropic organization)? Will third-party payments (such as insurance) be involved? What will the client be expected to contribute to the funding of services?

NEEDS ASSESSMENT

General information about the context (both community and organization) in which a program must function and information about the program's target population provides the program planner with a foundation for assessing service needs. As indicated above, needs assessments frequently focus on discrepancies between a desired level of service and the present condition. Planners should have a clear understanding of the rationale for selecting the desired condition. This selection might be based on an ideal (and perhaps unattainable) rehabilitation service system. Alternatively, the desired condition might be (1) based on the norm or what is available in other communities, or (2) a minimal level of service (Roth, 1990). Frequently rehabilitation service planners work with communities that desire minimal services, because those communities have very limited resources and histories of services.

Questions that might guide an assessment of need might include the following: Who will determine the desired level of service? Can that level of service be used as a standard for assessing existing services? Does that standard represent an ideal, a norm, or a minimal condition? Based on knowledge of existing resources and the other aspects of community context, is the desired level of service appropriate and realistic? What are the community's needs (the discrepancy between the desired and existing conditions)? Given the available resources, is it reasonable to expect that needs can be addressed through new (or changed) services?

This stage of planning involves the balance of needs and resources. If the process focuses too much on needs and does not adequately consider the availability of resources, then the plan developed may not be implemented because of insufficient resources. On the other hand, a process that is limited to planning services based on the use of existing resources is unlikely to expand or improve services and address the new needs identified in the assessment.

Anderson (1985) describes the difficulty of balancing needs and resources when planning community-based services, and highlights traps that hinder effective planning. He suggests that planners may be trapped by nebulous or incomplete assessments of need. A clear understanding of needs is required for effective planning. However, comprehensive needs assessments often reveal needs that surpass available resources. Thus planners can be trapped by "priority paralysis" if they are unable or unwilling to prioritize needs. Planners must also overcome the inertia associated with the use of existing resources. This resource rigidity must be addressed if new needs are to be served by existing resources that may be limited.

DEVELOPING PROGRAM OBJECTIVES

Objectives may be developed and described (1) in terms of what the planner expects the program to do (for example, to provide a particular kind or amount of rehabilitation services) or (2) in terms of outcomes or what the program's clients may be expected to do (for example, persons served will be able to function more independently). Planners may wish to develop both process objectives (what the program will do) and outcome objectives (what the program will accomplish). However, it is more important to focus on the persons served and to plan in terms of outcomes. Also, it is useful to develop objectives in terms of realistic deadlines and dates.

Questions such as the following may help plan program objectives: What needs or problems does the project aim to address or solve? For each need or problem, what is the program supposed to accomplish? How long will it take to accomplish each objective? As a result of the services that may be provided, what will clients be able to do or how will clients be different? How will the community be different? Are there likely to be undesired outcomes associated with the program?

PROGRAM PLANNING AND IMPLEMENTATION

To accomplish a program's objectives, services must be provided. Questions that may help design services include the following: For each program objective, what kind of services are to be provided? Who will provide services? What role will be played by professionals in specific disciplines (physical therapy, speech-language therapy, etc.)? Will there be interdisciplinary, multidisciplinary, or transdisciplinary service delivery? Will services cut across professional roles and organizational lines?

Given a particular community context and target population, there may be a need to plan services or activities with consideration of cultural taboos or beliefs about health, healing, and appropriate behavior. For example, in the Pacific Basin the gender of the service provider is an important cultural factor to be considered in the planning of rehabilitation services. Also, assistive devices and clinical tools must be culturally appropriate if they are to be effectively used.

Knowledge from the assessment of organizational context contributes to the planning of service delivery. Questions that may assist in planning services include: Who are the stakeholders in the program being planned and in the host organization? What is the level of stakeholder commitment to the program? Who will organize, manage, and administer service delivery? What will the relationships be among the new service program and established community programs and organizations? Will services be centralized (as in a clinic or hospital) or decentralized (as in community outreach)? Is there an established infrastructure to support program development? Are any of the services or related services currently available? If so, who provides them? Will current service providers be supportive or reactionary? Will current providers be incorporated into the new program?

Questions that may assist in personnel planning include: What kind of personnel will the program need and what roles will they play? Specifically, who will provide services? The scarcity of trained personnel can significantly limit the development of services in rural and remote communities. Are there appropriately trained personnel already in the area? Are there individuals who can be readily trained to provide services? Are resources for training personnel available?

Given knowledge of the community context and the target population, should service providers be from the same culture as their clients? If service providers are from other cultures, what provisions are there (1) to enhance the provider's knowledge of the culture(s) served and (2) to encourage cross-cultural sensitivity? Will the community and an organization accept change (e.g., an "outsider" providing services and a new service role)?

PROGRAM EVALUATION

Evaluation should be an integral part of every program. Planners and their stakeholders may have specific evaluation questions that they would like to answer. However, at a minimum, evaluation questions should address service delivery, outcome, and program impact. The following general evaluation questions may be helpful. First, are services being delivered as planned or intended? Second, are program objectives (outcomes) being accomplished? Third, are the needs or problems of the individuals for whom the program was intended being addressed? Is the program providing services desired by the community?

TWO EXAMPLES OF PROGRAM DEVELOPMENT

Examples of rehabilitation programs in the Pacific Basin are presented. First, a group of island-based rehabilitation programs that were established at about the same time and continue to be supported through training and technical assistance are briefly described. Second, the process of planning for the development of speech-language rehabilitation services in one Pacific Island community—American Samoa—is more fully described.

THE PACIFIC BASIN REHABILITATION TECHNICIAN PROGRAM

Background

The health directors for the rural, remote island communities in the U.S.-affiliated Pacific Islands identified the need for rehabilitation services. The Pacific Basin Rehabilitation Research and Training Center (PBRRTC) agreed to provide technical assistance for program development and technical training for the service providers. Once these individuals, called rehabilitation technicians, were in place and providing services, the plan was to gradually increase their range of skills.

Needs Assessment

Rehabilitation service needs were delineated by health directors for each of nine island communities located in the Pacific Basin. Directors of health used a service deficit model in their approach to assessing needs. Minimum standards for rehabilitation services were established and existing services were assessed in relation to the desired minimum standard. Three communities had developed services that approached the desired level of service. Six communities had little or no rehabilitation services at the time of the initial assessment.

Program Objectives

Initially, program objectives focused on service development, for example, to train one rehabilitation service provider from each community to provide basic, fundamental rehabilitation services. While program development has not addressed all of the rehabilitation needs in each of the communities, it has resulted in the provision of basic services. Over time, outcome objectives have been developed for each program. Those objectives address the needs of specific populations (e.g., persons with stroke), or service needs (e.g., more cost-effective prosthetics), or both.

Program Plans and Implementation

Service delivery models were developed with the involvement of administrators, service providers, representatives of the community, and organizations that provide training and technical assistance (e.g., PBRRTC). Each island has developed a model unique to its location, available resources, community support, and so forth. Two general hospital-based models have emerged: (1) a clinic staffed by rehabilitation technicians, who are Pacific Basin island-trained health care providers (e.g., nurses) who receive annual in-service training and have continuous access to technical assistance, and

(2) a therapy clinic staffed by a contract physical therapist with support from a rehabilitation technician. Training and technical assistance resources from the PBRRTC have been used to support programs based on either of the two models.

Evaluation

On an annual basis, health administrators, service providers, and PBRRTC staff evaluate each of the nine island-based rehabilitation programs. Evaluation information is then used to plan program improvement that addresses specific identified needs. A continuous cycle of assessment and improvement has been implemented.

Briefly, the four standard evaluation questions listed below are answered for the Pacific Basin programs as a group.

1. Are services being delivered as planned? Basic rehabilitation services are being provided as planned. Programs that use contract physical therapists have experienced difficulty in filling positions. However, island staff have provided continuity of service.

2. Are program objectives being accomplished? Information from each program indicates that programs are accomplishing their individualized objectives. Accomplishments include the development of services that, at one time, could only be obtained off-island. Data describing the number of persons served last year revealed a 30% increase over the previous year.

3. Are the needs of individuals for whom the program was intended being addressed? Programs were designed to meet the needs of persons with physical disabilities resulting from stroke, diabetes, trauma, and so forth. In general, the needs of persons with physical disabilities are being met. However, programs have not been effective in addressing the needs of children with disabilities or the needs of adults with cognitive rehabilitation needs and speech-language rehabilitation needs.

4. Is the program providing the services desired by the community? Programs are, for the most part, providing the desired services. However, effective service delivery has resulted in increased expectations in all island communities. Also, as indicated above, the needs of specific populations (e.g., children and those with speech-language impairments) are not being addressed. Thus, in each community program standards are being increased. Demands for additional and improved services include: (1) special education-related services for children with disabilities; (2) speech-language services; (3) increased staffing of hospital-based clinics; (4) the development of community-based service delivery strategies; and (5) disability prevention programs that focus on problems related to stroke and diabetes.

Development of Speech-Language Rehabilitation Services in American Samoa

Background

American Samoa, an unincorporated territory of the United States, is located some 2,300 miles southwest of Hawaii. Samoa is composed of five islands, Tutuila, Aunu'u, Ta'u, Ofu, Olosega, and an atoll with two islets named Rose Island, which collectively are situated on a land mass of 76 square miles. American Samoans are Polynesians. Most live on the island of Tutuila (53 square miles), which houses the only major medical facility, Lyndon Baines Johnson Tropical Medical Center (LBJ). Since the establishment of a U.S. naval base on Tutuila in 1900, the territory has been increasingly affected by Americanization. Some speculate that as the American influence has increased over the years, it has become a major contributor to the increasing prevalence of stroke. Changes in diet from fresh foods (obtained from daily fishing and farming) to the consumption of canned foods, which are high in salt and fat; stress from changing economic and employment patterns; and increases in the prevalence of hypertension and diabetes have all been cited as possible contributors (Hawaii Rehabilitation, Research, and Training Center, 1986).

While only about 7% of the 45,000 residents of Samoa are 55 years of age or older (American Samoa Economic Development Planning Office, 1990; Anderson, 1989), concern about stroke in this segment of the population has prompted recognition of the need for rehabilitation services. The LBJ Physical Therapy Department, when fully staffed, has two physical therapists (PTs), one occupational therapist (OT), and one rehabilitation technician. The Department of Vocational Rehabilitation (DVR) in Samoa is currently expanding its outreach services to include individuals who have suffered a stroke. The DVR works very closely with the Honolulu-based Pacific Basin Rehabilitation, Research, and Training Center (PBRRTC), which provides ongoing in-service training to medical professionals and allied health professionals in Samoa and other countries in the Pacific Basin (Anderson, 1989). The services are primarily targeted to enhance nursing care, medical rehabilitation, and vocational rehabilitation services for stroke patients.

These efforts are invaluable. However, available treatment options for patients with stroke-related impairments in communication and feeding are minimal. Deficits in these areas are typically managed by a speech-language pathologist. Until January 1993, Samoa had only one provider of speech-language pathology services for the entire territory. This person holds a bachelor's degree in general communications and a master's degree in special education. Her responsibilities include regular assessment and treatment of cases handled by the Department of Special Education, and more recently (as of September 1990) consultation services for LBJ and the DVR.

In January 1993, another Samoan returned to Samoa with a master's degree in speech-language pathology after being recruited and mentored by one of the authors (Gloriajean L. Wallace). Although this individual is employed by the Department of Special Education, she is qualified to provide direct and consultation services for individuals with communication and swallowing impairments secondary to stroke.

Because of the limited speech-language pathology services available in Samoa, patients with neurologically based communication and feeding impairments sometimes receive services from public health nurses and other health professionals who are not trained in speech-language pathology. Key community officials indicated an interest in exploring the need for expanding rehabilitation services available in Samoa. This interest provided the impetus for the needs assessment efforts, described below.

Needs Assessment

Data from the patient medical files at LBJ were examined to determine the annual incidence of stroke (Wallace, 1993). Seventy-four new stroke cases were identified over a 1-year period (June 1, 1989, to May 31, 1990). This included 29 adults who were admitted with a stroke diagnosis and who survived to the point of discharge (mean age 65 years; SD = 8.15), and 45 adults (mean age 68 years; SD = 13.35) who were recorded as suffering stroke-related fatality. Although individuals from a variety of ethnic backgrounds (including Korean, Tongan, European, Japanese, Chinese, Filipino, Micronesian, and Fijian) are treated at LBJ, only individuals of Samoan ancestry incurred new episodes of stroke during the initial period of data collection (June 1, 1989, to May 31, 1990). Primary risk factors for the reported episodes of stroke were hypertension and diabetes. The high stroke mortality rate in American Samoa is likely due to a combination of factors including the high incidence of hypertension and resulting hemorrhagic stroke, which results in mortality more often than occlusive stroke. LBJ Tropical Medical Center does not have a neurologist, a neurosurgeon, or a neuroradiologic diagnostic department. The unavailability of these services hinders efforts to provide early detection and prohibits the opportunity for timely medical management, particularly for individuals who have incurred hemorrhagic stroke.

Face-to-face field interviews were conducted to obtain information about the rehabilitation needs and available services for residents identified as having incurred stroke. These house-to-house surveys were conducted with individuals who had incurred stroke and their families. The surveys suggested that the Physical Therapy Department at LBJ was effective in making services available to all stroke patients who had difficulty with ambulation or using their extremities. Neither direct nor indirect speech-language pathology services were reported for the stroke patients who indicated that they had residual impairments in communication and swallowing (Wallace, 1993). DVR and LBJ staff assisted with all phases of data collection for the needs assessment.

Program Objectives

The results of the needs assessment were shared with staff at the DVR and LBJ, and with political officials in Samoa. A plan of action was developed with the following program objectives in mind:

1. Establishment of a multiagency stroke team to focus on the rehabilitation needs of the patient from the acute through the chronic stages of recovery (Wallace, 1995).
2. Development of a mechanism for ongoing training of team members on issues pertaining to the rehabilitation needs of stroke patients. Training will entail incorporating family and community members in the recovery and community re-entry process.
3. Government support for educational training of one master's-level speech-language pathologist who will serve as speech-language pathology rehabilitation consultant to the team. Until training of this individual is completed, services will be provided by the M.A.-level speech-language pathologist who is employed by the Department of Special Education on a consultation basis.
4. Community education about factors associated with the risk of stroke and stroke prevention.

Because of constraints on government finances, outside funding is currently being sought to help accomplish the above objectives, which are supported in concept by DVR and LBJ staff.

Development and implementation of activities to help meet these objectives are currently underway. One such activity is an annual LBJ-sponsored interdisciplinary workshop designed to provide nurses and other health care personnel with basic updated information on the management of communication and swallowing impairments that may occur after stroke. The workshop will be open to staff from LBJ, DVR, and the Department of Special Education. In addition to providing basic information about stroke rehabilitation, the workshop will provide an opportunity for organizing a multiagency stroke team and community-based stroke-related organizations such as the American Heart Association (InterAmerican Heart Division) and the National Aphasia Association. Development of community-based stroke-related organizations may be instrumental in future prevention efforts, which are important, given the high stroke mortality in Samoa and the preponderance of hypertension and diabetes in the Samoan population.

Evaluation

The success of the program will be gauged by information provided by pre- and post-workshop test scores, and the longevity, quality, and level of activity of the stroke team and stroke-related community-based organizations. Follow-up assessment will be conducted for each objective to be targeted. One aspect of this assessment will entail a follow-up review of the LBJ medical files to determine whether these efforts have resulted in a reduction in the annual incidence of stroke. Individuals identified as having incurred stroke would be surveyed to explore the scope and quality of services. The data would be compared to the previously collected data, reported earlier.

CONCLUSIONS

This chapter began with discussion of the challenges associated with developing rehabilitation services in rural and remote communities. Planning community-based rehabilitation services, like planning services for a client, needs to be a collaborative process that involves those who will be served as well as those who can contribute to service delivery. Service providers, because of their experience in planning services for individual clients, can be effective community planners. The process of planning services for individual clients can serve as a framework for planning community services; questions at each step in community planning can guide the process. By sharing this framework and a few experiences in planning rehabilitation services in rural and remote communities, we hope to have kindled an interest in serving rural and remote communities.

As everyone knows, there is no sure method for developing or improving community services. However, as Caplow (1976) suggests, there may be a "nearly magical" method for enhancing our capabilities to do so. According to Caplow, that magical enhancement can be achieved nine out of 10 times by providing an "intelligent emphasis on planning in a reasonably democratic spirit" (p. 22).

REFERENCES

American Samoa Economic Development Planning Office, Research and Statistics Division, American Samoan Government. (1990). *American Samoa statistical digest*. American Samoa: Author.

Anderson, D.D. (1985). Planning comprehensive community based service. In M.P. Brady & P.L. Gunter (Eds.), *Integrating moderately and severely handicapped learners* (pp. 47–62). Springfield, IL: Charles C. Thomas.

Anderson, D. (1989). *Pacific basin rehabilitation, research, and training center final report*. Cooperative Agreement #G0084C0001 from the NIDRR, Office of Special Education and Rehabilitative Services, U.S. Department of Education, Washington, D.C. (for period: October 2, 1984–February 28, 1989).

Caplow, T. (1976). *How to run any organization: Manual of practical sociology* (p. 22). Hinsdale, IL: Dryden Press.

Doezema, D., Skler, D.P., Roth, P.B., Rodolico, M.P., & Key, G. (1991). Development of emergency services in Costa Rica: A collaborative project in international health. *Journal of the American Medical Association, 265,* 188–190.

Elling, R.H. (1980). *Cross-national study of health systems: Political economics and health care.* New Brunswick: Transaction Books.

Hawaii Rehabilitation, Research, and Training Center (RRT). (1986). *Demographic data base and rehabilitation resources of Pacific Island nations.* (Report prepared by the RRT, NIDRR Cooperative Agreement #G0084C001). Honolulu: John A. Burns School of Medicine, Rehabilitation Hospital of the Pacific.

Lazarus, S.S., Page, C.M., & Barcome, D.F. (1984). Rehabilitation services in rural communities delivered by hospital based and local teams. *Archives of Physical Medicine and Rehabilitation, 65,* 383–387.

Maretzki, T.W. (1990). Health and medical provision. In R.W. Taylor (Ed.), *Handbook of the modern world: Asia and the Pacific.* New York: Oxford Facts on File.

Roth, J. (1990). Needs and the needs assessment process. *Evaluation Practice, 11,* 141–143.

Schneider, M.J., Leland, M., & Ferritor, D.E. (1986). Rural rehabilitation. In E.L. Pan, S.S. Newman, T. Backer, & C.L. Vash (Eds.), *Annual review of rehabilitation* (Vol. 5, pp. 217–252). New York: Springer Publishing Company.

Scriven, M., & Roth, J. (1990). Special feature: Needs assessment. *Evaluation Practice, 11,* 135–139.

Sue, D.W., Arredondo, P., & McDavis, R.J. (1992). Multicultural counseling competencies and standards: A call to the profession. *Journal of Counseling and Development, 70,* 477–486.

Wallace, G. (1993). Stroke and traumatic brain injury (Ma'i Ulu) in Amerika Samoa. *Hawaii Medical Journal, 52,* 234–250.

Wallace, G. (1995). Interagency programming for partnership to enhance the quality of life for individuals with communication and swallowing impairments in American Samoa. Workshop sponsored by the Department of Special Education, June, Pago Pago, American Samoa.

Chapter 19

Stroke Prevention: A Health Promotion Approach

Carolyn M. Mayo and Robert Mayo

The 1991 publication of *Healthy People 2000: National Health Promotion and Disease Prevention Objectives* by the U. S. Department of Health and Human Services (USDHHS) clearly established the nation's health care agenda for the remaining portion of this decade. Essentially, the plan of action for the 1990s and beyond is, as stated by Louis O. Sullivan, M.D., former Secretary of the USDHHS in his foreword to *Healthy People 2000*, to establish a way of thinking and being among the American citizenry that actively promotes responsible behavior and the adoption of lifestyles that are maximally conducive to good health. Sullivan notes that implementation of the objectives outlined in the document will result in three major accomplishments for the nation:

1. Dramatically cutting health care costs
2. Preventing the premature onset of disease and disability
3. Helping all Americans achieve healthier, more productive lives

Thus, health promotion has been placed in the forefront as a national issue to be addressed by individuals at all levels of society, including persons involved in the health care professions.

More often than not, academic training for speech-language pathologists includes a preponderance of coursework that focuses on the diagnosis and treatment of disease, disability, or illness, and associated communication deficits. Courses related to neurologic deficits due to stroke often take the form of discussions surrounding causes and forms of cerebrovascular accidents, the physical and physiologic consequences of stroke, and the diagnosis and treatment of stroke-related communication deficits such as aphasia or motor speech disorders. Seldom does there exist required or even elective courses that address concepts involving communicative well-ness or the prevention of communication disorders. This chapter intro-duces the speech-language pathologist to health promotion as a concept within this discipline and discusses strategies that may help speech-lan-guage pathologists develop a program that can help delay an initial or recurrent stroke in their patients and others, including themselves. By doing so, we superimpose a body of knowledge relevant to stroke preven-tion on the traditional "medical model" approach towards rehabilitation. Stated differently, the majority of health care practitioners, including speech-language pathologists, are trained to diagnose and treat a patient or client *after* an illness or disease has already occurred (the medical model), with emphasis on reducing the effects of the disability and restoring as much former function as possible (Marge, 1988). But the scope of speech-language pathologists' practice also includes preventing disorders of speech and language (American Speech-Language-Hearing Association [ASHA], 1990). Furthermore, the current national focus on health promo-tion (Fratalli, Cherow, & Cole, 1991; Jaynes & Williams, 1989; USDHHS, 1991) calls for speech-language pathologists to use a portion of their rou-tine clinical activity to engage in prevention activities to reduce the occur-rence or reoccurrence of diseases and disabilities that may lead to commu-nication deficits. Marge (1988) refers to this newly evolving role as promot-ing health within the context of rehabilitation.

This chapter does not discuss surgical methods of preventing strokes (e.g., carotid endarterectomy; extracranial-intracranial anastomosis) in at-risk individuals. Instead, we focus attention on those activities that speech-language pathologists can routinely perform to influence the behavior and lifestyle of at-risk individuals, whether or not they have previously experi-enced a stroke.

DEFINITIONS OF HEALTH PROMOTION

A review of the literature quickly indicates that a widely agreed on defini-tion of the term *health promotion* does not exist. Few current definitions suggest that individuals with disabilities benefit from health promotion pro-grams. But there are important exceptions. For example, Michael O'Donnell (1986), chief editor of the *American Journal of Health Promotion*, defines health promotion as "the science and art of helping people change their lifestyle to move toward a state of optimal health" (p. 4). He defines optimal health as a balance of physical, emotional, social, spiritual, and intellectual health. O'Donnell further suggests that lifestyle changes can be facilitated by combining strategies that enhance awareness, change behavior, and create environments that support good health practices. Of these strategies, he notes that establishing a supportive environment tends to have the greatest impact on producing permanent, long-lasting behavioral change.

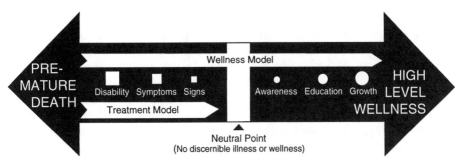

FIGURE 19–1. *The illness/wellness continuum. (From J.W. Travis and R.S. Ryan (Eds.). (1988). Wellness Workbook (2nd ed). Berkeley, CA: Ten Speed Press.)*

O'Donnell's concepts of wellness were adapted primarily from the work of John Travis, M.D., a trained physician and long-time proponent of promoting health within the context of the traditional medical model, including the rehabilitation process. In advancing his health promotion concepts, Travis (1972, 1981, 1988) captured the essence of his theory in what he described as the illness/wellness continuum (Figure 19.1). According to Travis, movement from the center to the left of the continuum shows a progressively worsening state of health, ultimately leading to the death of an individual. In contrast, movement to the right of center indicates increasing levels of health and well-being. The typical treatment model used by most health professionals moves the patient from the left of the continuum to the neutral point, where the symptoms of the disease have been alleviated. Travis also emphasizes that it is possible for a person to be physically ill and still be oriented toward wellness, or physically healthy while actually functioning from an illness mentality. For example, a disabled, sick, or dying person would typically fall on the left side of the continuum if only the physical dimension of his or her state of being were considered. However, if that same physically disabled individual takes responsibility for or maintains the locus of control of his or her life and is consciously engaged in the experience, he or she would definitely be placed on the right side of the continuum if emotional, intellectual, and spiritual dimensions were taken into account. Travis notes that this person's genuinely positive outlook would result in him or her facing to the continuum's right in the direction of high-level wellness. By contrast, a person who is physically in good health but is always complaining and worrying might be positioned to the right of the neutral point but is, in reality, facing toward the left—toward premature death. Thus, Travis purports that regardless of what point on the continuum a person might be assigned, what matters most is which direction he or she is facing. Speech-language pathologists and other health practitioners must involve themselves in holistic rehabilitation practices that maintain or shift the health paradigm of their patients in the direction of high-level wellness.

Health care professionals typically focus their attention on the left side of the continuum in an attempt to move patients toward the midpoint, where there is no discernible illness or wellness. At this midpoint, recovery is said to have reached "maximum benefits," and the patient is summarily dismissed from treatment. These same preconceptions of recovery and restoration of health are passed on to the patient. In contrast, the right end of the continuum represents a state of optimal health at which life satisfaction and resistance to disease or illness are maximized. Although O'Donnell briefly alludes to the potential benefits of health promotion activity in rehabilitating disabled individuals, Brandon (1985) notes that terms such as *wellness* and *health promotion* are typically not associated with the disabled individual or with the rehabilitation process. However, some practitioners do give credence to health promotion as a fundamental, integral part of rehabilitation. Goodstadt, Simpson, and Laranger (1987), for example, emphasize viewing rehabilitation holistically, directing patients beyond a symptom-free state and on a long-term path toward optimal wellness, by linking them to a health promotion network that ensures the continual enhancement of health following dismissal from treatment. Post-treatment continuation of health promotion efforts is important because research suggests that adults with disabilities resulting from neurologic impairment define "being healthy" more broadly than the simple *absence of illness*. Stuifbergen, Becker, Ingalsbe, and Sands (1990) report that while such individuals do not totally discount this aspect of being healthy, they place a stronger emphasis on functional, adaptive, and self-actualizing aspects of health.

Michael Marge, one of the foremost proponents of health promotion in the field of communication disorders (1984, 1988, 1990, 1991) and author of the Disabilities Prevention Act of 1991, notes the importance of including a comprehensive health promotion component in rehabilitation for disabled individuals. Marge defines *disability* as a dynamic condition that undergoes constant change from the moment of its acquisition. Marge also identified three types of prevention activities (1988) that were ultimately adapted by the American Speech-Language-Hearing Association (ASHA, 1988). Table 19.1 compares the definitions of these three forms of prevention based on statements by Marge and ASHA.

Traditionally, a speech-language pathologist's clinical activities center around tertiary prevention (i.e., assessment and management of neurogenic communication disorders). For the field to comply with the current national thrust to promote health and prevent disease, more efforts must be directed toward activities involving primary and secondary prevention. This includes but is not limited to the prevention of strokes.

EPIDEMIOLOGY AND RISK FACTORS OF STROKE

During his administration, President George Bush declared the 1990s as the "Decade of the Brain," emphasizing the need to foster joint activities between clinical and neuroscience communities and the National Institute

Table 19.1   Definitions of Primary, Secondary, and Tertiary Prevention According to Marge (1988) and ASHA (1988).

	Marge (1988)	*ASHA (1988)*
Primary preventions	The reduction of risk for disease or disability in susceptible or asymptomatic individuals. Approaches include interventions and behaviors that eliminate the cause or causes of disabilities before individual exposure.	The elimination or inhibition of the onset and development of a communication disorder by altering susceptibility or reducing exposure for susceptible persons.
Secondary preventions	The early identification and treatment of disease and disability in individuals who are displaying problems in the beginning phases of a condition. The major strategy used is screening of asymptomatic or susceptible populations.	The early detection and treatment of communication disorders. Early detection and treatment may lead to the elimination of the disorder or the retardation of the disorder's progress, thereby preventing further complications.
Tertiary prevention	Reducing the debilitating effects of a disability by intervention as soon as possible after the acquisition of the disability. The strategy used is the provision of a comprehensive intervention program to restore as much function as possible.	The reduction of a disability by attempting to restore effective functioning. The major approach is rehabilitation of the disabled individual who has realized some residual problem as a result of the disorder.

Source: Modified from M. Marge. (1988). Health promotion for persons with disabilities: Moving beyond rehabilitation. *American Journal of Health Promotion, 3*, 29–35; and American Speech-Language-Hearing Association. (1988). Position statement on the prevention of communication disorders. *ASHA, 30*, 90.)

of Neurological Disease and Stroke. These two entities were encouraged to join forces in moving ahead vigorously with research aimed at preventing and treating neurologic diseases, including stroke (Goldstein, 1990). The president's declaration was timely, given that stroke is the third leading cause of death in the United States, ranking only behind heart attack and cancer (American Heart Association, 1990; Nickens & Petersdorf, 1990).

In 1987, strokes killed about 149,200 people in the United States; the incidence of stroke was between 400,000 and 500,000 per year; and 2,060,000 persons had suffered a stroke at least once during their lives. Stroke and coronary heart disease kill more Americans than do all other diseases combined (American Heart Association, 1990). Stroke is also a major cause of disability in the United States. The Heckler Report (1985) noted that heart disease and stroke cause more deaths, disability, and economic loss in the United States than do any other acute or chronic diseases and are the leading cause of days lost from work. During the initial 30-day critical period following stroke, approximately one-third of stroke victims succumb to the disease. Despite a period of spontaneous recovery, when patients typically experience some gains in communicative, cognitive, and physical function, many survivors are left with a variety of disabilities that often require intensive rehabilitation.

The prevalence and incidence of strokes vary among age and sex cohorts. In general, strokes tend to occur more often in older people than in younger people, and about 30% more frequently in men than in women (American Heart Association, 1990). Research investigating the prevalence and incidence of stroke among racial and ethnic minority groups is sparse when compared with studies of whites. Data that do exist show that African-Americans have a considerably higher stroke mortality rate than do whites. In 1987, for example, the age-adjusted death rates for black men and women were 57.1 and 46.7 per 100,000 persons, respectively, compared to 30.3 and 26.3 for white men and women (USDHHS, 1990). Thus, African-Americans suffer "excess deaths" due to stroke. *Excess death* is defined as the difference between the number of deaths actually observed in a minority group and the number of deaths that would have occurred if members of the group died at the same rate for each age and sex cohort as the white population (Heckler, 1985).

Stroke mortality tends to be equal to or lower than that of the general U.S. population in the remaining three formally recognized racial and ethnic minority groups in the United States: American Indian/Alaska Natives, Hispanics (with the exception of younger Puerto Ricans in New York who exhibit a slightly higher incidence rate), and Asian/Pacific Islanders (Heckler, 1986). Geographic variations in stroke mortality also exist, with the highest level of stroke rates found among people living in the Southeast. Federal health officials have labeled this region of the country the "Stroke Belt."

Finally, it must be pointed out that, although stroke remains a leading killer, stroke mortality rates have been on the decline since the 1930s in both whites and nonwhites. Epidemiologic studies show an accelerated rate of decline in stroke mortality during the 1970s, with a slowdown in the rate of decline in the 1980s (Cooper, Sempos, Hsieh, & Kovar, 1990; Heckler, 1986). This decline in stroke mortality over the last two decades has been attributed to enhanced public awareness of the relationship between behavior and health outcomes, and sustained behavior change and participation of certain individuals, families, and communities in activities that promote health. (McGinnis, 1990).

Clinical trials and epidemiologic studies point to three major modifiable risk factors associated with stroke: hypertension (high blood pressure), cigarette smoking, and elevated cholesterol levels. Of the three, hypertension appears to be the most important risk factor (Heckler, 1986; Muir-Gray & Fowler, 1984; Nickens & Petersdorf, 1990). All three risk factors contribute to the narrowing of arterial walls, thereby creating a condition known as atherosclerosis, which may ultimately lead to stroke or coronary disease (Blankenhorn, 1984). However, these three primary risk factors are influenced by what Blankenhorn terms second-tier and third-tier risk factors. Second-tier factors enhance the opportunistic characteristics of primary risk factors in that they help create physical conditions conducive to stroke. These contributory factors include obesity, lack of exercise, diabetes mellitus, stress, episodic neurologic events, blood clotting factors, sickle cell disease, and immune system damage secondary to surgical procedures (e.g., heart transplantation) or more recently, acquired immune deficiency syndrome (AIDS). Substance abuse may also be a second-tier risk factor for stroke. The increased incidence of hemorrhagic and nonhemorrhagic stroke in middle-aged adults appears to decline when alcohol abuse is interrupted (Regan, 1990). Similarly, Gorelick (1990) notes that drug abuse should be among the possible causes of strokes, especially in young adults. With the current exception of AIDS, the aforementioned stroke risk factors are treatable or medically manageable conditions (Blankenhorn, 1984; Dyken et al., 1984). Third-tier factors (age, sex, race, and heredity) are not alterable by treatment. The health care provider must work around them.

Episodic neurologic events such as transient ischemic attack (TIA), reversible ischemic neurologic deficit (RIND), and partially reversible ischemic neurologic deficit (PRIND) are important warning signs of a possible future stroke. The consensus is that about half of all people who eventually suffer a stroke due to thrombosis, and a smaller but significant number who suffer a stroke due to embolism, experience such warning episodes. For example, one-third to one-half of persons who experience a TIA suffer a stroke within 5 years. Even more dramatic, possibly, is the fact that about one-half of these strokes occur within a year of the TIA and about one-fifth in the first month (Foley & Pizer, 1985). Episodic neurologic events are treatable through combinations of pharmacologic therapies, surgical interventions (Crowell & Jafar, 1990; Picone, Rosenbaum, Pettigrew, & Yatsu, 1990), and behavioral and lifestyle changes.

The reality facing the speech-language pathologist is that such activities are directed mostly toward individuals who have already experienced a stroke. Thus, the thrust of a health promotion program for poststroke patients and persons at risk for stroke involves developing a lifestyle and behavioral plan that reduces the occurrence or worsening of the three primary or related risk factors and, by so doing, forestall another stroke. Further, since insurance companies and other third-party payers continue to reimburse professionals to treat illness and disease rather than participate in health promotion activities, speech-language pathologists are forced to provide prevention services within the context of treatment. Fortunately, these two dichotomous activities are not mutually exclusive. Returning to Figure 19.1, the speech-language pathologist can act as a catalyst for returning the patient to the midpoint, where there is no discernible illness, while introducing the patient to clinical or community support that causes that individual to move even closer toward optimum health within the limitations of his or her disability.

HEALTH PROMOTION AND STROKE PREVENTION: VENUES AND ACTIVITIES

Patient Characteristics

Patients who are referred to a speech-language pathologist for assessment or treatment services commonly share certain prestroke and poststroke characteristics. Several of these characteristics include behavioral and lifestyle features that could reduce or enhance the likelihood that an individual patient will participate actively in a health promotion and stroke prevention program.

In general, the speech-language pathologist's health promotion and stroke prevention activities are directed toward patients who have previously experienced a left or right hemispheric cerebrovascular accident. On average, these patients are 45 years of age or older and exhibit aphasia and right hemiparesis of their upper and lower limbs. In the initial phase of recovery from stroke, these persons spend an average of 10 days in an acute-care hospital (Graves, 1991). Usually, such individuals have a history of atherosclerosis or high blood pressure and take a variety of prescribed medications (diuretics, anticoagulants, etc.) to reduce their chances of incurring another stroke. At the time of discharge from the acute-care setting, patients may be wheelchair-bound or able to ambulate with assistance from a cane or walker, and face several months of additional speech-language therapy as an inpatient at a rehabilitation hospital, as an outpatient, or at home.

The income and educational level of the patient will have played an important role in his or her health status before the stroke. In general, persons with fewer than 12 years of formal education and with annual incomes of less than $15,000 before a stroke suffer significantly more chronic diseases—conditions that increase their chances of having a stroke (Pincus, Callahan, & Burkhauser, 1987; Speake, Cowart, & Stephens, 1991). These same individuals are likely to accept little personal responsibility for their health status, viewing their health as "beyond their control." Conversely, patients who have attained higher educational and annual income levels tend to view their present and future health status as within their control (Speake et al., 1991), accept greater personal responsibility for improving their health status and will probably be more receptive to the speech-language pathologist's health promotion and stroke prevention activities.

The average patient at retirement age (i.e., age 65 years and older) will, prior to his or her stroke, have spent more than 50% of his or her free time watching television. However, older patients are likely to be only a little less active than younger people. Before a stroke, the average older patient spends more time walking than younger persons, spends time pursuing stress-reducing activities such as playing cards and other games, and invests him or herself to a greater extent in spiritual activities such as attending religious services (Robinson, 1991).

While several of these patient characteristics vary according to cultural background, prestroke access to and use of the health care system, and other factors, they do underscore the need for the speech-language pathologist to know more about the patient than simply his or her medical history and present diagnosis. Certainly, knowledge of the patient's prestroke and poststroke health status, course of recovery, and ability to communicate can be used to identify those conditions that place the patient at risk for another stroke, or that serve as barriers to full participation in a health promotion program. Equally important, however, is that the speech-language pathologist understands the patient's prestroke health locus of control (a measure of a person's belief that their health is determined by their own behavior or alternatively depends on luck, chance, or powerful others [Speake et al., 1991]), nutritional lifestyle, level of exercise, leisure pursuits, exposure to and management of internal and external stress, degree of support from the patient's family or significant others, cultural background, affiliation with community institutions, and personal and communication style before engaging the patient in a health promotion and stroke prevention program. Assessing the patient from such a holistic frame of reference largely determines whether the individual is a viable candidate for participation in a prevention program and, if so, provides the clinician with (1) targetable, functional goals for treatment as well as prevention activities, and (2) a large supply of personally relevant information that can be used to develop topics and themes for prevention activities (Aten, 1987; Pender, 1987, p. 4; Wallace & Canter, 1985).

Available instruments designed to assess an individual's health locus of control and health lifestyle include the Multidimensional Health Locus of Control Scale (Wallston, Wallston, & DeVillis, 1978) and the Health Promotion Lifestyle Profile (Walker, Sechrist, & Pender, 1987). A healthy lifestyle encompasses self-initiated actions that maintain or enhance wellness, self-actualization, and individual fulfillment (Speake et al., 1991). The Health Promotion Lifestyle Profile has proven useful for identifying an individual's past and present history of health practices associated with stress management, exercise, nutrition, health responsibility, self-actualization, and interpersonal support.

Presently, only one instrument provides the speech-language clinician with information about a stroke patient's prestroke personal and communication style. Swindell, Pashak, and Holland (1982) developed a family questionnaire that rates the patient's personal style in the areas of humor, flexibility, problem-solving, dependency, confidence, and so forth. The instrument also contains a checklist that allows the clinician to determine how the patient functions as writer, reader, speaker, listener, and nonverbal communicator— i.e., his or her "style" of communication. Preliminary data reported by Swindell et al. (1982) suggest a positive relationship between personal and communication style scores and recovery of language function. In addition to its value in planning patient treatment, the personal and communication style questionnaire can be used to identify those prestroke personal attributes and interpersonal styles unique to the stroke patient that, in turn, can be exploited within the context of the prevention program. For example, a patient with anomia and a "high" personal style score might be more receptive than an individual with a "low" personal style score to participating actively in a prevention program with the clinician. Further, if this same patient shows strong area scores on "Gesture/Writing," "Talking," and "Listening" on the communication style questionnaire, this finding might suggest that health promotion materials could be presented to the patient through the auditory channel and that he or she might use some combination of verbalization and gesture/writing to respond to the clinician, request help, protest, and so forth.

We have found in general that patients presenting with no more than mild to moderate aphasia can actively participate with the speech-language pathologist in health promotion activities cast within the context of the language treatment program.

Venues and Activities

Health promotion and stroke prevention activities can be carried out anywhere stroke patients are served by speech-language pathologists. These venues include hospitals, nursing care centers, community clinics, university clinics, adult day centers, and patients' homes. However, because most stroke rehabilitation services in the United States are probably provided within hospital settings, the speech-language pathologist is more likely to offer prevention services to stroke patients at a hospital. Over the last decade, community hospitals have become increasingly involved in health promotion efforts (McCormick, 1986; Pender, 1987). The number of speech-language pathologists employed in hospital settings has also increased over that time. Approximately 17% of speech-language pathologists report hospitals as their primary place of employment (ASHA, 1995).

Most of the present hospital-based health promotion programs for patients began as outgrowths of wellness programs for hospital employees. Pender (1987) and Sabatino (1989) note that a number of hospitals developed health promotion programs for patients to foster community good will with the hope that such attitudes would ultimately benefit the hospital. Economic considerations—the dwindling return to hospitals on the health care dollar, decreased average length of hospital stays, and reduced numbers of patient admissions—have also motivated hospitals to diversify their offerings to patients by providing programs such as health promotion.

Having established a role for speech-language pathology in health promotion, we now present suggested activities that the speech-language pathologist can pursue with poststroke patients and at-risk populations. These activities are divided into three categories: (1) patient-related activities, (2) community level activities, and (3) continuing education activities. Given the infancy of the health promotion movement in this country and within the field of communication disorders, this list is not exhaustive. Behavioral, environmental, and social factors play a well-known, significant role in the development of major chronic health problems (Pender, 1987). Thus, the prevention strategies provided below are designed to move the patient toward optimal health by: (1) helping the clinician and patient discover health-enhancing behaviors; (2) modifying sources of environmental stress, and internal and external barriers to good health; and (3) developing social networks (or strengthening existing ones) that will support the patient's continuous movement toward optimal health.

Patient-Related Activities

1. Reinforce the patient's active participation in controlling his or her behavior and lifestyle by encouraging the patient to (a) eat a healthful diet, concentrating on eliminating fat (saturated and unsaturated) and cholesterol; (b) reduce stress; (c) engage in classes or support groups that provide counseling and education on smoking cessation, and the elimination of drug and alcohol abuse; and (d) engage in an exercise program designed to increase cardiovascular fitness.

2. An example of a language treatment task that can be modified to encompass health promotion is presented below. This task requires the patient to sort life-like replicas or pictures of food into categories ranging from general ("food versus clothing") to specific ("nutritious foods").

> Level 1 Task: Separate food from clothing.
> Level 2 Task: Separate food into meal categories (e.g., breakfast, lunch, dinner food items).
> Level 3 Task: Separate food into nutritional categories (e.g., "foods that are good for you").
> Level 4 Task: Separate foods by personal favorites (e.g., "foods that you really like").
> Level 5 Task: Separate foods into categories that do or do not maintain the patient's health (e.g., "foods that your doctor wants you to cut back on").

3. A sample of a treatment session that incorporates promotion of health, in this instance physical exercise, is presented below. The patient, J.H., was a 57-year-old male with Broca's aphasia who exhibited moderate agrammatism, a mild auditory-comprehension deficit, and a mild impairment of gestural language. The patient's health promotion lifestyle profile indicated that until the time of his stroke, J.H. consumed a nutritious diet but did not take his blood pressure medication as prescribed. He obtained high personal style scores on the personal and communicative style questionnaire, particularly in the areas of humor, confidence, and flexibility. His communication style profile suggested strengths in the areas of drawing and

gesturing, listening, and talking. The theme of exercise, as presented in this example, is abstracted from a "promoting aphasics' communicative effectiveness" (PACE) (Davis & Wilcox, 1981) treatment session with J.H.

Materials: Pictures of people engaging in a variety of exercises
Task: Convey through any modality (verbal, gestural, writing/drawing) of the sender's choosing, a message describing the specific type of activity shown in a picture

Clinician (initiates message):	[*Gestures lifting a heavy weight.*]
J.H.:	Pumpin' up.
Clinician:	That's right. It looks pretty heavy.
J.H.:	[*initiates message*]: Whew! Bike ridin'.
Clinician:	Someone is riding a bicycle?
J.H.:	Yeah . . . Uh . . . No! Excise.
Clinician:	The person is riding an exercise bike?
J.H.:	Yeah!
Clinician:	Do you do that?
J.H.:	Yes Lordy!
Clinician:	How many miles are you up to now?
J.H.:	[*Gestures 4 miles by holding up four fingers.*]

4.   Encourage the hypertensive patient to take his or her medication regularly and faithfully. The hypertensive patient and family should also be encouraged to monitor blood pressure by purchasing and learning to use a sphygmomanometer (blood-pressure testing unit) to regularly assess blood pressure at home. Research shows that for those patients who have difficulty remembering to take their medication, self-recording and monthly home visits by a health professional help reduce blood pressure (Johnson, Taylor, Sackett, Dunnett, & Shimuzu 1978). The speech-language pathologist can design similar programs to help the stroke patient comply with the medical regimen established by the patient's physician.

5.   Develop an appraisal tool for communication wellness that focuses on primary and secondary risk factors that lead to stroke. Discuss results with patients and their family members and offer suggestions to minimize risks.

6.   Maintain a library for patients composed of written and audiovisual materials on health education and provide a list of community resources that can facilitate stroke reduction through exercise programs, diet and weight loss programs, and smoking and drug cessation programs for disabled or elderly patients.

7.   Use or develop educational materials that are appropriate to the cultural background and literacy level of the patients and support groups involved in patient care within the community.

8.   Engage the entire family and significant others (e.g., friends, religious and community leaders) in the process of the patient's recovery to

optimal health, by encouraging these individuals to participate in healthy lifestyle activities that support those of poststroke at-risk persons, and that foster the patient's ability and willingness to adhere to his or her medical, pharmaceutical, and rehabilitation regimen.

9. Query the patient to identify barriers to change. All individuals experience barriers to changing their behavior (Pender, 1987). Barriers may arise from within the patient (lack of motivation, fatigue, boredom, limited skills); from the family or significant other (family may encourage continuation of health-damaging behaviors, or actively discourage attempts at behavior change); or from the environment (lack of space or inappropriate setting, inclement weather, heavy traffic, high crime rate in which to carry out selected health promotion activities).

10. Help pass the locus of control and a sense of responsibility for establishing a healthy lifestyle to the patient. Patients who exhibit self-responsibility and self-control over their health status probably more readily invest themselves in health promotion activities.

Community-Level Activities

1. Develop a series of lectures or educational seminars and present them to community groups (e.g., churches, civic and professional associations). Topics might include communication wellness, stroke as a chronic disease that results in communicative deficits (aphasia, dysarthria, apraxia), and how to adapt behavior and lifestyle choices to minimize one's chances of suffering a stroke.

2. Develop, through the public relations office at your work site, broadcast and print ads to inform the community about minimizing communication deficits resulting from stroke.

3. Offer a risk appraisal for communication wellness as part of your screening activities during community-based or work site health fairs.

4. Establish individual health improvement contracts. These are useful for persons who are at risk but as yet do not have a chronic disease. A contractual health improvement plan identifies at least one negative behavior, sets goals for changing that behavior, and lists educational sessions and activities the person will attend or participate in.

5. Develop other health promotion and communicative wellness projects with professional colleagues at the local and state levels, and include a component on stroke prevention.

Continuing Education Activities

1. Enroll in continuing education or academic courses that focus on stroke epidemiology, health education, or public health and nutrition. These formal educational experiences can enhance a speech-language pathologist's knowledge and understanding of public health policy and health promotion

activities currently underway in the United States, especially those related to stroke outcome and prevention.

2.   Be knowledgeable about specific clinical measurements used to identify normal and abnormal blood pressure, normal and abnormal cholesterol and glucose levels, and what constitutes a healthy diet in general and for specific patients on a given caseload. Use this knowledge in promoting health with individual patients as well as during seminars presented to at-risk groups.

3.   Identify members of the health care team responsible for providing health promotion activities at your work site and in the community, and solicit their guidance or serve as a team member.

FUTURE DIRECTIONS

Health promotion appears to be here to stay. Current programs for adult populations are remedial, designed to correct destructive behaviors already learned. There is a growing interest, however, in health promotion for the younger population, which may lead to future health promotion activities being centered around maintenance and support for already acquired healthy lifestyles. We suggest that two major issues remain to be addressed in the field of health promotion: (1) a well-articulated research strategy that identifies the benefits and deficits associated with health promotion activities, and (2) strategies that economically reinforce and encourage both health care providers and their clients to engage in health-facilitating rather than health-damaging behaviors.

REFERENCES

American Heart Association. (1990). *1990 heart and stroke facts.* Dallas: Author.

American Speech-Language-Hearing Association. (1988). Position statement on the prevention of communication disorders. *ASHA, 30,* 90.

American Speech-Language-Hearing Association. (1990). Scope of practice, speech-language pathology and audiology. *ASHA, 32*(Suppl. 2), 1–2.

American Speech-Language-Hearing Association. (1995, January). [Demographic profile of the ASHA membership and affiliation for period of January 1, 1994, through December 31, 1994]. Unpublished data.

Aten, J. (1987). Functional communication treatment. In R. Chapey (Ed.), *Language intervention strategies in adults* (2nd ed., pp. 266–276). Baltimore: University Park Press.

Blakenhorn, D.H. (1984). *Preventive treatment of atherosclerosis.* Menlo Park: Addison-Wesley.

Brandon, J. (1985). Health promotion and wellness in rehabilitation services. *Journal of Rehabilitation, 51,* 54–58.

Cooper, R., Sempos, C., Hsieh, S.C., & Kovar, M.G. (1990). Slowdown in the decline of stroke mortality in the United States: 1978-1986. *Stroke, 21,* 1274–1279.

Crowell, R.M., & Jafar, J.J. (1990). Surgical revascularization for acute occlusion: Theoretical and practical considerations. In P.R. Weinstein & A.L. Faden (Eds.), *Protection of the brain from ischemia* (pp. 285–297). Baltimore: Williams & Wilkins.

Davis, G.A., & Wilcox, M.J. (1981). Incorporating parameters of natural conversation in aphasia treatment. In R. Chapey (Ed.), *Language intervention strategies in adult aphasia.* Baltimore: Williams & Wilkins.

Dyken, M.L., Wolf, P.A., Barnett, H.J.M., Bergan, J.J., Hass, W.K., Kannel, W.B., Kuller, L., Kurtzke, J.F., & Sundt, T.M. (1984). Risk factors in stroke: A statement for physicians by the subcommittee on risk factors and stroke of the stroke council. *Stroke, 15,* 1105–1111.

Foley, C., & Pizer, H.F. (1985). *The stroke fact book* (pp. 28–40). New York: Bantam Books.

Fratalli, C., Cherow, E., & Cole, L. (1991). Promotirg health for the nation. *ASHA, 33,* 30–35.

Goldstein, M. (1990). The decade of the brain: An era of promise for neurosurgery and a call to action. *Journal of Neurosurgery, 73,* 1–2.

Goodstadt, M.A., Simpson, R.I., & Laranger, P.O. (1987). Health promotion: A conceptual integration. *American Journal of Health Promotion, 2,* 58–63.

Gorelick, P.B. (1990). Alcohol and drug abuse: A current social peril. *Postgraduate Medicine, 88,* 171–174; 177–178.

Graves, E.J. (1991). *1989 Summary: National hospital discharge survey. Advance data from vital and health statistics; No. 199.* Hyattsville, MD: National Center for Health Statistics.

Heckler, M. (1985). *Executive summary report of the secretary's task force on black and minority health* (Vol. I, pp. 107–128). Washington, D.C.: U.S. Department of Health and Human Services.

Heckler, M. (1986). *Cardiovascular and cerebrovascular disease. Report of the Secretary's Task Force on Black and Minority Health* (Vol. IV, 1). Washington, D.C.: U.S. Department of Health and Human Services.

Jaynes, G.D., & Williams, R.M. (1989). *A common destiny: Blacks and American society.* National Research Council, Washington, D.C.: National Academy Press.

Johnson, A.L., Taylor, D.W., Sackett, D.K., Dunnett, C.W., & Shimuzu, A.G. (1978). Self-recording of blood pressure in the management of hypertension. *Canadian Medical Association Journal, 119,* 1034–1039.

Marge, M. (1984). The prevention of communication disorders. *ASHA, 26,* 29–33.

Marge, M. (1988). Health promotion for persons with disabilities: Moving beyond rehabilitation. *American Journal of Health Promotion, 3,* 29–35.

Marge, M. (1990). Future directions for disability prevention in America. *Proceedings of the Centers for Disease Control Annual Conference on Disability Prevention.* Atlanta, GA: Centers for Disease Control.

Marge. M. (1991). The challenge for communication sciences and disorders. *ASHA, 33,* 37–38.

McCormick, B. (1986). Hospitals gain savvy at selling worksite wellness. *Hospitals, 60,* 105–106.

McGinnis, J.M. (1990). Prevention in 1990: The state of the nation. *American Journal of Preventive Medicine, 6,* 1–5.

Muir-Gray, J.A., & Fowler, G. (1984). *Essentials of preventive medicine* (pp. 182–194). Boston: Blackwell Scientific Publications.

Nickens, H.W., & Petersdorf, R.G. (1990). Perspectives on prevention and medical education for the 1990's. *American Journal of Preventive Medicine, 6*(Suppl), 1–5.

O'Donnell, M.P. (1986). Definition of health promotion. *American Journal of Health Promotion, 1*, 4–5.

Pender, N.J. (1987). *Health promotion in nursing practice* (2nd ed., pp. 75–92, 277–278). Norwalk, CT: Appleton & Lange.

Picone, C.M., Rosenbaum, D.M., Pettigrew, L.C., & Yatsu, F.M. (1990). Anticoagulants and antiplatelet aggregation agents. In P.R. Weinstein & A.L. Faden (Eds.), *Protection of the brain from ischemia* (pp. 219–230). Baltimore: Williams & Wilkins.

Pincus, T., Callahan, L.F., & Burkhauser, R.V. (1987). Most chronic diseases are reported more frequently by individuals with fewer than 12 years of formal education in the age 18–64 United States population. *Journal of Chronic Diseases, 40*, 865–874.

Regan, T.J. (1990). Alcohol and the cardiovascular system. *Journal of the American Medical Association, 264*, 377–381.

Robinson, J.P. (1991). Quitting time. *American Demographics, 13*, 34–36.

Sabatino, F.G. (1989). The diversification success story continues: Survey. *Hospitals, 63*, 26–32.

Speake, D.L., Cowart, M.D., & Stephens, R. (1991). Healthy lifestyle practices of rural and urban elderly. *Health Values, 15*, 45–51.

Stuifbergen, A.K., Becker, H.A., Ingalsbe, K., & Sands, D. (1990). Perceptions of health among adults with disabilities. *Health Values, 14*, 18–26.

Swindell, C.S., Pashak, G.V., & Holland, A.V. (1982). A questionnaire for surveying personal and communicative style. In R. Brookshire (Ed.), *Clinical aphasiology conference proceedings*. Minneapolis: BRK Publishers.

Travis, J. (1975). Meet John Travis, doctor of wellbeing. *Prevention, 4*, 62–69.

Travis, J.W., & Ryan, R.S. (1988). *Wellness workbook (2nd ed.)*. Berkeley, CA: Ten Speed Press.

U.S. Department of Health and Human Services. (1990). *Heart disease and stroke: Resource list*. Washington, D.C.: Office of Disease Prevention and Health Promotion, National Health Information Center.

U.S. Department of Health and Human Services. (1991). *Healthy people 2000: National health promotion and disease prevention objectives* (Publication No. 91-50212). Washington, D.C.: U.S. Government Printing Office.

Walker, S.N., Sechrist, K.R., & Pender, N.J. (1987). The health-promoting lifestyle profile: Development and psychometric characteristics. *Nursing Research, 36*, 76–80.

Wallace, G.L., & Canter, G.J. (1985). Effects of personally relevant language materials on the performance of severely aphasic individuals. *Journal of Speech and Hearing Disorders, 50*, 385–390.

Wallston, K.A., Wallston, B.S., & DeVillis, R. (1978). Development of the multidimensional health locus of control (MHLC) scales. *Health Education Monographs, 6*, 160–170.

Chapter 20

Resource Guide for Aphasia and Stroke

Mary Boyle

Professionals striving to provide the best possible services to clients with aphasia must recognize the present era of information explosion. Futurists say that the volume of information now doubles every 2 years (Kiplinger, 1989), that 90% of the information available in the year 2000 is unknown today, and that graduates in the year 2000 will have been exposed to more information in that year than their grandparents were in a lifetime (Cannings, 1990). The thought of keeping pace with this rate of change is daunting. In the field of aphasia alone, speech-language pathologists are confronted with the need to stay abreast of advances in knowledge about the nature of aphasia and its assessment and treatment; knowledge about the relationship between language and other aspects of cognition; advances in neurology, neurophysiology, neuroimaging, and stroke; and knowledge about how language and other cognitive abilities change during normal aging.

Another change that will affect service provision is the increasingly interdisciplinary management of adult neurogenic disorders. A multitude of professional organizations represent these disciplines; often there are several organizations per discipline. Efforts to obtain the best possible services for clients will undoubtedly require effective collaboration with members of these organizations, which means that speech-language pathologists must be aware of who they are and what they do. There are also a growing number of consumer and volunteer organizations that may provide valuable support, advocacy, or other services for clients who are aphasic.

Legislation is another area that has a decided impact on clinicians' work in aphasia, since it is an important source of funding for treatment and research. Congress and state legislatures are struggling to stretch painfully limited resources to meet the needs of their constituencies. This means that the competition for government money to support research and services for the rapidly growing older segment of the population will become even more fierce. Speech-language pathologists not only need to be aware of legislative changes and how they affect the field, but must become proactive by trying to influence legislative changes that would be most beneficial for individuals with aphasia.

Finally, it is important to acknowledge that aphasia is an international problem. We must seek information about the research and services that exist in other countries, and share our knowledge in international forums. This means that we need to be aware of international journals, organizations, and agencies that are resources in this area.

This chapter serves as a resource guide for busy professionals who are trying hard not to be dismayed by the information explosion. The following sections contain sources for the latest information about aphasia, whether it pertains to theory, assessment, treatment, related disciplines, professional and volunteer organizations, legislation, or funding. Although it is certainly not an exhaustive listing, it serves as a convenient starting point for the aphasiologist who aims to stay on the cutting edge.

JOURNALS AND PERIODICALS

Acta Neuropathologica
Springer-Verlag
P.O. Box 2485
Secaucus, NJ 07094-2485

Age
American Aging Association
42nd and Dewey Avenue
Omaha, NE 68105

American Journal of Speech-Language Pathology
American Speech-Language-Hearing Association
10801 Rockville Pike
Rockville, MD 20852

Annals of Neurology
Little, Brown and Company
34 Beacon Street
Boston, MA 02108-1493

Aphasiology
Taylor & Francis, Inc.
1900 Frost Road, Suite 101
Bristol, PA 19007

Archives of Neurology
American Medical Association
515 North State Street
Chicago, IL 60610

Archives of Physical Medicine and Rehabilitation
W.B. Saunders Company
6277 Sea Harbor Drive
Orlando, FL 32887-4800

Brain
Oxford University Press
Walton Street
Oxford 0X2 6DP UK

Brain and Cognition
Academic Press
6277 Sea Harbor Drive
Orlando, FL 32887-4900

Brain and Language
Academic Press
1250 Sixth Avenue
San Diego, CA 92101-9665

British Journal of Disorders of Communication
Whurr Publishers Ltd.
196 Compton Terrace
London NI 2UN UK

Cognitive Neuropsychology
Lawrence Erlbaum Associates, Ltd.
27 Palmeira Mansions, Church Road
Hove, East Sussex BN3 2FA UK

Cognitive Rehabilitation
Neuroscience Publishers
6555 Carrollton Avenue
Indianapolis, IN 46220

Experimental Brain Research
Springer-Verlag
P.O. Box 2485
Secaucus, NJ 07094

Folia Phoniatrica et Logopaedica
S. Karger Publishers, Inc.
26 West Avon Road
P.O.Box 529
Farmington, CT 06085

Gerontology
S. Karger Publishers, Inc.
26 West Avon Road
P.O. Box 529
Farmington, CT 06085

International Journal of Neuroscience
Gordon Breach Science Publications Ltd.
1 Bedford Street
London WC2E 9PP UK

International Journal of Rehabilitation Research
Chapman & Hall
Department J, ITPS Ltd.
North Way
Andover, Hampshire
SP10 5BE UK

Journal of Communication Disorders
Elsevier Scientific Publishing Company, Inc.
Box 882 Madison Square Station
New York, NY 10159

Journal of Experimental Psychology
American Psychological Association
1400 North Uhle Street
Arlington, VA 22201

Journals of Gerontology
Gerontological Society of America
1275 K Street, NW, Suite 350
Washington, DC 20005-4006

Journal of Medical Speech-Language Pathology
Singular Pub. Group, Inc.
4284 41st Street
San Diego, CA 92105-1197

Journal of Memory and Language
Academic Press
6277 Sea Harbor Drive
Orlando, FL 32887-4900

Journal of Neurolinguistics
Pergamon Press Ltd.
Headington Hill Hall
Oxford OX3 0BW UK

Journal of Neurology
Springer-Verlag
P.O. Box 2485
Secaucus, NJ 07094-2485

Journal of Neurology, Neurosurgery, and Psychiatry
BMJ Publishing Group
Box No. 408
Franklin, MA 02038

Journal of Speech and Hearing Research
American Speech-Language-Hearing Association
10801 Rockville Pike
Rockville, MD 20852

Language and Cognitive Processes
Lawrence Erlbaum Assoc. Ltd.
27 Palmeira Mansions, Church Road
Hove, East Sussex, BN3 2FA UK

Neurology
Advanstar Communications, Inc.
131 West First Street
Duluth, MN 55802-2065

Neuropsychologia
Pergamon Press, Ltd.
Headington Hill Hall
Oxford OX3 0BW UK

Neuropsychology
Taylor & Francis, Inc.
1900 Frost Road, Suite 101
Bristol, PA 19007

Neuroscience
Pergamon Press, Ltd.
Headington Hill Hall
Oxford OX3 0BW UK

Psychological Bulletin
American Psychological Association
1400 North Uhle Street
Arlington, VA 22201

Seminars in Speech and Language
Thieme Medical Publishers, Inc.
381 Park Avenue South
New York, NY 10016

Topics in Language Disorders
Aspen Publishers, Inc.
200 Orchard Ridge Drive
Gaithersburg, MD 20878

Topics in Stroke Rehabilitation
Aspen Publishers, Inc.
200 Orchard Ridge Drive
Gaithersburg, MD 20878

PUBLISHERS OF TEXTBOOKS

Academic Press
Harcourt Brace Jovanovich, Publishers
6277 Sea Harbor Drive
Orlando, FL 32887-4900

ASHA Publications: American Speech-
Language-Hearing Association
10801 Rockville Pike
Rockville, MD 20852

Aspen Publishers, Inc.
200 Orchard Ridge Drive
Gaithersburg, MD 20878

B.C. Decker, Inc.
320 Walnut Street, Suite 400
Philadelphia, PA 19106

Butterworth-Heinemann
313 Washington Street
Newton, MA 02158-1626

Cambridge University Press
40 West 20th Street
New York, NY 10011

CIBA-GEIGY Corporation
Medical Education Division
P.O. Box 18060
Newark, NJ 07101

Elsevier Science Publishing Co., Inc.
Box 882 Madison Square Station
New York, NY 10159

Gallaudet University Press
800 Florida Avenue, NE
Washington, DC 20002-3695

Lawrence Erlbaum Associates, Inc.
365 Broadway
Hillsdale, NJ 07642

The MIT Press
55 Hayward Street
Cambridge, MA 02142-1399

Paul H. Brookes Publishing Co.
P.O. Box 10624
Baltimore, MD 21285

PRO-ED
8700 Shoal Creek Boulevard
Austin, TX 78758

Singular Publishing Group, Inc.
4282 41st Street
San Diego, CA 92105

Springer-Verlag
P.O. Box 2485
Secaucus, NJ 07094-2485

Thieme Medical Publishers, Inc.
381 Park Avenue South
New York, NY 10016

Williams & Wilkins
428 East Preston Street
Baltimore, MD 21202

NEWSLETTERS AND BOOKLETS

American Heart Association
7272 Greenville Avenue
Dallas, TX 75231-4596

Los Amigos Research and Education
Institute
Rancho Los Amigos Medical Center
12841 Dahlia Ave., Bldg. 306
Downey, CA 90242-4108

National Aphasia Association
P.O. Box 1887
Murray Hill Station
New York, NY 10156-0611

National Easter Seal Society
2023 West Ogden Avenue
Chicago, IL 60612

National Stroke Association
8480 East Orchard Road, Suite 1000
Englewood, CO 80111-5015

PROFESSIONAL ASSOCIATIONS

Academy of Neurologic Communication
Disorders and Sciences
Suite 300
1250 24th Street NW
Washington, DC 20037

American Association for International
Aging
1511 K Street, NW
Washington, DC 20005

American Heart Association
7272 Greenville Avenue
Dallas, TX 75231-4596

American Society on Aging
833 Market Street, Suite 511
San Francisco, CA 94103-1824

American Speech-Language-Hearing
Association
Special Interest Division, 2,
Neurophysiology and Neurogenic
Speech and Language Disorders
10801 Rockville Pike
Rockville, MD 20852

Associacion Nacional Pro Personas
Mayores
(National Association for Hispanic
Elderly)
2727 West 6th Street
Los Angeles, CA 90057

The Gerontological Society of America
1275 K Street NW, Suite 350
Washington, DC 20005

International Association of Logopedics
and Phoniatrics
c/o Sr. Marie DeMontfort Supple
School of Remedial Linguistics
Trinity College
Dublin 2, Republic of Ireland

National Black Association for Speech-
Language and Hearing
Neurogenics Special Interest Group
P.O. Box 50605
Washington, DC 2004-0605

National Caucus and Center on the Black
Aged
1424 K Street, NW
Washington, DC 20005

National Council on Aging
600 Maryland Avenue, SW
Washington, DC 20024

National Indian Council on Aging
P.O. Box 2088
Albuquerque, NM 87103

National Interfaith Coalition on Aging
9201 West Broward Boulevard
Plantation, FL 33324

National Pacific Asian Resource Center
on Aging
1341 G Street, NW
Washington, DC 20005

National Stroke Association
8480 East Orchard Road, Suite 1000
Englewood, CO 80111-5015

Society for Cognitive Rehabilitation, Inc.
P.O. Box 33548
Decatur, GA 30033-0548

CONSUMER AND VOLUNTEER ORGANIZATIONS

National Aphasia Association
P.O. Box 1887
Murray Hill Station
New York, NY 10156-0611

COMMUNITY, STATE, AND FEDERAL AGENCIES

Clearinghouse on the Handicapped
Office of the Asst. Sec. for Special
Education and Rehabilitation Services
U.S. Department of Education
400 Maryland Avenue, SW
Washington, DC 20202

Council of State Administrators of
Vocational Rehabilitation
1055 Thomas Jefferson St. NW
Washington, DC 20007

Health Care Financing Administration
U.S. Department of Health and Human
Services
200 Independence Avenue, SW
Washington, DC 20201

National Association of Area Agencies
on Aging
600 Maryland Avenue, SW
Washington, DC 20024

National Association of State Units on
Aging
600 Maryland Avenue, SW
Washington, DC 20024

Older American Volunteer Programs
ACTION
806 Connecticut Avenue, NW
Washington, DC 20525

The President's Committee on
Employment of the Handicapped
1111 20th St., NW, Suite 636
Washington, DC 20036

Social Security Administration
Altmeyer Building
6401 Security Boulevard
Baltimore, MD 21235

U.S. Dept. of Health and Human Services
330 Independence Avenue, SW
Washington, DC 20201

SOURCES FOR LEGISLATIVE INFORMATION

Governmental Affairs Division
American Speech-Language-Hearing
Association
10801 Rockville Pike
Rockville, MD 20852

House Education and Labor Committee
Subcommittee on Human Resources
U.S. House of Representatives
Rayburn House Office Building
Washington, DC 20515

House Select Committee on Aging
U.S. House of Representatives
House Office Bldg. Annex No.1
Washington, DC 20515

Senate Labor and Human Resources
Committee
Subcommittee on Aging, Family and
Human Resources
U.S. Senate
Washington, DC 20510

Special Committee on Aging
U.S. Senate
Dirksen Building
Washington, DC 20510

SOURCES FOR FUNDING

American Speech-Language-Hearing
Foundation
10801 Rockville Pike
Rockville, MD 20852

*Directory of Building and Equipment
Grants*
Research Grant Guides
P.O. Box 4970
Margate, FL 33063

Easter Seal Research Foundation
2023 West Ogden Avenue
Chicago, IL 60612

The Foundation Center (information on
private philanthropic foundations)
Reference Collections
• 79 Fifth Avenue
  New York, NY 10003
• 1001 Connecticut Avenue NW
  Washington, DC 20036
• Kent H. Smith Library
  1442 Euclid Avenue
  Cleveland, OH 44115
• 312 Sutter Street
  San Francisco, CA 94108
• Suite 150, Grand Lobby
  Hunt Building
  50 Hunt Plaza
  Atlanta, GA 30303

International Research and Exchanges
Board (IREX)
126 Alexander Street
Princeton, NJ 08540-7102

Handicapped Funding Directory
Richard M. Eckstein, Editor
Research Grant Guides
P.O. Box 4970
Margate, FL 33063

National Institute on Deafness and Other
Communication Disorders
Division of Communication Sciences
and Disorders
National Institutes of Health
Executive Plaza South, Suite 750
6120 Executive Boulevard
Rockville, MD 20852

National Institute on Disability and
Rehabilitation Research
Office of the Assistant Secretary for
Special Education and Rehabilitative
Services
U.S. Department of Education
400 Maryland Avenue, SW
Washington, DC 20202

NIH Guide for Grants and Contracts
Printing and Reproduction Branch
National Institutes of Health
Room B4BN08, Building 31
Bethesda, MD 20892

Profiles of Funding Sources
American Speech-Language-Hearing
Association
10801 Rockville Pike
Rockville, MD 20852

Rehabilitation Services Administration
Office of the Assistant Secretary for
Special Education and Rehabilitative
Services
U.S. Department of Education
400 Maryland Avenue, SW
Washington, DC 20202

Research Bulletin
American Speech-Language-Hearing
Association
10801 Rockville Pike
Rockville, MD 20852

World Rehabilitation Fund, Inc.
International Exchange of Experts and
Information in Rehabilitation (IEEIR)
Institute on Disability
6 Hood House
Durham, NH 03824

SOURCES FOR ASSESSMENT AND TREATMENT MATERIALS

Academic Communication Associates
P.O. Box 586249
Oceanside, CA 92058-6249

Communication Skill Builders
3830 East Bellevue
P.O. Box 42050-C55
Tucson, AZ 85733

Crestwood Company
6625 North Sidney Place
Milwaukee, WI 53209-3259

DLM
P.O. Box 4000
One DLM Park
Allen, TX 75002

Imaginart Communication Products
307 Arizona Street
Bisbee, AZ 85603

Lea & Febiger
428 E. Preston Street
Baltimore, MD 21202

LinguiSystems, Inc.
3100 4th Avenue
P.O. Box 747, Dept. HC
East Moline, IL 61244-0747

Parrot Software
P.O. Box 250755
West Bloomfield, MI 48325-0755

PRO-ED
8700 Shoal Creek Boulevard
Austin, TX 78757-6897

The Psychological Corporation
555 Academic Court
San Antonio, TX 78204-2498

The Riverside Publishing Company
8420 Bryn Mawr Avenue
Chicago, IL 60631

Slosson Educational Publications, Inc.
P.O. Box 280
East Aurora, NY 14052-0280

The Speech Bin
1965 Twenty-Fifth Avenue
Vero Beach, FL 32960

VNS Therapy Materials
Visiting Nurse Service, Inc.
1200 McArthur Drive
Akron, OH 44320

Wayne State University Press
The Leonard N. Simons Building
5959 Woodward Avenue
Detroit, MI 48202

Western Psychological Services
12031 Wilshire Boulevard
Los Angeles, CA 90025-1251

REFERENCES

Cannings, T. (1990). Toward 2000—The vision and the task. *CUE Newsletter, 12,* 10–13.
Kiplinger, A.H. (1989). *America in the global '90s.* Washington, D.C.: Kiplinger Books.

Appendix: Commonly Prescribed Drugs and Their Side Effects

Jeffrey S. Hecht

During the acute hospital stay, the rehabilitation phase, and later after discharge, patients are commonly on one or more medications. Unfortunately, side effects and drug interactions are common. Because patients come in different ages and sizes and with different chemical backgrounds, they may respond to the same medication in different ways. All medications have the potential for undesirable side effects that may influence the patient's progress with rehabilitation.

This appendix lists the names of several medications that are commonly seen while treating patients with aphasia. These include medications to reduce the risk of recurrent ischemic or embolic stroke, such as aspirin, warfarin (Coumadin), or ticlopidine (Ticlid). A physician may include medications to reduce risk factors for stroke, such as antihypertensives, antihyperlipidemics, and oral hypoglycemics. There may be medications to reduce the risk of brain damage early after stroke, such as adrenocorticoids or mannitol. On the other hand, medications may be used to treat late effects of stroke, such as depression, epileptic seizures, insomnia, or spasticity. Patients with stroke commonly have problems with constipation and infection, such as bronchitis, pneumonia, and urinary tract infections. The attentive speech pathologist may play an important role in advising the physician if there is a significant decline in functional ability. This may be due to a side effect of a medication (such as an accumulation of benzodiazepine or anticonvulsant in the bloodstream) or may be due to a late effect of stroke, such as infection that needs treatment.

COMMONLY PRESCRIBED MEDICATIONS

Note: Generic names are boldface with side effects listed; brand names are in regular type.

Angiotensin-converting enzyme (ACE) inhibitors (Capoten, **captopril, enalapril, lisinopril,** Prinivil, Vasotec, Zestril): Used to treat high blood pressure and heart failure. Side effects: appetite loss, change in taste sensation, constipation, bronchial spasm, cough, swelling, itching, rash, dizziness, low blood pressure, rapid or slow pulse, chest pain.

Acetaminophen (Anacin-3, Darvocet-N, Datril, Excedrin, Tylenol): Side effects: rare; causes liver damage in overdose.

Acetazolamide (Diamox): Used to reduce cerebral edema, treat epilepsy, treat glaucoma, and promote fluid loss. Side effects: tingling of lips and fingers, hearing changes, stomach upset; see **Diuretics.**

Adapin (**doxepin; see Antidepressants, tricyclics**)

Adrenocorticoids (Decadron, **dexamethasone, methylprednisolone, prednisone,** Solu-Cortef, Solu-Medrol, etc.): Used to reduce swelling in the brain. Used topically for rashes. Side effects: acne, fluid retention, poor wound healing, stomach upset, and ulcers. Inform physician if there is a history of blood clots, diabetes, glaucoma, heart disease, peptic ulcer, or tuberculosis.

Alpha-adrenergic blockers (Hytrin, Minipress, **prazosin, terazosin**): Used to treat hypertension and avoid heart failure by relaxing and expanding walls of the blood vessels. Also used to relax muscles in the bladder neck to improve voiding. Common side effects: Anticholinergic—dizziness, drowsiness, weakness, vivid dreaming, rapid heart beat, low blood pressure— sometimes even causing black-out spells with the first dose; bladder accidents; inability of the erect penis to relax.

Amitriptyline (see **Antidepressants, tricyclics**): Side effects:　see **Anticholinergics**; overeating.

Analgesics: Medications used to treat pain, from mild to severe.

Antacids (Amphojel, Maalox, Mylanta, Tums): Used to treat "heartburn" and stomach upset by neutralizing acid in the stomach and esophagus.

Antiarthritics: Used to treat arthritis, including aspirin, gold, nonsteroidal anti-inflammatory drugs, and others.

Antiasthmatics (Alupent, **aminophylline,** Brethine, Bronkosol, Theo-dur, **theophylline,** Ventolin): Used to prevent and relieve bronchial spasm, wheezing, or asthma.

Anticholinergics: Used to slow overactive bladder function. Many drugs used for other problems have anticholinergic side effects. Side effects: dry mouth, dry eyes, blurred vision, constipation, nausea, vomiting, difficulty urinating, fatigue, headaches, insomnia, confusion, hallucinations, rapid pulse. Problems with asthma, bronchitis, glaucoma, heart disease, liver disease, myasthenia gravis, peptic ulcers, or prostate may be worsened.

Anticoagulants (oral types: Coumadin, **dicumarol, warfarin sodium**): Used to reduce the recurrence of embolic and, sometimes, thrombotic stroke; commonly used in atrial fibrillation. Side effects: bleeding. Bleeding may be obvious or hidden, such as stomach bleeding showing up as dark stools. This class interacts with many other classes to affect the ease of bleeding as well as the drug's other effects. **Heparin** is an anticoagulant given intravenously or by injections. Its primary side effect also is bleeding. Other side effects: dark stools or urine, easy bruising, fatigue, fever, hair loss, nausea, sore throat, rash, yellow jaundice.

Anticonvulsants (**carbamazepine**, Depakene, Depakote, Dilantin, Paradione, **phenobarbital, phenytoin**, Tegretol, **valproic acid**): Used to treat and prevent epileptic seizures. Side effects: dizziness, drowsiness, interactions with other medications, rash. See specific drug for other side effects.

Antidepressants, monamine oxidase inhibitors (isocarboxazid, Marplan, Nardil, **pargyline**, Parnate, **phenelzine, tranylcypromine**): Rarely used to treat depression. Side effects: see **Anticholinergics**; dangerously high blood pressure if interacting with other drugs, dizziness, swelling. There are many foods with which these react to produce hypertension.

Antidepressants, tricyclic (**amitriptyline**, Desyrel, **doxepin**, Elavil, Endep, **fluoxetine, nortriptyline**, Pamelor, Prozac, **sertraline, trazodone**, Zoloft): Commonly used to treat depression, pain due to nerve damage, and sometimes bed wetting or insomnia. Side effects: see **Anticholinergics**; fatigue, change in appetite or weight, constipation, dizziness, drowsiness, confusion, dry mouth, headache, tremors, hallucinations, insomnia, irregular heart beats, itching, rash, seizures, sore throat, yellow jaundice due to effect on the liver. See specific drug for additional effects. It may take 3 weeks to obtain a significant effect from the medication. There may be interactions with several other types of medications.

Antiemetics (Compazine, Dramamine, Phenergan, Reglan, Vistaril): Used to treat motion sickness, nausea, and vomiting. Side effects: see **Anticholinergics**; drowsiness, abnormal eye or facial movements.

Antifungals: A varied group used to treat fungal infections of the skin or within the body. They may have a few side effects when used topically (on the skin) but many side effects when used for severe internal infections.

Antihistamines (Atarax, Benadryl, **chlorpheniramine, diphenhydramine**, Seldane, and many others): Primarily used to treat allergies, itching, rashes, and insomnia.

Antihyperlipidemics (cholestyramine, Colestid, **colestipol,** Lopid, Mevacor, **niacin, nicotinic acid,** Questran, Zocor): A variety of drugs used to treat elevated cholesterol and triglycerides to lower the risk of recurrent strokes. Side effects: while digestive symptoms are common, drowsiness is not. Some require close monitoring for toxicity.

Antihypertensives: A wide variety of drugs used to treat high blood pressure. Primary groups include ACE **inhibitors, alpha blockers, beta blockers, calcium channel blockers, diuretics, vasodilators.**

Anti-inflammatory medications (see **aspirin, NSAIDs, adrenocorticoids**)

Antipruritics (see Antihistamines): Used to treat itching.

Antipsychotics (chlorpromazine, Haldol, **haloperidol,** Mellaril, Navane, **thioridazine, thiothixene,** Thorazine; see **Phenothiazines**): Used to reduce severe anxiety, agitation, and psychotic behavior. Side effects: see **Anticholinergics**; abnormal movements of face, limbs, or tongue; constipation, dizziness, drowsiness, interactions with many drugs, jaundice, restlessness.

Antipyretics (acetaminophen, aspirin, Tylenol): Used to treat fever.

Antispasmodics (Bentyl, **dicyclomine**): Used to treat bladder spasms, intestinal cramp, and irritable bowel. Side effects: see **Anticholinergics**.

Antispasticity medications (see **baclofen, benzodiazepines,** Dantrium): A group of medications used to reduce muscle cramps and spasms.

Anxiolytics (see **Antipsychotics, Benzodiazepines**): Used to reduce anxiety and nervousness.

Aspirin (Anacin, Bayer, Bufferin, Ecotrin, Empirin, and many others; also a component in various combination medications): Used to reduce the risk of stroke and myocardial infarct as well as reducing inflammation and pain of various types. Side effects: black stools, heartburn, indigestion, nausea, stomach pain, ulcers, vomiting, ringing in the ears. Rare, but dangerous, are severe allergic reactions and, in children, Reye's syndrome (confusion, coma, kidney and liver damage).

Ativan (**lorazepam**; see **Benzodiazepines**)

Axid (**nizatidine**): Uses and side effects: see **H₂-Blockers**.

Baclofen (Lioresal): Used to relieve muscle cramps and spasms; sometimes used to reduce hiccoughs or pain. Side effects: confusion, dizziness, drowsiness, light-headedness, nausea, numbness and tingling, rash, weakness of muscles.

Barbiturates (phenobarbital, secobarbital, and others): A group of strong sedatives used also for treatment of epilepsy. They are very sedating.

Benzodiazepines (alprazolam, Ativan, Dalmane, **diazepam**, Doral, **flurazepam**, Halcion, Librium, **lorazepam, quazepam**, Restoril, Serax, **temazepam, triazolam**, Valium, Xanax). Used as mild tranquilizers for anxiety, nervousness, and tension; for muscle spasm; and for acute treatment of epileptic seizures.

Beta blockers (Corgard, Inderal, **nadolol, propranolol**, Tenormin, and others): Used to lower blood pressure, stabilize an irregular heartbeat, reduce angina, reduce the frequency of migraine headaches, and reduce agitation after head injury. Side effects: cold hands and feet, constipation, depression, diarrhea, dizziness, drowsiness, dry eyes or mouth, fatigue, nausea, low blood pressure, slow pulse, tingling of hands and feet, weakness. **This medication should not be stopped suddenly, as it may precipitate a heart attack**.

Bumetanide (Bumex): See **Diuretics**; a strong "fluid" pill used to reduce fluid retention (edema). Side effects: cramps, dehydration, fatigue, irregular heartbeats, unsteadiness, weakness.

Bupropion (see Wellbutrin)

Butazolidin (**phenylbutazone**; see **NSAIDs**)

Calan (**verapamil**; see **Calcium Channel Blockers**)

Calcium channel blockers (Calan, Cardizem, **diltiazem**, Isoptin, **nifedipine**, Procardia, **verapamil**): Used to prevent angina attacks and hypertension by reducing spasm of blood vessels. Also used to stabilize irregular heartbeats. Side effects: constipation, dizziness, nausea, headache, swelling, slow heart rate, low blood pressure, shortness of breath, fatigue, rash, soreness and swelling of the breasts.

Carbamazepine (Apo-Carbamazepine, Mazepine, Tegretol): Used to treat and prevent epileptic seizures. Side effects: blurred vision, nausea, vomiting, diarrhea, confusion, slurred speech, headache, rash, sensitivity to sunlight. A rare side effect is a lowering of blood counts, causing easy bleeding or bruising, excessive fatigue, sore throat, and fever. Alcohol increases the sedation.

Capoten (**captopril**; see **ACE inhibitors; Antihypertensives**)

Cardizem (**diltiazem**; see **Calcium channel blockers**)

Cimetidine (Tagamet): Uses and side effects: see **H$_2$-Blockers**.

Ciprofloxacin (Cipro): Side effects: abdominal pain, diarrhea, headache, nausea, rash, vomiting.

Clinoril (**sulindac**; see **NSAIDs**)

Corgard (**nadolol**): Uses and side effects: see **Beta Blockers**.

Coumadin (**warfarin sodium**): Used to prevent and treat blood clots. See **Anticoagulants**. It is to be taken 1 hour before or 2 hours after eating. It interacts with many foods and other medications.

Cozaar (**losartan**): Used to treat high blood pressure. Side effect: dizziness.

Dalmane (**flurazepam**): Uses and side effects: see **Benzodiazepines**. With prolonged use for insomnia, it can accumulate, causing overdose and excessive sedation during the day.

Dantrolene sodium (Dantrium): Used to relieve muscle spasticity caused by stroke. Side effects: abdominal pain, appetite loss, blurred vision, confusion, constipation, depression, diarrhea, difficulty with erection or emptying the bladder, headache, hepatitis, insomnia, rapid pulse, rash, sore muscles and back. It should not be used by people with liver disease such as cirrhosis or hepatitis.

Decadron (**dexamethasone phosphate**): Uses and side effects: see **Adrenocorticoids**. Commonly used after stroke or head injury to reduce brain swelling.

Depakene (see **Valproic acid**).

Depakote (see **Valproic acid**).

Desyrel (**trazodone**): Uses and side effects: see **Antidepressants, tricyclic**.

Diazepam (Valium; see **Benzodiazepines**)

Dicumarol (See **Anticoagulants**)

Didronel (**etidronate disodium**; see **Diphosphonates**)

Dilantin (**phenytoin**): Used to prevent and treat epileptic seizures. It is also used to stabilize irregular heartbeats. Side effects: blurred vision, bruising, confusion, constipation, diarrhea, dizziness, drowsiness, hallucinations, headaches, increased body or facial hair, jumping movements of the eyes (nystagmus), nausea, rash, slurred speech, staggering, swollen gums, vomiting. Many of these side effects are signs of overdose. The medication interacts with many other drugs and vitamins to cause other side effects.

Diphosphonates (Didronel): Used to prevent or treat heterotopic ossification (HO). HO is the abnormal formation of bone in areas that usually have only muscle. It usually occurs around joints and can restrict motion and cause pain. Also known as myositis ossificans, it can be seen following head injury or, rarely, stroke. This medication is also used to treat osteoporosis (thinning of the bones). Side effects: constipation, diarrhea, stomach upset, and, rarely, rash and swelling. No food should be eaten within 2 hours of dosing.

Dipyridamole (Persantine): Used to reduce the risk of stroke after heart surgery or in patients with artificial heart valves. It is of equivocal benefit in ischemic stroke. Side effects: dizziness, headache, flushing, rash, nausea, cramps, weakness, hypotension.

Diuretics (Bumex, Dyazide, **furosemide, hydrochlorothiazide**, Lasix, Maxzide, **triamterene**): Water pill used to reduce fluid retention (edema) and treat high blood pressure (hypertension). Side effects: blurred vision, bleeding or bruising, dizziness, fatigue, low blood pressure, rash, light-headedness, nausea, vomiting, weakness, stomach pain, thirst, yellow jaundice. There may be interactions with other drugs.

Doral (**quazepam**; see **Benzodiazepines**)

Doxepin (Adapin, Sinequan; see **Antidepressants, tricyclic**)

Elavil (**amitriptyline**; see **Antidepressants, tricyclic**)

Famotidine (Pepcid; see **H₂-Blockers**)

Fluoxetine (Prozac; see **Antidepressants, tricyclic**)

Flurazepam (Dalmane; see **Benzodiazepines**): Promoted for sleep. May accumulate and cause sedation if used regularly.

Furosemide (Lasix; see **Diuretics**)

H₂-Blockers (**cimetidine, famotidine**, Pepcid, **ranitidine**, Tagamet, Zantac): Used to treat and prevent peptic ulcers by reducing acid production by the stomach. Side effects: breast swelling or soreness in men, confusion, decreased sex drive or impotence, diarrhea, dizziness, hair loss, muscular pains. Rare side effects that necessitate calling the doctor right away: unusual bleeding or bruising, unusual fatigue, fever, sore throat. Can interact with many other medications and usually increase their effects.

Haloperidol (Haldol; see **Antipsychotics**)

Hydrochlorothiazide (Dyazide, Maxzide; see **Antihypertensives; Diuretics**)

Hytrin (**terazosin**; see **Alpha Blockers; Antihypertensives**)

Ibuprofen (Advil, Motrin, Rufen; see **NSAIDs**)

Indomethacin (Indocin; see **NSAIDs**)

Insulin (Regular, Lente, Ultralente, NPH, Humulin): Injectable medication used to control diabetes.

Isoptin (**verapamil**; see **Calcium Channel Blockers; Antihypertensives**)

Lasix (**furosemide**; see **Diuretics**): If patient is allergic to sulfa drugs, he or she may also be allergic to this strong fluid pill.

Lorazepam (Ativan; see **Benzodiazepines**)

Mannitol: An injectable medication used to reduce brain swelling (cerebral edema) in the early stages after head injury or stroke.

Meclomen (**meclofenamate**; see **NSAIDs**)

Methylprednisolone (Depo-Medrol, Depo-Predate, Medrol Acetate; see **Adrenocorticoids**)

Metoclopramide (Reglan): Used to speed passage of food through the stomach and reduce nausea. Side effects: confusion, drowsiness, jerking movements of face, head muscle spasms, tremors.

Minipress (**prazosin**; see **Alpha Blockers; Antihypertensives**)

Mysoline (**primidone**; see **Anticonvulsants**)

Nabumetone (Relafen; see **NSAIDs**)

Naproxen (Naprosyn; see **NSAIDs**)

Nitrofurantoin (Macrodantin): Commonly used for bladder/urinary tract infections. Commonly colors urine a brown or rusty color. Side effects: diarrhea, nausea, vomiting, chest pain or breathing difficulty, numbness or tingling of skin or limbs, unusual weakness or fever.

Nitroglycerine (glyceryl trinitrate, Nitro-Bid, Nitro-Dur): Used to prevent or treat angina attacks of heart pain. Side effects: dizziness, flushing, bad headaches, nausea, vomiting, rash, low blood pressure.

Norfloxacin (Noroxin)

NSAIDs (nonsteroidal anti-inflammatory drugs) (Advil, Butazolidin, Clinoril, **diclofenac, diflunisal,** Dolobid, Feldene, **ibuprofen,** Indocin, **indomethacin, meclofenamate,** Meclomen, **mefenamic acid,** Motrin, **nabumetone,** Naprosyn, **naproxen, phenylbutazone, piroxicam,** Relafen, Rufen, Sulindac, Tolectin, **tolmetin,** Voltaren): Used as a general pain reliever as well as to treat the stiffness, swelling, and joint pain of arthritic conditions. Some must be taken several times daily, some once daily. Side effects: abdominal pain, constipation, heartburn, nausea, stomach upset, ulcers, dizziness, headache, fluid retention. Prolonged use is more likely to cause stomach problems and may lead to kidney problems. **Phenylbutazone** causes more blood problems, including fatal aplastic anemia (failure of the bone marrow to produce blood cells) than the other drugs. **Diclofenac** causes more liver problems than the other drugs.

Nystatin (Mycostatin, Milstat): Used to treat fungus infections such as thrush involving the mouth or throat. Side effects: diarrhea, nausea, vomiting, stomach pain.

Oxazepam (Ox-Pam, Serax; see **Benzodiazepines**)

Pepcid (**famotidine**; see **H₂-Blockers**)

Persantine (see **Dipyridamole**)

Phenobarbital (see **Anticonvulsants**): Used to prevent or treat epileptic seizures. Side effects: confusion, dizziness, drowsiness, depression, slurred speech, diarrhea, nausea, vomiting, rash, swelling of the eyelids, muscle or joint pain. There are many interactions with other medications, many producing dangerous oversedation. Alcohol should be avoided.

Phenytoin (see **Anticonvulsants**; Dilantin): Used to prevent or treat epileptic seizures.

Prazepam (Centrax; see **Benzodiazepines**)

Prednisolone (see **Adrenocorticoids**)

Prednisone (see **Adrenocorticoids**)

Primidone (Mysoline, Sertan; see **Anticonvulsants**)

Prinivil (**lisinopril**; see **ACE inhibitors**)

Procardia (see **Nifedipine**)

Quazepam (Doral; see **Benzodiazepines**)

Reglan (see **Metoclopramide**)

Restoril (**temazepam**; see **Benzodiazepines**)

Sertraline (Zoloft; see **Antidepressants, tricyclic**)

Sinequan (**doxepin**; see **Antidepressants, tricyclic**)

Steroids (see **Adrenocorticoids**)

Sulcralfate (Carafate): Used to treat peptic ulcers by coating the ulcer site and protecting it from stomach acid. Side effects: abdominal pain, constipation, indigestion, nausea, vomiting, dizziness, sleepiness, rash. It will absorb other medications, so it should be taken 1 hour before meals and at bedtime, and at least 2 hours apart from other medications.

Sulfa drugs (**sulfamethoxazole**, Bactrim, Gantrisin, Septral, **sulfisoxazole**): For those who are very allergic, some sulfa drugs that are not antibiotics include **disulfiram** (Antabuse), **furosemide** (Lasix), and **sulfonurea** drugs used for treatment of diabetes. Side effects of the antibiotics include appetite loss, diarrhea, nausea, vomiting, dizziness, headache, rash, peeling, blistering, painful urination, unusual bruising, fatigue, sore throat, or fever—which could reflect an effect on the blood count. They can increase the effects of alcohol.

Sulindac (Clinoril; see **NSAIDs**)

Tagamet (**cimetidine**; see **H$_2$-Blockers**)

Tegretol (**carbamazepine**; see **Anticonvulsants; Carbamazepine**)

Tetracycline: Side effects: abdominal pain, diarrhea, nausea, vomiting, headaches, sore mouth and tongue, itching around rectum and genitals due to development of a fungal (yeast) infection. It may make the skin extra sensitive to sun. It can interact with other drugs and foods.

Theophylline (Slo-Phyllin, Theo-Dur, Theolair): Used for bronchial asthma. Side effects: seizures, anxiety, confusion, irregular heartbeat, stomach upset. It is better absorbed if taken on an empty stomach but can be taken with food to lessen stomach upset.

Ticlopidine hydrochloride (Ticlid): Used to reduce platelet aggregation and, in turn, reduce the risk of stroke. Side effects: nausea, weakness, rash, sore throat or fever, reduction in white blood cell count.

Trazodone (Desyrel; see **Antidepressants, tricyclic**)

Trimethoprim (Bactrim, Septral, Trimpex): Side effects: headache. See physician if rash, breathing trouble, blue lips, or blue skin develops.

Valium (**diazepam**; see **Benzodiazepines**)

Valproic acid (Depakene, Depakote; see **Anticonvulsants**): Used to treat and prevent epileptic seizures. Side effects: irregular menstruation, depression, emotional changes, headache, incoordination, rash, hair loss, nausea, vomiting, abdominal pain, easy bruising or bleeding, liver damage, lethargy, weakness. It can interact with other anticonvulsants to change their effect and with several other medications.

Vasotec (**enalapril**; see **ACE inhibitors**)

Verapamil (Calan, Isoptin; see **Antihypertensives; Calcium channel blockers**)

Voltaren (**diclofenac**; see **NSAIDs**)

Warfarin sodium (Coumadin; see **Anticoagulants**)

Wellbutrin (**bupropion**): Used to treat depression. Its side effects are similar to the tricyclic antidepressants, but there are less anticholinergic and sedative effects as well as less sexual dysfunction. It does not affect heart rate or cause weight gain. Other side effects include appetite loss, constipation, dizziness, headache, insomnia, psychotic reactions, seizures, and weight loss. The incidence of seizures is higher than with the tricyclic antidepressants.

Xanax (**alprazolam**; see **Benzodiazepines**)

Zantac (**ranitidine**; see **H$_2$-Blockers**)

Zestril (**lisinopril**; see **ACE inhibitors**)

Ziac (**bisoprolol fumarate,** and **hydrochlorothiazide**): Used to treat high blood pressure. Side effects: dizziness or light-headedness, swelling of the ankles or feet, unusual thirst or fatigue, muscle pain or weakness, difficulty breathing, or an unusually slow or irregular heartbeat.

Zoloft (**sertraline**; see **Antidepressants, tricyclic**)

Index